D0337642

ETHICS IN HEALTH SERVICES MANAGEMENT

FOURTH EDITION

by

KURT DARR, J.D., Sc.D., FACHE
THE GEORGE WASHINGTON UNIVERSITY
WASHINGTON, D.C.

HEALTH PROFESSIONS PRESS

Baltimore • London • Winnipeg • Sydney

HEALTH
PROFESSIONS
PRESS

Health Professions Press, Inc.
Post Office Box 10624
Baltimore, Maryland 21285-0624

www.healthpropress.com

Second printing, August 2007

Typeset by International Graphic Services, Newtown, Pennsylvania.
Manufactured in the United States of America by
Versa Press, Inc., East Peoria, Illinois.

Certain case studies in this book are based on well-known news accounts
and use real names and details as reported in the media. Others are based
on real stories, but names and identifying details have been changed to
protect identities. Still other case studies are composite or fictional
accounts that do not represent the lives or experiences of specific individuals, and no implications should be inferred.

Library of Congress Cataloging-in-Publication Data

Darr, Kurt.
  Ethics in health services management / by Kurt Darr.—4th ed.
    p.   cm.
  Includes bibliographic references and index.
  ISBN 13:978-1-878812-99-5, ISBN 10:1-878812-99-8
  1. Health services administration—Moral and ethical aspects.
2. Medical ethics. [DNLM: 1. Health Services Administration—
ethics—Case Reports. 2. Ethics, Medical—Case Reports.] I. Title
RA394.D35 2005
174'.2—dc22   2004014261

British Library Cataloguing in Publication data are available from the
British Library.

ETHICS IN
HEALTH SERVICES
MANAGEMENT

Contents

About the Author vii
Preface ix
Acknowledgments xi

Introduction 1

Section I   Identifying and Solving Ethical Problems
Chapter 1   Considering Moral Philosophies and Principles 15
Chapter 2   Resolving Ethical Issues 35

Section II   Guiding Ethical Decision Making
Chapter 3   Developing Organizational Values, Vision,
            and Mission 53
Chapter 4   Codes of Ethics in Health Services 75
Chapter 5   Organizational Responses to Ethical Problems 93

Section III   Administrative Ethical Issues
Chapter 6   Conflicts of Interest and Fiduciary Duty 123
Chapter 7   Ethical Issues Regarding Organization and Staff 143
Chapter 8   Ethical Issues Regarding Patients and Community 175

Section IV   Biomedical Ethical Issues
Chapter 9   Consent 211
Chapter 10   Dying and Death 229
Chapter 11   Patient Autonomy and the Paradigm
            of Physician-Assisted Suicide 259

Section V   Emerging Ethical Issues
Chapter 12   Ethics in Marketing and Managed Care 283
Chapter 13   Ethics in Resource Allocation 303
Chapter 14   Social Responsibility 329

Appendix A   Organizational Philosophies and
            Mission Statements 349
Appendix B   Ethical Codes 359
Select Bibliography 373
Index 379

About the Author

Kurt Darr, J.D., Sc.D., FACHE, is Professor of Hospital Administration in the Department of Health Services Management and Leadership at The George Washington University. He holds a Doctor of Science from The Johns Hopkins University and a Master of Hospital Administration and a Juris Doctor from the University of Minnesota.

Professor Darr completed his administrative residency at Rochester (Minnesota) Methodist Hospital and subsequently worked as an administrative associate at the Mayo Clinic. After being commissioned in the U.S. Navy, he served in administrative and educational assignments at St. Albans Naval Hospital and Bethesda Naval Hospital. He completed postdoctoral fellowships with the Department of Health and Human Services, the World Health Organization, and the Accrediting Commission on Education for Health Services Administration.

Dr. Darr is a fellow of the American College of Healthcare Executives and a member of the District of Columbia and Minnesota Bars. He is a mediator in the Superior Court of the District of Columbia and serves on a panel of mediators for the American Health Lawyers Association.

Professor Darr educates in the areas of health services ethics, management theory, hospital organization and management, quality improvement, and application of the Deming method in health services delivery. In addition, he is a consultant and educator to hospital ethics committees. Professor Darr has authored and edited several books used in undergraduate and graduate health services management programs and numerous articles on various health services topics.

Preface

The fourth edition of *Ethics in Health Services Management* continues the intention of the first three. It seeks to help students of health services management and nascent and experienced managers of health services organizations hone their skills in applied managerial and biomedical ethics. It is hoped that by providing a methodology for identifying and solving ethical problems and proposing tools to guide ethical decision making, the reader will become a more effective problem solver. As previously, brevity and organization have been watchwords.

Numerous cases and vignettes are included—a dozen more than in the third edition. Many come from the author's personal experience; others are based on information from colleagues or reports in the popular press and professional literature. Some are fully analyzed for the reader's scrutiny and critique. Others invite the reader's dissection and offer an opportunity to identify the ethical issues and consider their solution. All offer lessons in normative and applied ethics.

Ready answers are available neither in managerial nor ethical problem solving. As in medicine, the "cookbook" approach is inadequate because it fails to account for the nuances of fact, setting, and personalities that vary with each situation. Were ready answers available, most of the challenge and much of the satisfaction in solving them would be gone from a manager's professional life.

Virtue ethics is given much more attention in this edition. The principles of respect for persons, beneficence, nonmaleficence, and justice, however, continue to do most of the heavy lifting in terms of the duties and relationships managers have to the patients, staff, and profession. The virtues supplement and have the advantage of offering managers specific attributes and characteristics that should be instilled in those who would be virtuous managers.

It cannot be overstressed that one's personal ethic is key. Plato said the unexamined life is not worth living; his pupil, Aristotle, a bit snidely perhaps, added that the unplanned life is not worth examining. These aphorisms are useful guides to us as managers. We cannot be effective as managers (or, likely, as human beings) without having a lodestar by which to navigate our personal and professional lives. The moral certainty of a well-developed personal ethic is an essential element of personal and professional success. It is hoped that the fourth edition will benefit those examining or reconsidering their personal ethic.

This reorganized, updated, and enhanced fourth edition includes 14 chapters in five sections. Section I sets the framework for identifying and solving ethical problems. It includes discussion of the moral philosophies and derivative principles, as supplemented by the virtues, and a methodology for solving ethical problems. Section II identifies the importance of the organizational philosophy—its values, complemented by managers' personal ethic and supported by professional codes. In addition, organizational responses to ethical issues are identified. Section III considers administrative ethical issues, including conflicts of interests and the organization's ethical obligations to patients, staff, and the community, as guided by managers whose moral agency makes them the organization's conscience. The ethical issues arising from human immunodeficiency virus/acquired immunodeficiency syndrome (HIV/AIDS) have been reorganized from a freestanding chapter and integrated into Chapters 7 and 8 to make them more relevant to health services managers. The shrillness that marked earlier discussions of HIV/AIDS has diminished; the managerial and ethical implications continue, however, and raise some of the most perplexing problems health services managers face.

Section IV addresses major biomedical ethical issues including consent, dying and death, and patient autonomy as expressed through the paradigm of physician-assisted suicide. The role of managers is emphasized. Section V considers ethical issues relating to marketing and managed care, resource allocation, and the social responsibility of health services organizations. These areas are at the same time new, emerging, and continuing. Now in separate chapters, consideration of resource allocation and social responsibility has been substantially enhanced to reflect greater organizational and societal concern. Appendices include valuable resource material; a detailed index makes the book user friendly and enhances its value as a reference.

The genesis of this book lies 20 years in the past. Each edition has been written in an environment that presented seemingly insurmountable challenges to those who manage among the most important organizations in American society. As managers are called upon to do more with less, compete aggressively but fairly, meet an increasingly oppressive regulatory and payment environment, and provide a broader range of services, it is hoped that this fourth edition will provide a measure of help in their work. If so, I will have accomplished my goal.

Acknowledgments

This book was conceived as a vehicle to assist health services managers to identify and solve the numerous and complex ethical issues they confront. This goal came to fruition with the first edition in 1987. Publication of the second edition only 4 years later was a response to the rapid pace of change in the health services field. Subsequent editions have built on the first two.

Preparing and publishing four editions of a book necessitates assistance from many individuals and organizations. Those instrumental in preparing the first three editions have my continuing thanks. My late colleague and friend, Robert G. Shouldice, D.B.A., was helpful in preparing the managed care section in the first two editions. I hope he is at peace. For the fourth edition thanks are owed Soo Bang for reviewing and improving the information on institutional review boards. Robert Burke, Acting Chair of the Department of Health Services Management and Leadership, and Ruth Katz, Dean of the School of Public Health and Health Services, both at The George Washington University, have been supportive as they have striven to create an environment that stresses research and writing. A special thanks is owed Donald Lehman, Executive Vice President for Academic Affairs, and Stephen Joel Trachtenberg, President of The George Washington University, for approving the sabbatical that enabled me to prepare the manuscript.

Research and other assistance for this edition were provided by Kathleen Anne Flavin, Megha Kachalia, and Madeline Helen Smith, who worked industriously and cheerfully, often under demanding time constraints. They have my appreciation and best wishes for every future success.

At Health Professions Press, Mary Magnus, Director of Publications and patient taskmaster, was consistently encouraging and helpful. She has my gratitude. Nicole Schmidl's constructive editorial assistance improved the manuscript in numerous ways. I thank her.

To Anne

INTRODUCTION

Two themes underlie *Ethics in Health Services Management*: the autonomy, primacy, and protection of the patient* and the health services manager as moral agent and leader of the health services organization.

This book is intended to assist health services managers develop a personal ethic and gain an understanding of administrative and biomedical ethical issues, and it suggests a methodology for solving the problems that these issues raise. The emphasis is on normative ethics (*what should be done*). Some attention is paid to descriptive ethics (*what is actually done*) and metaethics (*study of ethical systems*) because they assist in understanding normative ethics. The theories of ethical relativism and ethical nihilism are not considered. Ethical relativism holds that there are no absolutes and that all answers to ethical questions are morally correct, depending on circumstances and culture. Nihilists consider no choice correct. These theories neither help managers meet the needs of patients, staff, and organizations nor aid them in resolving ethical problems. Furthermore, ethical relativism and nihilism do not help the manager formulate and reconsider a personal ethic.

For the health services manager, a personal ethic is a moral framework for relationships with employees, patients, organization, and community. In these relationships, the manager is not, and cannot be, a morally neutral technocrat. The manager is a moral agent—someone who morally affects and is morally affected by what is done or not done. This places special emphasis on misfeasance, malfeasance, and nonfeasance. Management's decisions are not value free; in a moral sense, they affect the organization's environment and are touched by them.

---

*To ease reading, *patient* is used to describe anyone served by a health services organization.

1

The patient relies on the health services organization and its staff to perform services unique in society. Managers' responsibilities to patients take precedence over their fiduciary duty to their organizations. Protecting the patient is more than providing safe surroundings and competent staff. It is more than licensure, accreditation, and compliance. It is more than a surplus at the end of the fiscal year. The manager is the organization's conscience. This responsibility is exemplified by the organization's willingness, prompted and led by management, to recognize the inherent human dignity of the patient and do so through effective programs that make this recognition a reality. It means using effective consent forms and procedures and ascertaining that all who have contact with patients are qualified and work for the patient's good. It means not considering patients as adversaries and not deserting them should something go wrong in the care process. An organization that has done its best can face the consequences of an error honestly, mitigate the injury, and find a fair solution. The loop is closed when management determines the cause of the problem, prevents or minimizes the probability of its recurrence, and strives to continuously improve quality. At times justice requires a decision process that prospectively includes the criteria of cost–benefit analysis and utilitarianism (*the greatest good for the greatest number*). Even here, the organization recognizes the dignity and worth of people as yet unserved or only partially served.

How does the health services organization develop and implement a "just" policy? How does it strive to treat patients as equals and work to serve their interests? Implementation of a just policy begins with the organizational philosophy,* which should explicitly state the nature of the relationship between patient and organization. This philosophy should reflect the view that the patient is autonomous and is entitled to be treated with respect and dignity. In a sense, there is a contract—an implicit but verifiable understanding between patient and provider, grounded in mutual trust and confidence. It recognizes that whenever possible, patients retain control of their lives.

Once enunciated, the organization's philosophy must be reflected in all derivative mission and vision statements, policies, procedures, and rules, but especially in relationships with patients and community. If not operationalized, the organization and its managers will be judged cynical about themselves and those they serve. This cynicism is easily recognized by

---

**Organizational philosophy* is used as a generic concept to include values, core values, shared values, ministry, healing ministry, philosophy, or similar terms used to convey the philosophical framework in which services are delivered.

staff and, in turn, will be reflected in staff's relationship with patients. Staff may not succumb to the negative implications of this inconsistency, but it will be an underlying, festering incongruity nonetheless.

A major participant in developing and maintaining the appropriate relationship with patients is the physician,* necessarily a primary actor. Physicians must respect decisions made by a patient or an appropriate proxy. The roles of physician and organization are complementary, but the organization remains morally (ethically) accountable for the physician's activities.

CONCERN ABOUT ETHICS

Ethics is a word used frequently in health care. Questions are asked daily about making the ethically right choice. Seemingly straightforward and value-free management decisions have ethical implications for patients, staff, organization, community, and society. Many decisions that cause ethical dilemmas are the result of the continuing revolution in biology and technology. Fiscal constraints, competition, and new means of delivering services exacerbate existing ethical problems and raise new ones. Beyond these causes is an enhanced level of awareness resulting from the research and writing of ethicists and the work of government commissions on experimentation and bioethics.

Ethical dilemmas occur when decision makers are drawn in two directions by competing courses of action that are based on differing moral frameworks, varying or inconsistent elements of the organizational philosophy, conflicting duties or moral principles, or managers who have an ill-defined sense of right and wrong. For example, staff members may be asked to follow rules they consider inappropriate or unjust, or two moral principles may conflict with one another. A nurse's duty to preserve life clashes with the patient's wishes not to be kept alive artificially. Another source of ethical dilemmas is the existence of two compelling, ethically defensible positions on an issue such as the possible conception of a genetically defective infant. Required genetic screening and counseling for people at risk conflict with individual autonomy. Conclusions vary when decision makers put different weight on various principles, such as personal liberty

---

*To ease reading, *physician* includes medical doctors and other practitioners of the medical and healing arts licensed to independently treat patients (e.g., dentists, nurse midwives, clinical psychologists, podiatrists, chiropractors). Such persons are often known as *licensed independent practitioners (LIPs)*.

or privacy competing with societal interests and economic considerations. Ethical decisions are also affected by politics, laws, and regulations. Reasonable persons could differ as to the ethically "right" result on some issues. For virtually all ethical issues, however, one answer almost always emerges as morally superior. Ethical problems are often characterized as *dilemmas* because that emphasizes the difficulty of finding the morally best solution. Solving ethical problems may be demanding, but few are properly labeled dilemmas.

Are laws and regulations the problem or the solution? Some perceive that ethical problems arise because laws or regulations fail to guide actions. Others perceive that laws force organizations and managers to act in ways that cause ethical problems. Depending on the issue and facts, both views may have merit. Even when there are external rules, decision makers in organizations must decide when the rules apply, how they are interpreted, and whether to obey them. In fact, by designating and clarifying rules, there is less middle ground, the ethical problems are starker, and solving them may be more difficult. Some people may ignore the rules and apply a personal ethic. Others will apply rules dogmatically, choosing not to think about the underlying philosophy or resulting ethical issues. Conversely, some ethical problems occur because no external rules assist decision makers. For others, there is no consensus as to what the rules should be. A further complication is that some ethical problems have developed more quickly than the ability of the health services field or society to solve them.

ETHICS DEFINED

Defining ethics is difficult because it can have several meanings. For philosophers, ethics is the formal study of morality. Sociologists see ethics as the mores, customs, and behavior of a culture. For physicians, ethics means meeting the expectations of profession and society and interacting with patients in certain ways. Health services managers should consider ethics a special charge and a responsibility to patients, organization and staff, to themselves and profession, and, ultimately but less directly, to society. Managers are confronted with the normative question "What ought I to do?"

Distinctions often blur, but ethical problems may be divided into administrative and biomedical. Biomedical ethical problems involve individual patients or groups of patients in their relationships with one another or with providers and organizations. Depending on the issue, the manager is involved less directly in biomedical ethical problems. Beyond biomedical ethical problems, some of which become dilemmas that receive great media attention, is the need to identify and solve management problems with ethical dimensions. Administrative ethical problems involve manager and profession, organization, patients, and society. Administrative ethical issues less frequently involve competing, ethically defensible choices. Solving these problems is usually a matter of recognition and resolve—doing what is morally right.

SOURCES OF LAW

The relationship between law and ethics (morality) is dynamic. Thus, it is useful to begin a book about ethics by briefly reviewing development of law. Every organized society has a code or system of laws that distinguishes acceptable behavior from unacceptable behavior and establishes penalties for transgressors. *Law* may be defined as a system of principles and rules of human conduct prescribed or recognized by a supreme authority. This definition includes criminal and civil law. In contrast, ethics is the study of standards of moral judgment and conduct. For individuals this is the personal ethic. For a profession it is the guiding system or code of ethics.

The moral underpinnings in criminal law are especially clear in reflecting society's sense of right and wrong, or its ethics (morality). In a democratic society laws are said to derive from and reflect the views of justice and fairness held by the majority. This is less true in civil law, which governs relations among individuals and includes torts and contracts. The common law tradition of the United States means that a great deal of law is based on the precedents of judicial opinions. Civil law emphasizes predictability, stability, and property rights.

In a democracy, laws are thought to reflect the moral values of most people, but substantial minorities may hold contrary views and consider a law or government action so unjust that they risk the penalties of breaking it. An historical example is the 18th Amendment to the U.S. Constitution. Adopted in 1919, it prohibited manufacture, sale, or transportation of intoxicating liquors. Violation was widespread until the amendment's repeal in 1933. Contemporary examples are draft resistance during the Vietnam war, common disregard of roadway speed limits, and marijuana use.

Some cultures regarded the law as a gift from the gods. Plato's *Republic* postulated the ideal state as one based on rational order and ruled by philosopher-kings. Plato considered written law a regrettable oversimplification that could not take into account the differences and conditions in parties and situations involved in legal disputes. He believed that it was best to have a philosopher apply an unwritten law. His own experience proved this theory impossible, and he accepted a written law administered without regard to the circumstances of the individuals involved.[1, 2] This concept of a rule of law, not of men, became established in Anglo-American legal tradition. However, because of the absurd results that can occur when civil law is applied without considering the situations of the parties, the concept of unwritten law preferred by Plato was continued, but in a limited manner. Parallel court systems developed in the common law; civil actions could be brought in either. Some states have courts of equity that hear cases in which fairness is the primary concern; most, however, have merged law and equity into one court system.

Because of the link between societal views of right and wrong and the law, morality is reflected in all types of law, whether formal or nonformal. A leading jurisprudent, Edgar Bodenheimer, identified formal sources of law as constitutions, statutes, executive orders, administrative regulations, ordinances, charters and bylaws of autonomous or semiautonomous bodies, treaties, and judicial precedents. Nonformal sources of law have not received an authoritative, or at least articulated, formulation and embodiment in a formalized legal document. These sources include standards of justice, principles of reason and consideration of the nature of things (*natura rerum*), equity for individuals, public policies, moral convictions, social trends, and customary law.

Bodenheimer's inclusion of the charters and bylaws of autonomous and semiautonomous bodies in the list of formal sources of law has significance for health services management. Such documents include the articles of incorporation and bylaws of the organization. General references to the organizational philosophy and mission may be included in both but will appear in expanded form in other documents. These are key. Medical staff bylaws and rules and regulations also reflect the organizational philosophy and mission and must be consistent with them.

In addition to their importance in reflecting the philosophy and mission, the charter and bylaws are an organization's basic laws. Persons affected by the organization—employees, physicians, patients—look to them for guidance. Some formal laws, such as the medical staff bylaws, detail the rights and obligations of physicians. Should a legal controversy develop, courts and other reviewing bodies look to these documents as sources of formal law.

Bodenheimer's definition of formal law is broad enough to include professional codes of ethics. A code can be effectively implemented only when interpreted and enforced. Such activities guide a code's application and related decision making, give it dynamism and life, and ensure the important virtues of consistency and predictability.

RELATIONSHIP BETWEEN ETHICS AND LAW

For professions, ethics is much more than obeying the law. The law is but the minimum standard of morality established by society to guide interactions among individuals and between them and government. The law governing one's relationships includes few positive duties. Only in unique situations is one person obliged to aid another, for example. The law concentrates on prohibitions—the "thou shalt nots." Professions are bound by the law but have a higher calling, one that includes numerous positive duties to patients and society and to one another.

Positive duties are not exclusive to professions. Individuals may hold themselves to a standard obligating them to aid others or work on their behalf. In many respects this positive duty means practicing the Golden Rule: "Do unto others as you would have them do unto you." This duty is far more demanding than merely refraining from interfering with someone or enacting a law that protects one person from another.

As noted previously, it is paradoxical that law both prevents and causes ethical problems. Choices must be made whether a public law exists. Absent public law, managers rely on the formal law of the organization, such as statements of the organizational philosophy (its ethic/values) and mission. Also important in guiding decision making is the informal law present in the manager's personal ethic. Public law may not be determinative in solving a problem. Even when it is clear, ethical problems may remain. An example is the U.S. Supreme Court decision that a woman has an unfettered constitutional right to an abortion during the first trimester of pregnancy. The controversy over the morality (ethics) of abortion continues.

Statutes, court decisions, and codes of ethics are formal sources of law, but the latter affect only members of an identified group, usually one of voluntary association. Belonging to an association may not be completely voluntary because colleagues have expectations and demands, employers may consider memberships important in judging qualifications, and better-informed consumers ask questions and express views about an individual's professional memberships. At root, however, participating in professional groups is voluntary.

Licensure is ubiquitous for clinical personnel. Of health services managers, only nursing facility managers must be licensed. Including ethical standards in licensing statutes gives them the force of law. This does not, however, relieve the professional association of the need to regulate members' behavior, to the point of adopting more stringent guidelines. Groups whose codes are not reflected in statutes or regulations bear a heavier burden. Their codes are only private statements of acceptable behavior; monitoring must be done by the groups themselves. A profession's obligation to protect and serve society greatly heightens its need to monitor members and is a hallmark of a profession.

In disciplinary proceedings pursuant to a licensing statute, the actions of public regulatory bodies are distinct from those of private groups. If a license is necessary to belong to a group, expulsion may follow delicensure; expulsion usually occurs only after a separate hearing and review process by the professional group.

The relationship between law and ethics might seem to be one to one: anything lawful is ethical and vice versa. This may not be true, however. Most important is that the law states the minimum expected from members of society; it contains few positive duties. Professions expect members to comply with the law but often add substantially to this standard. The result is that the professional code of ethics may require an action that the law does not. For the professional, then, performing (or not performing) a particular activity may be legal but unethical.

The relationship between law and ethics is shown in Figure 1, a model developed by Henderson. It shows a succession of events leading to corporate decisions being scrutinized by the public and a determination whether they are legal and/or ethical. This judgment is necessarily after the fact, despite management's efforts to predict consequences of a decision. The model suggests that for many corporate actions it cannot be known with certainty whether those who finally judge the decision will consider it legal (as determined by law enforcement officials) or ethical (as determined by the profession or the general public). This consideration adds a high degree of uncertainty to decision making inside and outside health services. It is usually easier to predict whether an action will be judged legal than to predict whether it will be perceived as ethical.

The matrix by Henderson shown in Figure 2 shows the combinations of legal, illegal, ethical, and unethical. In Quadrant I, managers act legally and ethically.

Quadrant II includes decisions that are ethical but illegal. The American College of Healthcare Executives' Code of Ethics requires affiliates to comply with all laws and regulations. Given this broad prohibition, it is virtually impossible for health services managers to justify as ethical an act that is illegal. There are exceptions, however. For example, it is morally

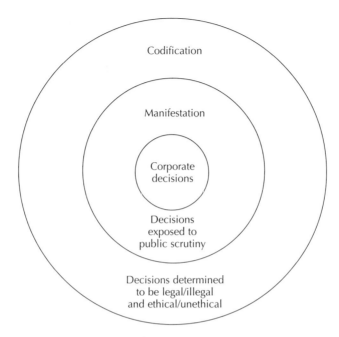

Figure 1.   The relationship between law and ethics. (Reprinted from "The Ethical Side of Enterprise" by V.E. Henderson, *MIT Sloan Management Review, 23,* 1982, pp. 37–43, by permission of the publisher. Copyright © 1982 by Massachusetts Institute of Technology. All rights reserved.)

justifiable to break the law to prevent greater harm or injury. Someone who engages in civil disobedience or breaks other laws must be prepared to suffer the penalties imposed.

Quadrant III includes decisions that are unethical but legal. It incorporates the concept that ethical standards, especially those of a profession, hold the member to a higher standard than does the law. Examples include failing to take reasonable steps to protect the patient from incompetent medical care and preventing manager self-aggrandizement at the expense of patients.

Quadrant IV includes activities that are illegal and unethical. Embezzlement falls into this quadrant, as does ignoring local fire safety requirements or filing false Medicare or Medicaid reports.

It is important to stress the dynamic between law and ethics: each affects and is affected by the other. Professional codes and conduct reflect society's perceptions of a profession as well as that profession's self-image. To the extent that law codifies society's need to protect itself and regulate conduct, licensure laws further clarify what is expected of a profession. Morality reflected in the law evolves but likely lags behind private morality

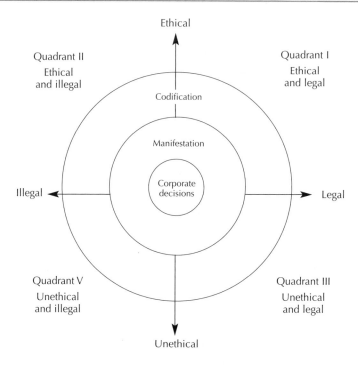

Figure 2. A matrix of possible outcomes concerning the ethics and legality of corporate decisions. (Reprinted from "The Ethical Side of Enterprise" by V.E. Henderson, *MIT Sloan Management Review, 23,* 1982, pp. 37–43, by permission of the publisher. Copyright © 1982 by Massachusetts Institute of Technology. All rights reserved.)

and ethics. In this regard, the law leads some subsets of society but follows others.

CONCLUSION

Gandhi said, "Noncooperation with evil is as much a duty as cooperation with good." Edmund Burke said, "The only thing necessary for the triumph of evil is for good men to do nothing." Both philosophies are germane to health services, especially to its managers. Understanding and meeting their ethical obligations are essential.

Contemporary demands on health services organizations and managers may seem inconsistent with the often-idealized statements found in codes of ethics. Managers must recognize their responsibility, however, and strive to transform the ideal into reality. Managers see themselves and are seen by others as moral agents with a critical role in the organization and its efforts to serve, protect, and further the interests of patient and community.

There is ample evidence of ethical and legal problems in the world of business. Despite occurring less often and having less impact on the economy and society, there have been enough ethical and legal misadventures in the health services management field to know that it faces important challenges. A number of these misadventures are described in the book. There is much of concern beyond the scandals and illegality, however. What about a manager's relationships with persons served by the organization or its staff? Managing health services organizations will always be among the most demanding work in society. No one said it would be easy; few in the field expect kudos for their work. But we raise the pride of profession and self and meet our responsibilities when we act as moral agents whose primary duty is to protect patients' interests and further their care. This is the continuing challenge of health services management.

NOTES

1. Edgar Bodenheimer. (1974). *Jurisprudence: The philosophy and method of the law* (p. 6). Cambridge, MA: Harvard University Press.
2. A useful discussion of Plato's political philosophy is found in Jeremy Waldron. (1995). What Plato would allow. In Ian Shapiro & Judith Wagner DeCew (Eds.), *Theory and practice: Nomos XXXVII* (pp. 138–178). New York: New York University Press.

IDENTIFYING AND SOLVING ETHICAL PROBLEMS

Chapters 1 and 2 present information basic to identifying, understanding, analyzing, and solving administrative and biomedical ethical problems. A generic background and methodology are developed and applied to the case of Baby Boy Doe. The nature of ethical problems evolves and new types appear, but the framework and process described here have continued usefulness for managers.

Chapter 1 identifies and discusses moral philosophies and derivative principles—a background essential to analyzing and solving administrative and biomedical ethical problems. Understanding the philosophies and derivative principles, supplemented by virtue ethics, is key to managers developing a vibrant and robust personal ethic.

The theory and application of a generic problem-solving method are part of management education. The methodology detailed in Chapter 2 builds on that generic skill to enable managers to more readily identify, analyze, and resolve ethical problems. Managers should read the discussion of moral philosophies and the derivative principles, supplemented by virtue ethics, within the context of their problem-solving education and experience as well as their personal ethic.

Solving administrative ethics cannot be exclusive to managers, nor can biomedical ethical problems be exclusive to physicians. Meeting an organization's ethical imperative is vital and is inextricably linked to successfully meeting its mission and objectives. Managers who act only as technocrats ignore their role as moral agents. Moral agency requires each of us to be morally accountable for nonfeasance, misfeasance, and malfeasance. Managers must participate fully in solving ethical problems. It is too important to be left to others.

CHAPTER 1

CONSIDERING MORAL PHILOSOPHIES AND PRINCIPLES

W hat are the sources of ethical guidelines? How do they help us identify and act on the morally correct choice? Philosophers, theologians, and others grapple with such questions. The tradition of ethics in medicine dates from the ancient Greeks. Throughout the 20th century and into the 21st century, managers and nurses have formally sought to clarify, establish, and sometimes enforce ethical standards. Their codes and activities incorporate philosophies about the ethical relationships of providers to one another, to patients, and to society. For managers, the appropriate relationship with the organization employing them is an added dimension to their codes.

A natural starting point for discussing ethics and understanding how to resolve ethical problems is to review the moral philosophies that have had a major influence on western European thought and values. Among the most prominent of these philosophies are utilitarian teleology; Kantian deontology; natural law as formulated by Thomas Aquinas; and the work of 20th-century American philosopher John Rawls, as the latter part of the 20th century saw renewed interest in virtue ethics and casuistry. In addition, the ethics of care is considered briefly.

Principles derived from these moral philosophies provide the framework or moral (ethical) underpinnings for delivery of health services by organizations. These principles will assist managers (and health services caregivers) in honing a personal ethic. The derivative operative principles are respect for persons, beneficence, nonmaleficence, and justice. Virtue ethics is used to supplement the principles when they lack the rigor in analyzing or solving ethical problems.

The following case about Baby Boy Doe actually happened. State and federal law would prevent it today. Its simplicity and starkness make it a useful paradigm against which to apply the moral philosophies and derivative principles discussed in this chapter.

Baby Boy Doe

In 1970, a male infant born at a major East Coast medical center was diagnosed with mental retardation and duodenal atresia (the absence of a connection between the stomach and intestine). Surgeons determined that although the baby was very small, the atresia was operable, with a high probability of success. The surgery would not alter the baby's mental retardation, but would permit him to take nourishment by mouth.

The baby's parents decided to forego the surgery—something they had the legal right to do—and over the course of the following 2 weeks the infant was left to die from dehydration and starvation. No basic determination of the extent of mental impairment had been made, nor could it have been, at the time the infant died. Neither hospital personnel nor state family and social services sought to aid him.

This case sends a shudder through most people. Feelings alone, however, are insufficient. If managers are to be effective in addressing and solving—or, preferably, preventing—such problems, they must identify and understand the issues involved, know the roles of staff and organization, and apply guidelines for ethical decision making. Following a discussion of moral philosophies and ethical principles, the case of Baby Boy Doe is analyzed.

MORAL PHILOSOPHIES

Utilitarianism

Utilitarians are consequentialists: They evaluate an action in terms of its effect rather than the action's intrinsic attributes. Synonymous with utilitarians are teleologists (from the Greek, *telos*, meaning end). Utilitarianism has historical connections to hedonism (Epicureanism), which measured morality by the amount of pleasure obtained from an act or a rule as to how to act—greater pleasure was equated with greater morality. This theory was refined by two 19th-century philosophers, Jeremy Bentham and John Stuart Mill. Mill's elaboration of utilitarianism was the most complete. Unlike Bentham, Mill sought to distinguish pleasures (the good) on qualitative grounds. Questions about the superiority of certain pleasures, such as listening to a piano concerto, were to be answered by consulting a person of sensitivity and broad experience, even though requiring such judgments diminished the objectivity of utilitarianism. Mill stressed individual freedom. In *On Liberty*, he noted that freedom is requisite to producing happiness and that this makes it unacceptable for the privacy of any group or individual to be infringed in significant ways.

In determining the morally correct choice, utilitarians ignore the means of achieving an end and judge the results of an action by comparing the good produced by a particular action to the good produced by alternatives or the amount of evil avoided. Modified utility theory is the basis for the cost–benefit analysis commonly used by economists and managers. "The greatest good for the greatest number" and "the end justifies the means" are statements attributable to utilitarians. However, these statements are only crude gauges of utilitarianism, inappropriately applied without qualification.

Utilitarianism is divided into *act utility* and *rule utility*. Both measure consequences, and the action that brings into being the most good (understood in a nonmoral sense) is deemed the morally correct choice.

Act utilitarians judge each action independently, without reference to preestablished guidelines (rules). They measure the amount of good, or (nonmoral) value brought into being, and the amount of evil, or (nonmoral) disvalue avoided by acting on a particular choice. Each person affected is counted equally, which seems to assign a strong sense of objectivity to this moral philosophy. Because it is episodic and capricious, act utilitarianism is incompatible with developing and deriving the ethical principles needed for codes of ethics and a personal ethic. Therefore, it receives no further attention.

Rule utilitarians are also concerned only with consequences but have prospectively considered various actions and the amount of good or evil brought into being by each. These assessments are used to develop rules (guidelines) for action, because it has been determined that, on average, certain rules produce the most good and result in the least evil. Therefore, these rules determine the morally correct choice. The rules are followed for all similar situations, even if sometimes they do not produce the best results. The rule directs selection of the morally correct choice. Rule utilitarianism assists in developing moral principles for health services management.

Deontology

Deontologists adhere to a formalist moral philosophy (in Greek, *deon* means duty). The foremost proponent of deontology was Immanuel Kant, an 18th-century German philosopher. Kant's basic precept was that relations with others must be based on duty. An action is moral if it arises solely from "good will," not from other motives. According to Kant, good will is that which is good without qualification. Unlike utilitarians, deontologists view the end as unimportant, because, in Kant's view, persons have duties to one another as moral agents, duties that take precedence over the consequences of actions. Kantians hold that certain absolute duties are always in force. Among the most important is respect, or the Golden Rule ("Do unto others as you would have them do unto you"). Kant argued that all persons have this duty; respect toward others must always be paid.

Actions that are to be taken under the auspices of this duty must first be tested in a special way, a test Kant termed the *categorical imperative*. The categorical imperative requires that actions under consideration be universalized. In other words, if a principle of action is thought to be appropriate, a determination is made as to whether it can be consistently applied to all persons in all places at all times. There are no exceptions, nor can allowances be made for special circumstances. If the action under consideration meets the test of universality, it is accepted as a duty. The action fails the test if it is contradictory to the overriding principle that all persons must be treated as moral equals and are, therefore, entitled to respect. Truth telling is a prominent example of a duty that meets the categorical imperative.

For the Kantian deontologist, it is logically inconsistent to argue that terminally ill persons should be euthanized because this amounts to the self-contradictory conclusion that life can be improved by ending it. Similarly, caregivers should not lie to patients to improve the efficiency of health care delivery; such a policy fails the test of the categorical imperative because it treats patients as means to an end—efficiency—rather than moral equals. The Golden Rule is the best summary of Kant's philosophy. Kantian deontology gives no consideration to results or consequences. This does not mean that managers must ignore consequences, but that the consequences of an action are neither included nor weighed in ethical decision making.

Natural Law

Mill defined morally right actions by the happiness or nonmoral value produced. Kant rejected all ethical theories based on desire or inclination. Unlike Mill and Kant, natural law theorists contend that ethics must be based on concern for human good. They also contend that good cannot be defined simply in terms of subjective inclinations. Rather, there is a good for human beings that is objectively desirable, although not reducible to desire.[1] Natural law holds that divine law has inscribed certain potentialities in all things, which constitute the good of those things. In this sense, the theory is teleological because it is concerned with ends. Natural law is based on Aristotelian thought as interpreted and synthesized with Christian dogma by St. Thomas Aquinas (1225–1274).[2]

The potentiality of human beings is based on a uniquely human trait, the ability to reason. Natural law bases ethics on the premise that human beings will do what is rational, and that this rationality will cause them to tend to do good and avoid evil. Natural law presumes a natural order in relationships and a predisposition by rational individuals to do or to refrain from doing certain things. Our capability for rational thought enables us to discover what we should do. In that effort, we are guided by a partial notion of God's divine plan that is linked to our capacity for rational thought. Because natural law guides what rational human beings do, it serves as a basis for positive law, some of which is reflected in statutes. Our natural inclination directs us to preserve our lives and to do such rational things as avoid danger, act in self-defense, and seek medical attention when needed. Our ability to reason shows that other human beings are like us and therefore entitled to the same respect and dignity we seek. A summary statement of the basic precepts of natural law is "do good and avoid evil." Using natural law, theologians have developed moral guidelines about medical services that are described in Chapters 10 and 11.

Rawls's Theory

Moral philosopher John Rawls, who died in 2002, espoused a hybrid theory of ethics that has applications in health services allocation and delivery. His theories were expounded in his seminal work, *A Theory of Justice*, originally published in 1971. They are redistributive in nature, and the philosophical construct that he used results, with some exceptions, in egalitarianism in health services.

Rawls's theory uses an elaborate philosophical construct in which persons are in the "original position," behind a veil of ignorance. Such persons are rational and self-interested but know nothing of their individual talents, intelligence, social and economic situations, and the like. Rawls argues that persons in the original position behind a veil of ignorance will identify certain principles of justice. First, all persons should have equal rights to the most extensive basic liberty compatible with similar liberty for others (the *liberty principle*). Second, social and economic inequalities should be arranged so that they are both reasonably expected to be to everyone's advantage and attached to positions and offices open to all (the *difference principle*).[3] According to Rawls's theory, the liberty principle governing political rights is more important and precedes the difference principle, which governs primary goods (distributive rights), including health services.

Rawls argued that hypothetical rational and self-interested persons in the original position will reject utilitarianism and select the concepts of right and justice as precedent to the good. Rawls concluded that rational self-interest dictates that one will act to protect the least well off because (from the perspective of the veil of ignorance) anyone could be in that group. He termed this *maximizing the minimum position (maximin)*.

When applied to primary goods, one of which is health services, Rawlsian moral theory requires egalitarianism. *Egalitarianism* is defined to mean that rational, self-interested persons may limit the health services available to people in certain categories, such as particular diseases or age groups, or limit services provided in certain situations. It is also rational and self-interested for persons in the original position not to make every good or service available to everyone at all times.

Rawls's theory permits disproportionate distribution of primary goods to certain groups but only if doing so benefits the least advantaged. This is part of the difference principle and justifies elite social and economic status for persons such as physicians and health services managers if their efforts ultimately benefit the least advantaged members of society.

Casuistry and the Ethics of Care

Casuistry   Many historical definitions of casuistry are not flattering. They include a moral philosophy that uses sophistry and encourages rationalizations for desired ethical results, uses evasive reasoning, and is quibbling. Despite these unflattering definitions and a centuries-long hiatus, advocates of casuistry see it as a pragmatic approach to understanding and solving problems of modern biomedical ethics. *Casuistry* can be defined as a kind of case-based reasoning in historical context. A claimed strength is that it avoids excessive reliance on principles and rules, which it is argued provide only partial answers and often fall short of comprehensive guidance for decision makers.

A significant effort to rehabilitate casuistry was undertaken by Jonsen and Toulmin,[4] who argued that

Casuistry redresses the excessive emphasis placed on universal rules and invariant principles by moral philosophers. . . . Instead we shall take seriously certain features of moral discourse that recent moral philosophers have too little appreciated: the concrete circumstances of actual cases, and the specific maxims that people invoke in facing actual moral dilemmas. If we start by considering similarities and differences between particular types of cases on a practical level, we open up an alternative approach to ethical theory that is wholly consistent with our moral practice.

At its foundation casuistry is similar to the law in which court cases and the precedents they establish guide decision makers. Beauchamp and Walters[5] stated that

In case law, the normative judgments of a majority of judges become authoritative, and . . . are the primary normative judgments for later judges who assess other cases. Cases in ethics are similar: Normative judgments emerge through majoritarian consensus in society and in institutions because careful attention has been paid to the details of particular problem cases. That consensus then becomes authoritative and is extended to relevantly similar cases.

In fact, this process occurs in organizations when ethics committees, for example, develop a body of experience with ethical issues of various types—their reasoning uses paradigms and analogies.

Clinical medicine is case focused as, increasingly, is management education. This development has made it natural to employ a case approach in health services. Traditionally, ethics problem solving in health services has applied moral principles to cases—from the general to the specific, or deductive reasoning. Classical casuists, however, used a kind of inductive reasoning—from the specific to the general. They began by stating a paradigm case with a strong maxim (e.g., "thou shalt not kill") set in its most obvious relevance to circumstances (e.g., a vicious attack on a defenseless person). Subsequent cases added circumstances that made the relevance of the maxim more difficult to understand (e.g., if defense is possible, is it moral?) Classical casuists progressed from being deontologists to teleologists and back again, as suited the case, and adhered to no explicit moral theory.[6] Jonsen[7] argued that modern casuists can profitably copy the classical casuists' reliance on paradigm cases, reference to broad consensus, and acceptance of probable certitude (defined as assent to a proposition but acknowledging that its opposite might be true). Casuistry has achieved a prominent place in applied administrative and biomedical ethics. Increasing numbers of cases and a body of experience will lead to consensus and greater certainty in identifying morally right decisions.

Ethics of Care   Medicine is based on caring, the importance of which is reflected historically and in contemporary biomedical ethics. "Care" focuses on relationships; in clinical practice, this means relationships between caregivers and patients. Effective management also depends on relationships between managers and staff and through them to patients. As the ethics of care evolves, it may be more applicable to management; at this point, however, it applies almost exclusively to clinical relationships.

The interest in the ethics of care beginning in the 1980s has been attributed to the feminist movement.[8] Its proponents argue that various interpersonal relationships and the obligations and virtues they involve "lack three central features of relations between moral agents as understood by Kantians and contractarians, e.g., Rawls—it is intimate, it is unchosen, and is between unequals."[9] Thus, the ethics of care emphasizes the attachment of relationships rather than the detachment of rules and duties.

A clear link to virtue ethics exists in that the ethics of care focuses on character traits such as compassion and fidelity that are valued in close personal relationships. It has been suggested that the basis for the ethics of care is found in the paradigmatic relationship between mother and child. It is claimed that this paradigm sets it apart from the predominantly male experience, which often uses the economic exchange between buyer and seller as the paradigmatic human relationship and, which it is argued, characterizes moral theory, generally.[10]

A leading exponent of the ethics of care, Carol Gilligan,[11] argued that unlike traditional moral theories, the ethics of care is grounded in the assumption that

> Self and other are interdependent, an assumption reflected in a view of action as responsive and, therefore, as arising in relationships rather than the view of action as emanating from within the self and, therefore, "self-governed." Seen as responsive, the self is by definition connected to others, responding to perceptions, interpreting events, and governed by the organizing tendencies of human interaction and human language. Within this framework, detachment, whether from self or from others, is morally problematic, since it breeds moral blindness or indifference—a failure to discern or respond to need. The question of what responses constitute care and what responses lead to hurt draws attention to the fact that one's own terms may differ from those of others. Justice in this context becomes understood as respect for people in their own terms.

Similar to virtue ethics and the renewed interest in casuistry, the ethics of care is a reaction to the rules and systems building of traditional theories. Its proponents argue that the ethics of care more closely reflects the real experiences in clinical medicine and of caregivers who are expected to respond with, for example, warmth, compassion, sympathy, and friendliness, none of which fits well into a system of rules and duties. "Ethical problems are considered in a contextual framework of familial relationships and intra personal relationships combined with a focus on goodness and a reflective understanding of care."[12]

Virtue Ethics

Western thought about the importance of virtue can be traced to Plato but more particularly to Aristotle.[13] Like natural law, virtue ethics is based on theological ethics but does not focus primarily on obligations or duties. As with casuistry, virtue ethics is receiving increased attention. Some of this attention results from a perception that traditional rule—or principle-based moral philosophies—deal inadequately with the realities of ethical decision making. That is to say, rules (as derived from moral principles) take us only so far in solving ethical problems; when there are competing ethical rules or situations to which no rules apply, something more than a coin toss is needed. This is where virtue ethicists claim to have a superior moral philosophy. Rule utilitarians and Kantian moral philosophies provide principles to guide actions, thus allowing someone to decide how to act in a given situation. By contrast, virtue ethics focus on what makes a good person rather than on what makes a good action.[14]

Contemporary authors Pellegrino and Thomasma[15] have argued that virtue ethics has three levels. The first two are 1) observing the laws of the land and 2) observing moral rights and fulfilling moral duties that go beyond the law. The third and highest level is the practice of virtue.

> Virtue implies a character trait, an internal disposition habitually to seek moral perfection, to live one's life in accord with a moral law, and to attain a balance between noble intention and just action. . . . In almost any view the virtuous person is someone we can trust to act habitually in a good way—courageously, honestly, justly, wisely, and temperately.[16]

Thus, virtuous managers (or physicians) are disposed to the right and good that is intrinsic to the practice of their profession and will work for the good of the patient. As Pellegrino noted, "Virtue ethics expands the notions of benevolence, beneficence, conscientiousness, compassion, and fidelity well beyond what strict duty might require."[17]

Some virtue ethicists argue that as with any skill or expertise, practice and constant striving to achieve virtuous traits (good works) improves one's ability to be virtuous. Other virtue ethicists argue that accepting in one's heart the forgiveness and reconciliation offered by God (faith) "would lead to a new disposition toward God (trust) and the neighbor (love), much as a physician or patient might be judged to be a different (and better) person following changed dispositions toward those persons with whom . . . (they) are involved."[18]

As noted, the virtues are character traits, a disposition well entrenched in the possessor. The fully virtuous do what they should without any struggle against contrary desires.[19] Most of us are less than fully virtuous, however. We are continent—we have need to control a desire or temptation to do otherwise than be virtuous. Another way to describe a virtue is that it is a tendency to control a certain class of feeling and to act rightly in a certain kind of situation.[20]

Plato identified only four cardinal virtues: wisdom, courage, self-control, and justice.[21] Aristotle expanded these four virtues in ways that need not concern us. Beauchamp and Childress identified five "focal virtues" that are appropriate for health professionals: compassion, discernment, trustworthiness, integrity, and conscientiousness.[22] Virtues appropriate for health services managers include those selected by Plato and Beauchamp and Childress, and several more that can be added, including honesty, punctuality, temperance, friendliness, cooperativeness, fortitude, caring, truthfulness, courteousness, thrift, veracity, candor, and loyalty. The goal of the virtuous manager is to achieve a mean between a virtue's excess and its absence. For example, courage is a virtue, but its excess is rashness; its absence is cowardice. Another example is friendliness. In excess, it is obsequiousness; its absence is sulkiness. Neither extreme is acceptable in the virtuous manager.[23] A way to understand the virtues is to identify the vices or character flaws managers should avoid. These include being irresponsible, feckless, lazy, inconsiderate, uncooperative, harsh, intolerant, dishonest, selfish, mercenary, indiscreet, tactless, arrogant, unsympathetic, cold, incautious, unenterprising, pusillanimous, feeble, presumptuous, rude, hypocritical, self-indulgent, materialistic, grasping, short sighted, vindictive, calculating, ungrateful, grudging, brutal, profligate, disloyal, and so on.[24]

All people should live virtuous lives, but those in the caring professions have a special obligation to do so, which is to say that virtuous managers and physicians are not solely virtuous persons practicing a profession. They are expected to work for the patient's good even at the expense of personal sacrifice and legitimate self-interest.[25] Virtuous physicians place the good of their patients above their own and seek that good unless pursuing it imposes injustice on them or their families or violates their conscience.[26] Thus, virtuous physicians place themselves at risk of contracting a deadly infectious disease to comfort and treat their patients, and they provide large amounts of uncompensated treatment even though it diminishes their economic circumstances. Similarly, virtuous managers place the good of the patient (through the organization) above their own. This means that they speak out to protect the patient from harm because of incompetent care, even though doing so risks their continued employment, and they work the extra hours that are needed to ensure that needed services are provided, despite a lack of commensurate remuneration.

Summary

The moral philosophies described in this section span a spectrum. Health services managers are likely to be eclectic in selecting those that become part of the organization's philosophy and those that will influence the content of their personal ethic, as well as its reconsideration and evolution. Most important is that managers recognize that a basic understanding of moral philosophies is vital.

LINKING THEORY AND ACTION

Ethical theories are drawn from abstractions that are often stated broadly. Principles developed from these theories establish a relationship and suggest a course of action. Rules can be derived from the principles; the specific judgments and actions to be applied are the final result. Figure 3 was developed by Beauchamp and Childress to demonstrate the relationship between ethical theories (moral philosophies) and actions implementing decisions.

Ethical theories do not necessarily conflict. Diverse philosophies may reach the same conclusion, albeit through different reasoning, by various constructs, or by focusing divergent criteria (e.g., the rule utilitarian's use of ends versus the Kantian's use of duty). The principles discussed here, supplemented by various of the virtues, are considered crucial and should be reflected in the organization's philosophy and the personal ethic of health services managers.

Linking ethical theories and derivative principles permits the development of usable guidelines. To aid in that process, this discussion identifies

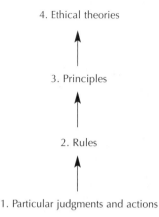

4. Ethical theories

3. Principles

2. Rules

1. Particular judgments and actions

Figure 3.   Hierarchy of relationships. (From Beauchamp, T.L., & Childress, J.F. [1983]. *Principles of biomedical ethics* [2nd ed., p. 5]. New York: Oxford University Press. Reprinted by permission.)

four principles that provide a context for managing in health services environments: 1) respect for persons, 2) beneficence, 3) nonmaleficence, and 4) justice. Utility is sometimes treated as a distinct principle, but that construct is somewhat artificial and potentially confusing. Here, utility is included as an adjunct to the principle of beneficence.

Respect for Persons

The theories discussed in this chapter support the conclusion that respect for persons is an important ethical principle. This principle has four elements. The first, autonomy, requires that one act toward others in ways that allow them to be self-governing—to choose and pursue courses of action. To do so, a person must be rational and uncoerced. Sometimes patients are or become nonautonomous (e.g., some persons with physical or cognitive disabilities). They are owed respect nonetheless, even though special means are required. Recognizing the patient's autonomy is the reason that consent for treatment is obtained, and it is a general basis for the way in which an organization views and interacts with patients and staff.

Autonomy is in dynamic tension with paternalism, the concept that one person knows what is best for another. Paternalism is an established tradition in health services. The earliest evidence of it is found in the Hippocratic oath, which directs physicians to act in what they believe to be the patient's best interests. Stressing autonomy does not eliminate paternalism, but paternalism should be limited to certain situations.

The second element of respect for persons is truth telling, which requires managers to be honest in all activities. Depending on how absolute a position is taken, this element prohibits fibs or white lies, even if they are told because it is correctly believed that knowing the truth would harm someone. The morality of insisting that patients be told the truth may also be problematic, depending on the circumstances. Some patients would suffer mental and physical harm if told the truth about their illnesses. In doing so, physicians would not meet their obligation of *primum non nocere*, or "first, do no harm." The modern expression of this concept is nonmaleficence, which is discussed later in the chapter.

Confidentiality is the third element of the principle of respect for persons. It requires managers as well as clinicians to keep what they learn about patients confidential. Morally justified exceptions to confidentiality are made, for example, when the law requires that certain diseases and conditions be reported to government. For managers, the obligation of confidentiality extends beyond patients. It applies to information about staff, organization, and community that becomes known to them in the course of their work.

The fourth element of respect for persons is fidelity: doing one's duty or keeping one's word. Sometimes this is called "promise keeping." We treat persons with respect when we do what we are expected to do or what we have promised to do. Fidelity enables managers to meet the principle of respect for persons. Here, too, if exceptions are made, they cannot be made lightly. Breaking a promise must be justified on moral grounds; it must never be done merely for convenience or self-interest.

Beneficence

Like respect for persons, the principle of beneficence is supported by most of the moral philosophies described previously, although utilitarians would require it to meet the consequences test they apply. Beneficence is rooted in Hippocratic tradition and in the history of the caring professions. Beneficence may be defined as acting with charity and kindness. Applied as a principle in health services, beneficence has a similar but broader definition. It suggests a positive duty, as distinct from the principle of nonmaleficence, which requires refraining from actions that aggravate a problem or cause other negative results. Beneficence and nonmaleficence may be viewed as opposite ends of a continuum.

Beauchamp and Childress[27] divided beneficence into two categories: 1) providing benefits and 2) balancing benefits and harms (utility). Conferring benefits is firmly established in medical tradition, and failure to provide them when one is in a position to do so violates the moral agency of both clinician and manager. Balancing benefits against harms provides a philosophical basis for cost–benefit analysis, as well as other considerations of risks balanced against benefits. In this sense it is similar to the principle of utility espoused by the utilitarians. However, here, utility is only one of several considerations and has more limited application.

The positive duty suggested by the principle of beneficence requires organizations and managers to do all they can to aid patients. A lesser duty exists to aid those who are potential rather than actual patients. This distinction and its importance vary with the philosophy and mission of the organization and whether it serves a defined population, as would a health maintenance organization. Thus, under a principle of beneficence, the hospital operating an emergency department has no duty to scour the neighborhoods for individuals needing its assistance. However, when they become patients, this relationship changes.

The second aspect of beneficence is balancing the benefits and harms that could result from certain actions. This is a natural consequence of a positive duty to act in the patient's best interests. Beyond providing benefits in a positive fashion, one cannot act with kindness and charity when risks outweigh benefits. However it is interpreted, utility cannot be used to justify overriding the interests of individual patients and sacrificing them to the greater good.

Nonmaleficence

The third principle applicable to managing health services organizations is nonmaleficence. Like beneficence, it is supported by most of the ethical theories discussed previously (it must meet the consequences test to claim utilitarianism as a basis). Nonmaleficence means *primum non nocere*. This dictum to physicians is equally applicable to health services managers. Beauchamp and Childress[28] noted that although nonmaleficence gives rise to specific moral rules, neither the principle nor the derivative rules can be absolute because it is often appropriate (with the patient's consent) to cause some risk, discomfort, or even harm in order to avoid greater harm or to prevent a worse situation from occurring. Beauchamp and Childress included the natural law concepts of extraordinary and ordinary care and double effect in the principle of nonmaleficence. (These concepts are considered later in this chapter under the subheading titled "Application of the Principles and Virtues.") Nonmaleficence also leads managers and clinicians to avoid risks, unless potential results justify them.

Justice

The fourth principle, justice, is especially important for administrative (and clinical) decision making in resource allocation, but it applies to areas of management such as human resources policies as well. What is just, and how does one know when justice has been achieved? Although all moral philosophies recognize the importance of achieving justice, they define it differently. Rawls defined justice as fairness. Implicit in that definition is that persons get what is due them. But how are fairness and "just desserts" defined? Aristotle's concept of justice, which is reflected in natural law, is that equals are treated equally, unequals unequally. This concept of fairness is used commonly in policy analysis. Equal treatment of equals is reflected in liberty rights (e.g., universal freedom of speech). Unequal treatment of unequal individuals is used to justify progressive income taxation and redistribution of wealth: It is argued that those who earn more should pay higher taxes. This concept is expressed in health services delivery by expending greater resources on individuals who are sicker and thus in need of more services.

These concepts of justice are helpful, but they do not solve the problems of definition and opinion, which are always troublesome. Macro- and microallocation of resources have received extensive consideration in the literature, but there is little agreement as to operational definitions. Each organization must determine how its resources will be allocated. An essential measure of whether organizations and their clinicians and managers are acting justly is that they consistently apply clear criteria in decision making.

Summary

Philosophers call respect for persons, beneficence, nonmaleficence, and justice *prima facie* (at first view, self-evident) principles or *prima facie* duties. None is more important; none has greater weight. Health services managers are expected to meet all four. A principle can be violated only with clear moral justification, and then negative results must be minimized. Virtue ethics holds a special place in the work of managers, and the virtues are applied to supplement and complement the *prima facie* duties.

MORAL PHILOSOPHY AND THE PERSONAL ETHIC

This examination of moral philosophies and derivative principles provides a framework for developing a personal ethic and subsequently analyzing ethical problems. Like philosophers, managers are unlikely to agree with all elements of a moral philosophy and make it their own. Most managers are eclectic as they develop and reconsider their personal ethic. In general, however, the principles and virtues described here are essential to establishing and maintaining appropriate relationships among patients, managers, and organizations, and they should be part of the ethic of health services managers and the value system of the organizations they manage. It should be stressed that the four derivative principles may appropriately carry different weights, depending on the ethical issue being considered. The principle of justice requires, however, that there be a consistent ordering and weighing when the same types of ethical problems are considered.

Application of the Principles and Virtues

How do the principles and virtues identified and discussed in the preceding section and their underlying moral philosophies assist in solving ethical problems in cases such as Baby Boy Doe (see p. 16)? The principle of respect for persons implies certain duties and relationships, including autonomy. Nonautonomous persons, however, must have decisions made for them by a surrogate. The parents of Baby Boy Doe, a nonautonomous person, had to make decisions on behalf of their son. Surrogates cannot exercise unlimited authority, especially when it is uncertain that a decision is in the patient's best interests. If the infant's and parents' interests differ, caregivers (including managers) are duty bound under the principles of beneficence and nonmaleficence to try to persuade parents to take another course of action. Such efforts by caregivers and managers should have been attempted for Baby Boy Doe.

Extending the principles of beneficence and nonmaleficence, it is acceptable for the organization to seek legal intervention and obtain permission to treat an infant against the parents' wishes. The moral compulsion to do so is especially great when the parents are not acting in the child's best interests, but this moral duty should be exercised only as a last resort. Courts intervene under the theory of *parens patriae* to permit a hospital or social welfare agency to stand *in loco parentis* (in the role or in place of a parent). Courts take this step reluctantly because of the common law tradition that gives parents control over reproductive and family matters, including decisions about infant children. As noted, although it is an element of beneficence, utility is not an overriding concept that permits trampling on the rights of the person, as happened to Baby Boy Doe.

Intervention has limits. Absent an emergency, treating the infant against the parents' wishes without a court order is unethical because it breaks the law. If persons caring for the infant cannot continue to do so because of their personal ethic, they should be permitted to withdraw. The option to remove oneself from a situation that is ethically intolerable should be reflected in the organization's philosophy and policies.

In applying the principle of nonmaleficence, one must consider whether the ethically superior choice would have been to shorten Baby Boy Doe's life through active euthanasia. This consideration raises the question of the moral difference between killing and letting die. Some argue that the identical results make them morally indistinguishable. The analysis cannot end there, however; to do so ignores critical aspects of medical decision making.

When caregivers apply the principle of nonmaleficence, they refrain from doing harm, which includes minimizing pain and suffering. Asking caregivers dedicated to preserving life to end it will cause significant role conflict. Furthermore, physicians and nurses in such roles are on a slippery slope that may lead to more exceptions and increasing use of positive acts to shorten lives that are deemed by someone to be not worth living.

The concept of extraordinary care is a part of the principle of nonmaleficence that developed from natural law. *Ordinary care* is treatment that is provided without excessive expense, pain, or inconvenience and that offers reasonable hope of benefit. Care is *extraordinary* if it is available only in conjunction with excessive expense, pain, or other inconvenience or if it does not offer any reasonable hope of benefit.[29] With no reasonable hope of benefit, *any* expense, pain, or inconvenience is excessive. Beauchamp and Childress[30] concluded that the "ordinary-extraordinary distinction thus collapses into the balance between benefits and burdens, where the latter category includes immediate detriment, inconvenience, risk of harm, and other costs." For Baby Boy Doe, there was hope of benefit, even though correcting the atresia would not reverse his mental retardation. Surgery would have given Baby Boy Doe a normal life for someone with his cognitive abilities. That benefit justifies the use of treatment involving significant expense, pain, and/or inconvenience.

Justice is the final principle to be applied, a principle that was previously noted to have rather divergent definitions. Rawls defined justice as fairness. Applied to the case of Baby Boy Doe, one could conclude that the result was just. Fairness is arguably compatible with an enlightened self-interest expressed by persons in the original position behind a veil of ignorance—the Rawlsian philosophical construct. Rational persons could decide that no life is preferable to one of significantly diminished quality, even though this arguably limits the liberty principle, which Rawls considered ultimately important.

For a Kantian or an adherent to natural law, the outcome in the Baby Boy Doe case is abhorrent because the infant was used as a means rather than as an end. Conversely, rule utilitarians would find the result accept-able. Other definitions of justice produce different conclusions. For exam-ple, if justice is defined as getting one's just desserts, it is clear that Baby Boy Doe fared badly. Applying an even cruder standard—that individuals equally situated should be treated equally—it is clear that if an adult had been in a similar situation, the necessary treatment would have been rendered. For Baby Boy Doe, the results of applying the principle of justice are uncertain.

The final regulations about infant care published by the U.S. Depart-ment of Health and Human Services (DHHS) in April 1985 focus on beneficence and nonmaleficence. In implementing the Child Abuse Amendments of 1984 ([PL 98-457], amending the Child Abuse Prevention and Treatment Act of 1974 [PL 93-247]), DHHS placed no weight on the parents' traditional right to judge what should be done for infants with cognitive and/or physical impairments and life-threatening conditions. The potential problem caused by parents who may not fully understand the implications of the diagnosis (of both the impairments and the life-threatening conditions) and the effects of their decision is obviated by the regulations because medical criteria applied by a knowledgeable, reasonable physician are used. Quality of life criteria cannot be considered. The preliminary regulations to implement the law made specific reference to a case similar to that of Baby Boy Doe and stated that appropriate medical treatment had to be rendered. The final regulations contain no examples, however. Nevertheless, it is likely that DHHS will view narrowly any decisions to forego treatment of infants with impairments and life-threat-ening conditions. Specifics of the regulations are discussed in Chapter 10.

As with most governmental efforts to regulate ethical decision making, these regulations are likely to be modified in the future. From an ethical standpoint, it is more important to bear in mind the moral considerations that should underlie public policy than to be preoccupied with the seman-tics of a particular enactment.

Implications for Management

What are the implications of cases like that of Baby Boy Doe for health services managers? Such events place a heavy burden on caregivers. What-ever the decision, these cases split the staff. The resulting controversy diminishes morale. In addition, criticism may be leveled against manage-ment, governance, and medical staff by individuals who question the moral-ity of the decision and the organization's role in it. In extreme cases, legal action may ensue.

It is crucial that the health services organization implement a view (a philosophy) about matters such as these that is reflected in its policies and procedures. This means the organization has explicitly formulated a course of action—a plan—that it will take when confronted with such problems. Having a philosophy in place permits a deliberate response rather than one that is reactive, inadequately considered, or governed by (rather than governing) events. At the very least, the organization must consider these issues prospectively and within the constraints of its organizational philosophy.

Paradoxically, prior to the 1984 Child Abuse Amendments, the health services organization could legally do to Baby Boy Doe what the parents could not. Had the parents taken the infant home and allowed him to starve and dehydrate until he died, it is likely that they would have been charged with child neglect or some degree of homicide or manslaughter. However, the organization did not face the same liability. In fact, had it surgically repaired the atresia without parental consent it would have committed battery on the infant for which it could have been sued for civil damages and for which the staff charged criminally. Criminal charges are unlikely, but the hospital is legally obligated to obtain consent from the parents or legal guardian for a minor when no emergency exists.

CONCLUSION

This chapter helps the manager develop a personal ethic and stimulates the organization to formulate a philosophy. Few managers will disagree as to the importance of the principles of respect for persons, beneficence, nonmaleficence, justice, and various other complementary virtues. However, not all managers will embrace unequivocally the principles and underlying moral philosophies discussed here. It is even more unlikely that they will agree about their weighing or priority. Chapter 2 suggests a methodology that managers can use in solving ethical problems.

NOTES

1. Robert Hunt & John Arras, Eds. (1983). *Issues in modern medicine* (2nd ed., p. 27). Palo Alto, CA: Mayfield Publishing.
2. Edgar Bodenheimer. (1974). *Jurisprudence: The philosophy and method of the law* (Rev. ed., pp. 23–24). Cambridge, MA: Harvard University Press.
3. John Rawls. (1971). *A theory of justice* (p. 60). Cambridge, MA: Belknap Press.
4. Albert R. Jonsen & Stephen Toulmin. (1988). *The abuse of casuistry: A history of moral reasoning* (p. 13). Berkeley, CA: University of California Press.

5. Tom L. Beauchamp & LeRoy Walters, Eds. (1994). *Contemporary issues in bioethics* (4th ed., p. 21). Belmont, CA: Wadsworth Publishing.
6. Albert R. Jonsen. (1986). Casuistry and clinical ethics. *Theoretical Medicine*, 7, p. 70.
7. *Ibid.*, p. 71.
8. Beauchamp & Walters, p. 19.
9. Annette C. Baier. (1987). Hume, the women's moral theorist? In Eva Feder Kittay & Diana T. Meyers, Eds. *Women and moral theory* (p. 44). Totowa, NJ: Rowman & Littlefield.
10. Virginia Held. (1987). Feminism and moral theory. In Eva Feder Kittay & Diana T. Meyers, Eds. *Women and moral theory* (p. 111). Totowa, NJ: Rowman & Littlefield.
11. Carol Gilligan. (1987). Moral orientation and moral development. In Eva Feder Kittay & Diana T. Meyers, Eds. *Women and moral theory* (p. 24). Totowa, NJ: Rowman & Littlefield.
12. James J. Finnerty, JoAnn V. Pinkerton, Jonathan Moreno, & James E. Ferguson. (2000, August). Ethical theory and principles: Do they have any relevance to problems arising in everyday practice? *American Journal of Obstetrics and Gynecology 183*(2), 301–308.
13. Virtue Ethics. (2003, July 18). *Stanford encyclopedia of philosophy*. Retrieved December 18, 2003, from http://plato.stanford.edu/entries/ethics-virtue
14. Virtue ethics contrasted with deontology and consequentialism. (2003, November 17). *Wikipedia: The free encyclopedia*. Retrieved November 30, 2003, from http://en.wikipedia.org/wiki/Virtue_ethics
15. Edmund D. Pellegrino & David C. Thomasma. (1988). *For the patient's good: The restoration of beneficence in health care* (p. 121). New York: Oxford University Press.
16. *Ibid.*, p. 116.
17. Edmund D. Pellegrino. (1994). The virtuous physician and the ethics of medicine. In Tom L. Beauchamp & LeRoy Walters, Eds. *Contemporary issues in bioethics* (4th ed., p. 55). Belmont, CA: Wadsworth Publishing.
18. Frederick S. Carney. (1978). Theological ethics. In Warren T. Reich, Ed., *Encyclopedia of bioethics: Vol. 1* (pp. 435–436). New York: The Free Press.
19. Virtue Ethics.
20. William David Ross. (1995). *Aristotle* (6th ed., p. 209). New York: Routledge.
21. *Ibid.*
22. Tom L. Beauchamp & James F. Childress. (2001). *Principles of biomedical ethics* (5th ed., pp. 32–37). New York: Oxford University Press.
23. *Ibid.*, p. 210.
24. Virtue Ethics.
25. Pellegrino & Thomasma, p. 121.
26. Pellegrino, p. 53.
27. Tom L. Beauchamp & James F. Childress. (1989). *Principles of biomedical ethics* (3rd ed., p. 195). New York: Oxford University Press.
28. *Ibid.*, p. 122.
29. Gerald Kelly. (1951, December 12). The duty to preserve life. *Theological Studies*, p. 550.
30. Beauchamp & Childress, p. 153.

CHAPTER 2

RESOLVING
ETHICAL ISSUES

Managers are problem solvers. It is the reason they are hired—organizations without problems do not need managers. Some problems burst on the scene. Something is no doubt amiss when a wildcat strike occurs among the nursing staff or when the local newspaper attacks the organization editorially. Other problems are hard to uncover and often provide no clear evidence or warning. They must be identified and treated early; undetected, they will grow and may threaten the organization's survival (i.e., "a stitch in time saves nine"). Solving them is similar to detection and early treatment of cancer.

Successful managers possess highly developed conceptual and problem identification skills. Preventing (if possible) or identifying and solving ethical problems with the least disruption to the organization are as critical as solving management problems affecting personnel or finances. Ethical problems have implications for traditional management areas, and traditional management problems have ethical dimensions. It is important to note in using this comparison that the techniques and skills employed in solving ethical problems have many similarities to those needed to solve management problems. Problem solving is a generic process that applies to both.

IDENTIFYING ETHICAL PROBLEMS

Often, managers believe that they are inadequately prepared to recognize ethical problems and even less able to solve them. This view understates the typical manager's credentials and ability. Identifying ethical issues that could become problems is primarily a matter of mind-set, attitude, and application of common sense when reviewing or analyzing a situation. Identifying an ethical problem and its dimensions is often less difficult than developing and implementing morally acceptable alternative solutions.

Developing and implementing solutions are more likely to require assistance from within the organization or even from outside it.

Managers who see their function only as solving problems of staffing, directing, budgeting, controlling, organizing, coordinating, integrating, and planning need increased sensitivity to ethical issues more than postgraduate education in philosophy. Methodologies similar to those used to solve traditional management problems can be used to solve ethical problems, whether they are administrative or biomedical. (This generic process is examined later in the chapter.) However, traditional management issues often overshadow and may even overwhelm the ethical dimensions that invariably accompany them. In addition, the ethical dimensions of managerial problems can be subtle, which complicates initial identification and solution.

Using authority delegated by the governing body, managers represent the organization. As considered in Chapter 3, the organization's philosophy provides a general context for the manager's activities and decision making. The presence of an organizational philosophy, however, does not eliminate the manager's need to have a personal ethic. A personal ethic provides managers with a framework for decisions and permits greater refinement of principles, rules, and particular judgments (as well as actions or nonactions) than is likely in the statement of philosophy developed by the typical health services organization. It bears repeating that each human being is a moral agent whose actions, nonactions, and misactions have moral consequences. Morally unacceptable conduct cannot be excused because someone was following orders or policy, regardless of their source. Orders from lawfully constituted authorities, such as courts, pose a special problem. Moral agents who consider such orders unjust or immoral may engage in civil disobedience, but in doing so they must be prepared to bear societally imposed sanctions. The ethical (moral) implications of acts must be considered independently.

Occasionally, there may be conflict between the organization's ethic, as expressed in its philosophy, and the manager's personal ethic. The organization is a bureaucracy and the manager must carefully consider the implications of acquiescing to its values. This follows from the concept of moral agency. Often, it seems easier to "go along to get along" than to risk one's position by speaking out. Professional dissent or whistleblowing are rare, despite evidence that sharp or dishonest practices, criminal behavior, or activities that pose a danger to the public are not uncommon in organizations, even those in the health services field. Managers must recognize both the distinction between and the integration of an organizational and a personal ethic. They must not perform their daily tasks with little thought about the ethical context or implications of what they do, fail to do, or do badly.

In terms of the problem-solving methodology described later, the organization's philosophy and the individual's personal ethic are vital. They provide the framework and context in which the manager functions and they enhance sensitization to and identification and solution of ethical problems so that managers can approach these problems as they would traditional management problems.

Another technique that may be useful in identifying ethical problems is the ethics audit. Conducted much like a financial audit, the ethics audit allows the organization to compare actual with desired performance using a set of criteria. Even small increases in some measures should warn managers of ethical problems: patient complaints, incident reports, and legal actions; employee grievances, resignations, terminations, and wrongful discharge complaints; medical staff complaints and resignations; problems with suppliers and other vendors; and adverse publicity. The ethics audit should include three steps. First, analyze key documents (e.g., vision, mission, and values statements) and their operationalization in policies and procedures, with special attention paid to issues such as uncompensated care, confidentiality, consent, conflicts of interest, and sexual harassment. Second, survey representative board members, managers, physicians, employees, volunteers, and community residents and organizations to determine whether actual performance matches that desired. Third, address deficiencies through education or other appropriate strategies.[1] Compliance or noncompliance with laws and regulations raises other ethical (and legal) issues.

Administrative Ethical Issues

Leadership is essential in management. It includes setting goals, establishing direction, and guiding the organization. These activities are more ethics sensitive than are many routine managerial activities. Day-to-day activities (i.e., transactional leadership) seem less tied to values, but even these are based on earlier decisions rooted in ethical principles, whether or not those principles are identified and expressly stated. However management functions are interpreted, human beings cannot escape their role as moral agents. Managers set a tone and establish a context for the organization and staff. They can neither avoid scrutiny of their personal ethic nor its congruence with the organization's philosophy.

Managers hold positions of trust, which may not be used for personal advantage or personal aggrandizement. Managers must not act in any ways that raise the slightest hint of wrongdoing. If one seeks to be an effective leader, these are essential elements of a personal ethic. Actions (and nonactions and misactions) should be judged by applying the ethical principles and virtues discussed in Chapter 1. Another effective way to clarify the pragmatic effect of an action is to step back and view what is being done or contemplated as though one were an outsider. One should ask oneself, "How would the public and my colleagues see this decision?" This "as seen through the eyes of others" or "light of public scrutiny" standard for judging managerial decisions is helpful. A cynic's standard is not useful—meeting it is impossible because cynics see problems when it is unreasonable to do so. Skepticism is a useful criterion for managers to apply as they seek to understand how their actions might be interpreted. A standard of discovery is unacceptable because the concept of "if you don't get caught, it's okay" negates the need for ethics and substitutes deviousness and deceit.

In a way quite different from a personal ethic or an organization's philosophy, the law is a baseline of what is considered ethical. The Introduction noted that laws provide useful comparisons; however, they guide us only partially because the law is a minimum standard of conduct and no manager is effective by meeting minimum requirements. The manager qua leader must set an example that substantially surpasses what is expected of others. Professional codes also guide conduct and provide frames of reference. Codes have a more demanding level of performance than the law but should not be seen as incorporating all expectations of ethical performance.

Is it persuasive to argue that where one stands on administrative ethics depends on where one sits? Does the concept of "rank hath its privileges" apply to managing health services? Many senior managers act as to suggest that they believe it does. One readily finds situations in which subordinates are reprimanded for behavior unpunished at the upper echelons. Here, it is "do as I say, not as I do" or "what is good for the goose is not good for the gander." Few will fail to distinguish words from actions. This double standard sends staff a clear message of cynicism and inconsistency and greatly diminishes the manager's ability to lead.

Managers can become sensitive to administrative ethical issues in several ways. They should be voracious readers of the popular press and professional literature because what happens elsewhere could become a problem for them. Codes of ethics are valuable guides to understanding the concerns of the profession and parameters of acceptable action. Asking whether the Golden Rule is being met will help identify ethical problems. Not to be forgotten is intuition and hunch, which form that sixth sense that something is wrong. Both can be nurtured to alert managers to the presence of ethical problems.

Identifying ethical problems means focusing on the principles of respect for persons, beneficence, nonmaleficence, and justice, as complemented by the virtues; asking if the actions contemplated violate them; and determining whether the violation is justified by special circumstances. A questioning mind permits managers to consider the situation further or seek assistance, as appropriate. Identifying administrative ethical problems requires attention to detail and constant vigilance.

Biomedical Ethical Issues

All contemplated and actual interactions with patients present potential sources of ethical problems, which range from paternalism to consent and from truth telling to decisions at the end of life. Managers may feel uncomfortable and out of place working to solve biomedical ethical problems. They should not. *Medicine and the clinician provide key information that assists in making informed ethical decisions, but the decision itself is ethical (moral), not clinical.* The distinction between clinical and ethical aspects of biomedical decision making is critical and is one managers must not forget. Managers will gain confidence with greater experience and exposure to biomedical ethical issues. Their participation is needed because increased medical staff–administration interaction results in a more effective and efficient organization and because all biomedical problems have administrative dimensions. Thus, the manager's involvement is critical.

Managers do not supersede clinicians but are important to preventing or solving a wide range of biomedical ethical problems through actions including serving on institutional ethics committees and institutional review boards and participating in resource allocation decisions. In addition, managers are key in developing the processes and operationalizing the policies, procedures, and rules that implement the organization's philosophy.

As noted in the section on administrative ethics issues, managers need not take postgraduate courses in philosophy or ethics to identify the presence of potential problems, although such courses might be helpful. Primarily, identifying potential ethical problems requires sensitization, an inquiring mind, and a reasonably well-developed personal ethic. Questions such as the following are useful in identifying biomedical ethical problems:

- "Is there a clearly enunciated value system reflected in the organization's culture?"

- "Is there an institutional ethics committee to resolve ethical issues?"

- "Is this patient being treated as I would wish to be?"

- "Is the patient protected from unnecessary risk?"

- "Does the consent process adequately inform the patient about the treatment contemplated?"

As with all problem solving, asking the right questions may be the most important part of the process.

A key role for managers is stimulating the medical staff and other caregivers to develop the expertise to prevent or effectively address biomedical ethical problems. To do so, caregivers must be availed of procedures and rules to follow. Here, the manager's role as a catalyst is much the same as that played in traditional administrative activities. Regrettably, codes of administrative ethics provide limited guidance in addressing biomedical ethical issues.

SOLVING PROBLEMS

Unresolved ethical problems exact the same destructive effect on an organization as do problems involving personnel, finance, or the medical staff. Therefore, it is imperative that managers possess a methodology for solving these problems. This poses difficulties, however, because few managers are formally trained in ethics. Ethical issues may seem more subtle than management problems, and because managers tend to be pragmatic, they are less inclined to grapple with nuances. Sometimes ethical problems are combined with and overshadowed by administrative issues. Furthermore, managers may consider ethical issues less important than other problems, perhaps because they do not comprehend their potentially devastating effect. These obstacles are surmountable, however.

In 1910, the American educator and philosopher John Dewey wrote in his book *How We Think* that problem solving comprises three stages: identifying the problem, identifying the alternatives, and determining which alternative is best. Implicitly or explicitly, successful managers use a similar process. The stages of the process include identifying the problem in terms of both the current manifestation (which may be only a symptom) and the underlying cause, developing alternative solutions and the decision criteria to judge them acceptable, unacceptable, or optimal; preparing an implementation plan for the solution selected; and developing a means to evaluate the solution, once implemented.

Philosophers use a similar methodology, *moral reasoning*, to analyze ethical problems. Its components are surprisingly similar to the manager's problem-solving methodology:

- *Analyzing*—separating the overall structure of a problem in a particular case into its major components
- *Weighing*—assessing the strengths and weaknesses of various alternatives that could be used in solving the problem by balancing them against one another
- *Justifying*—providing a compelling and sufficient moral reason that appeals to an established moral principle, such as "always tell the truth" [any such principle must be compatible with the organization's philosophy and the manager's personal ethic]
- *Choosing*—selecting one or more of the available alternatives, preferably on the basis of a position that can be and has been shown to be justified
- *Evaluating*—reexamining the choices and their justifications, identifying unanswered questions, and relating decisions about one particular case to similar cases[2]

Problem solving can be divided into two basic types:

> The specific focus on problem solving is rooted in two broad models, the rational and the heuristic. Problem definition is addressed differently by each. The rational model (sometimes identified with programmed decisions) assumes that one is faced with a specific problem and focuses primarily on a search for the optimal solution.
>
> Operations research, for example, is primarily a quantitative expression of this approach applied to a wide range of management issues. In the hospital, it includes problems such as work scheduling, e.g., developing a computer program that maximizes the preferred work schedule of a large number of nurses, or a PERT chart used to schedule the construction of a new building. These and similar problem-solving techniques are important for an organization, and help it to establish patterns for problem solving.
>
> The heuristic model (sometimes identified with nonprogrammed decisions, or a learning model) acknowledges that some problems may be more diffusely defined, poorly structured, and are often not routine. It focuses upon an iterative process of dealing with problem definition, as well as solution. Heuristic general problem-solving techniques have been suggested for training administrators. Heuristic problem-solving approaches which are quantitative and computer-based have been advocated.[3]

The distinctions between the rational and heuristic models suggests that solving ethical problems is heuristic. First, however, process and substance components must be separated, and ethical problems that recur and have similar features must be distinguished from those that are unique and unlikely to recur. Process components are more amenable to analysis and solution by the rational model than are substance (content/issue) components. Ethical problems that recur and have similar features are also more amenable to using the rational model. Even here, however, implementing the process may uncover unique or subtle problems of substance, such as relative authority of different individuals in the decision-making process. The two problem-solving theories are not mutually exclusive, and the heuristic model often benefits from using a rational model for parts of the analysis. Thus, problem solvers should not choose one model to the exclusion of the other.

Graduate programs in health services administration and business administration teach problem solving. Such methodologies are useful in solving ethical problems and are similar to the generic problem-solving model in Figure 4. The model is shown in two dimensions, but should be conceptualized with time as the third dimension. In this respect, the model is like a corkscrew: While the process cycles from problem analysis to evaluation of results, the whole activity is moving through time.

In Figure 4, problem analysis begins when the manager objectively or intuitively finds something amiss. Commonly, in solving management problems, it is here that actual results deviate from desired or expected results or a situation occurs that demands an organizational response. Examples of developments requiring management's attention include a rapid decrease or increase in outpatient admissions, increased turnover among staff in a department, more uneaten food returned from patient rooms or the cafeteria to dietary, or an announcement that competing emergicenters are opening or closing. Some of these potential problems are foreseen through analysis of routinely collected data; others are apparent only when they occur. Obvious and defined problems are more likely to be amenable to the rational model than the heuristic.

Similarly, the ethical dimensions of some situations are apparent. If a patient is diagnosed as being in a persistent vegetative state (PVS), an ethical problem having both clinical and administrative dimensions exists. An ethical problem is also present when the organization lacks an effective consent process. In such situations heuristic problem solving is not the most effective methodology.

A potential administrative and biomedical ethics problem needs a solution only when the problem solver determines that it must be solved. Sometimes, before an ethical problem can be resolved, it disappears (e.g., the patient in PVS cannot be resuscitated after cardiac arrest). The problem is gone but not because it was solved.

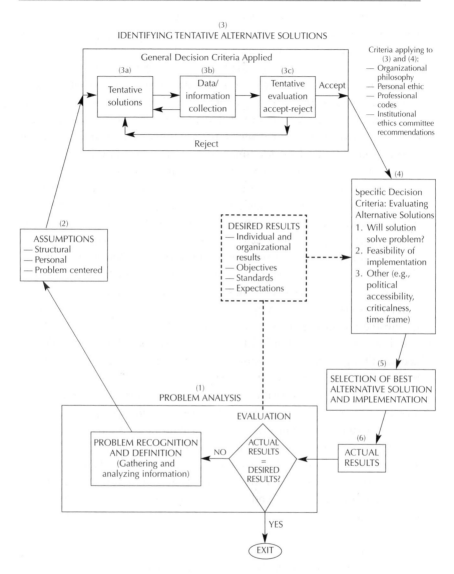

(3)
IDENTIFYING TENTATIVE ALTERNATIVE SOLUTIONS

General Decision Criteria Applied

(3a) Tentative solutions → (3b) Data/information collection → (3c) Tentative evaluation accept-reject → Accept

Reject

Criteria applying to (3) and (4):
— Organizational philosophy
— Personal ethic
— Professional codes
— Institutional ethics committee recommendations

(4)
Specific Decision Criteria: Evaluating Alternative Solutions
1. Will solution solve problem?
2. Feasibility of implementation
3. Other (e.g., political accessibility, criticalness, time frame)

(2)
ASSUMPTIONS
— Structural
— Personal
— Problem centered

DESIRED RESULTS
— Individual and organizational results
— Objectives
— Standards
— Expectations

(5)
SELECTION OF BEST ALTERNATIVE SOLUTION AND IMPLEMENTATION

(1)
PROBLEM ANALYSIS

EVALUATION

PROBLEM RECOGNITION AND DEFINITION (Gathering and analyzing information)

NO → ACTUAL RESULTS = DESIRED RESULTS?

(6)
ACTUAL RESULTS

YES

EXIT

Figure 4.   Schema for solving ethical problems. (From Longest, B.B., Jr., Rakich, J.S., & Darr, K. [2000]. *Managing health services organizations and systems* [4th ed., p. 323]. Baltimore: Health Professions Press; adapted by permission.)

Berry and Seavey[4] argued that problem definitions "are fundamentally subjective [and] . . . are not objective, concrete realities; they are perceptions of reality." This statement is correct as it bears on perceptions of cause and effect but must be qualified when applied to certain situations. For example, several unexplained deaths in a nursing facility are a fact and will be defined by a manager as a problem that needs solving. Perceptions (subjectivity) vary in determining the cause or in identifying the underlying situation (problem) that may be the cause. Views of problems and their solutions are affected by the positions held and responsibilities of the individuals involved. Nursing service is likely to provide a different explanation of the deaths than would management.

Context is far more important in solving problems that are primarily ethical than when solving management problems with few ethical dimensions. The context of ethical problems is the organization's philosophy and mission interpreted and applied by a manager who is a moral agent with a personal ethic. Once an ethical problem has been recognized and defined as a problem needing a solution, it must be understood. The information about its extent and character may be available in existing data or special efforts may be required to obtain it. Managers solving ethical problems will experience data deficits similar to those they confront when solving other problems.

Box 2 in Figure 4 asks managers to identify assumptions about the problem, personal implications and views, and the structure within which the problem arises. Staff were undoubtedly affected by the case of Baby Boy Doe, and it is reasonable to assume that in similar cases, staff will become depressed and angry and morale will decline. One may also assume that few staff members will be so upset that they will resign, turn to a union, or refuse to work in the nursery. Assumptions such as these require judgment by managers and may result in a decision to ignore the situation (i.e., not define it as a problem requiring a solution), which is what occurred in the case of Baby Boy Doe. The hospital accepted the parents' directives and determined there was either no problem that required a solution or that the solution was to do nothing. Such a result is dependent on the organization's philosophy and the individual manager's personal ethic. Choosing to do nothing is always an option, if it meets the decision criteria. This may be the best alternative in some situations. However, it must never be the choice by default.

Preliminary review of options occurs in Box 3, in which alternative solutions are identified and assessed. Here, decision makers may brainstorm creative solutions. Managers solving administrative or biomedical ethical problems must be mindful of the organization's philosophy as well as their personal ethic. Unless the constraints of the context can be changed, solutions falling outside them must be discarded. Arbitrarily ignoring or applying these constraints creates inconsistencies and discontinuities that eventually cause serious problems for the organization and the manager. Other, more general criteria are also applied in such instances.

Alternative solutions that pass this preliminary screening are subject to detailed assessment. This assessment compares each option against specific decision criteria. Examples of these criteria are shown in Box 4 of Figure 4: time available to solve the problem, real costs of all kinds (e.g., political, financial, reputation), opportunity costs, feasibility of implementation, adequacy of solving the problem, and benefits derived. Applying more specific criteria results in better solutions and outcomes. A primary benefit of greater specificity in the process is that managers must review, analyze, and be as precise as possible, both in defining the problem and in selecting the alternative that best solves it. This is a useful exercise because it hones management decision making. A more sophisticated approach is to weight or assign relative values to decision criteria because some are more important than others.

Prior to and after selecting the alternative, the manager must consider implementation and evaluation. A common failing is that great effort is put into developing a solution and beginning implementation. Then, managers are distracted by other problems. The result is that the solution flounders before it is fully implemented. Implementing the solution should receive as much attention as selecting it. Evaluation must be included in the solution so that difficulties can be identified and timely corrective action can be taken. Corrective actions are a subset of the problem-solving process and may involve the same or similar steps.

This ethical problem-solving methodology is useful for decision making by one manager, by management as a group, by governing body committees, or by specially established committees, such as institutional ethics committees, infant care review committees, or institutional review boards. It is effective for solving one problem, considering guidelines for a class of problems, or developing a process to bring a similar methodology to bear on solving individual problems or groups of problems. Regardless of the source of decision making, once the process is established and policies (which have gone through a similar problem-solving process) have been formulated and implemented, operating procedures and rules will be established. This means that an issue such as consent has been considered and that the ethically acceptable policies, procedures, and processes have been identified and implemented. The desired result is that many ethical problems will be prevented. Exceptions and special attention will be necessary when the facts differ sufficiently from the assumptions implicit in the policy and procedures derived from it.

In this regard it is unnecessary to distinguish administrative from biomedical ethical problems. Because both types of problems are certain, policies should be adopted prospectively. The derivative procedures and rules will cover the majority of predictable, recurring ethical problems. That is why, for example, a governing body adopts a conflict of interest policy applicable to itself and management staff. Despite the usefulness of policies and procedures, problems occur in interpreting and applying them and because unique ethical issues arise. It bears repeating that the problem-solving model discussed previously is usable on two levels: general policy development and consideration of individual cases.

Although in most ways implementing solutions to administrative or biomedical ethical problems is the same as it is for management problems, some distinctions are noteworthy. One is that ethical issues often involve high levels of emotion. Examples are situations that suggest a manager has acted unethically (administrative ethics) or that a patient's view of life and death has been violated or challenged (biomedical ethics). Thus, managers and staff who work to solve ethical problems must exercise greater sensitivity to human factors and must understand that they are not dealing with units of production or ordinary services. Another distinction is that administrative and, especially, biomedical ethical issues often have the potential for significant legal consequences. Although all health services organizations should apply a standard that is much higher than the minimum set by the law, mistakes do occur, and occasionally, there are problems that bring in lawyers. Yet another distinction is that negative public relations consequences may occur inside and outside the organization.

DEVELOPING A PERSONAL ETHIC

Health services managers begin their careers as adults who at least have an implicit personal ethic. In developing that ethic managers have been affected by a host of influences beyond their own introspection, including family and friends, religious principles and teachings, secular education, and the law. It is in this context that adults become managers and that a personal ethic about management emerges. For some managers their personal ethic may be only an intuitive sense of right and wrong, with no identifiable source or explicitly defined code of conduct.

Developing a personal ethic necessitates introspection and self-examination. Questions such as the following are helpful: "Who am I?", "How do I view certain actions or activities?", "What do I consider unethical?", and "What is morally right or wrong?" Understanding and grappling with questions such as these are critical as managers search for the "right" answer to ethical problems. Both new and experienced health services managers use numerous sources to develop and refine their personal ethic. Chief among them are professional codes of ethics; organization values and culture; educational socialization; and association and pressure of peers, subordinates, and superiors.

In selecting the principles to be included in a personal ethic, managers should apply the criteria of comprehensiveness, consistency, and coherence and ask themselves the following questions:

- Do the principles apply to the broadest possible range of ethical issues?

- How useful and applicable are they in solving ethical problems?

- Do they use the scientific method in terms of exactness, systemization, and predictability?

- Are the ethical concepts clear and consistent?

- Are they in conflict with or consistent with other knowledge or life experiences?

- Are they reasonably adaptable to a changing world?

Although the criteria of comprehensiveness, consistency, and coherence are not applied with the rigor employed by a moral philosopher, they should be used when developing, judging, or reconsidering a personal ethic and when analyzing the ethics of others or disputing their reasoning or conclusions. In developing and reconsidering one's personal ethic it is useful to paraphrase Plato, who said that the unexamined life is not worth living.

The moral philosophy of casuistry has special relevance in the manager's efforts to hone a personal ethic. Casuistry's emphasis on cases and the reiterative nature of cases and similar events provides special assistance in terms of a personal ethic. Virtue ethics has a unique role here, too. The virtues noted in Chapter 1 should be included in a personal ethic and reexamining whether one is a virtuous manager will reinforce or highlight a need for further attention.

In addition to the manager's personal ethic, the organization's philosophy is vital to ethical decision making. It is tempting to say that the personal ethic is and ought to remain the most important factor. However, one cannot ignore the realities of bureaucratic life. Some sectarian health services organizations seek complete congruence between a manager's personal ethic and the organization's ethic by hiring no one above mid-level management who is not an adherent to that faith. The wisdom of such a policy is examined later. Suffice to say that in modern, complex health services organizations a significant and undesirable potential for discontinuity exists between the philosophy of the organization and that of its managers. However, the extent to which these philosophies *must* be identical, or even congruent, is unclear. It is likely that the organization's philosophy and the values expressed in its culture will have a greater impact on development of the personal ethic of a younger, less experienced manager. Like everyone else, managers can become set in their ways.

CONCLUSION

In solving problems, successful managers implicitly or explicitly use a methodology similar to that outlined in Figure 4. Effectively solving ethical problems requires the same attention and a similar approach. Managers cannot ignore ethical problems, and they must be prepared to participate in solving them. This does not mean that health services managers supersede physicians or other clinical staff when biomedical ethics are involved. It is critical, however, to separate the technical and clinical dimensions from the ethical. It does mean that in an effort to operationalize the principles and virtues developed in Chapter 1, managers must participate effectively in solving ethical problems of all types. It is the nature of the job that managers serve as team leaders and catalysts. Serving as the organization's conscience is consistent with the manager's role as moral agent in a position of ethical leadership. In terms of administrative ethics, the manager's role is preeminent but not to the exclusion of physicians.

Successful managers have a well-developed personal ethic and a clear perspective on administrative and biomedical ethical issues. This ethic has been defined by drawing from a wide variety of sources. A personal ethic cannot be chiseled in stone, and it can be expected to evolve over time. Although one's basic view of the world is likely to remain relatively stable, experience, maturation, and technological developments do affect one's personal ethic.

NOTES

1. Paul B. Hofmann. (1995, November/December). Performing an ethics audit. *Healthcare Executive, 10*(2), p. 47.
2. Frank Harron, John Burnside, & Tom Beauchamp. (1983). *Health and human values* (p. 4). New Haven, CT: Yale University Press.

3. David E. Berry & John W. Seavey. (1984, March/April). Reiteration of problem definition in health services administration. *Hospital & Health Services Administration, 29*(2), p. 58.

4. *Ibid.*, p. 59.

GUIDING ETHICAL
DECISION MAKING

A significant problem with applied administrative and biomedical ethics is that numerous written and unwritten factors influence a manager's behavior. These factors are a blend of intellect, experience, education, and relationships. The common result is a too-often ill-defined personal code of conduct. A poorly defined personal ethic combined with tolerance for varying views may cause managers to believe that there is no one best answer to questions of administrative and biomedical ethics. Lacking a well-defined personal ethic, managers haven't a lodestar to guide them as they seek to answer the continuing question of normative ethics "What ought I to do?" The mind-set of a personal ethic helps them filter vague, contradictory guidance and to do the shaping rather than being shaped.

Key to a well-defined, robust personal ethic is self-analysis and introspection. Questions such as "Who am I?", "What is my bottom line?", and "For how long will I tolerate certain behaviors?" must be asked by managers who wish to understand and hone their personal ethic. Plato asserted that the unexamined life is not worth living. This is also true of a personal ethic.

Managers of health services organizations are community leaders ex officio. This prominence raises for managers (and the profession, generally) questions of the demarcation between private and professional lives. Private conduct breaching the profession's code of ethics may result in disciplinary action. Beyond the tension between managers' private and professional lives is that between a manager's personal ethic and the organization's philosophy. Philosophy and mission guide development and implementation of policies, procedures, and rules. An important question for individuals and organizations is the need for congruence between the organization's philosophy and the manager's personal ethic.

Chapters 3 and 4 suggest development and content of an organizational philosophy and examine its importance in the delivery of services.

Codes of ethics and their role in guiding health services managers and in helping them develop a personal ethic are examined. The dynamic between the organization's philosophy and the manager's code is analyzed.

Assistance for managers and organizations in solving ethical problems is identified in Chapter 5. Specialized committees that focus on different types of ethical problems and other means of obtaining assistance are suggested. As leader and moral agent, the manager acts to prevent, identify, and solve ethical problems.

CHAPTER 3

DEVELOPING ORGANIZATIONAL VALUES, VISION, AND MISSION

Managers confront a variety of moral and symbolic issues in health services organizations. This chapter focuses on the organization's need to identify and adopt values and principles—a philosophy. It is within the context of this philosophy that a vision and a mission are developed. The vision statement presents the goals the organization seeks to achieve. The mission statement describes its specific activities. Defining the philosophy prospectively resolves conflicts among competing values. The sequence of philosophy–vision–mission is the theoretical ideal. The reality is that more likely the mission is defined first or that it evolves from historical activity in the context of an implicit, rather than explicit, philosophy. The concept of "visioning" in health services organizations was first used in the 1980s and continues to the present. It is the rare health services organization that does not have a framed copy of its values, vision, and mission hanging in the lobby. This chapter describes the importance of identifying the moral values and principles that provide a context for the vision and mission statements and the necessity of reflecting these values across the organization.

Mission (and vision) is necessarily limited by, and is a function of, the physical location, size, resources, and other aspects of the organization's internal and external environments. These factors can usually only be affected over time. A significant change in these factors requires review of the mission, many of whose elements directly relate to the moral values and principles identified by the organization's governance and management. The decision of a nongovernmental acute care hospital not to perform abortions, for example, is derived from a determination that such services are incompatible with its moral values and principles. Offering abortion services raises other questions, the answers to which must be consistent with the organization's position on abortion. For example, is performing abortions compatible with legally required efforts to provide medically indicated treatment to live aborted fetuses? Some organizations avoid these questions and the attendant ethical implications by simply adhering to the law—they offer all legal services. This equates legality and morality. Such an approach only partially solves the problem, however, because the law is poorly developed in a number of areas in which administrative and biomedical ethical problems arise.

Although a governing body may adopt a statement of philosophy with certain values and principles, this is no indication that the staff agrees. Generally, staff in organizations pay little attention to such matters; the health services field is no exception. Many staff may not know the organization's philosophy, despite reasonable efforts to communicate it. Even if the philosophy is understood, many members make no commitment to it. If little attention is paid to the organization's stated moral values and principles (philosophy), it is not surprising that even less attention is paid to what should have been said but was not. For such staff, the organization is only a place to work. They do their work and are unconcerned about what the governing body and senior management say is the context for or the goals of service delivery. Absent significant discontinuity—when even sabotage is possible—staff rarely overtly challenge what is being done. If a challenge is made, the results tend to be negative rather than positive in outcome and effect.

Consideration must be given to how much more effective the organization could be were it built on a clearly understood system of shared values and goals. Adequately communicated to and accepted by staff, a resource-supported goal as simple as "getting the caring back into curing" could reap rewards for the organization through improved efficiency and patient care and relations. Moving staff in the same direction—a direction known in advance and recognized as important in the organization—will positively affect staff attitude, productivity, and effectiveness.

DEVELOPING AN ORGANIZATIONAL PHILOSOPHY

The starting point for an organization to prevent and, if necessary, solve ethical problems is its philosophy. The statement of philosophy identifies values and principles reflecting the moral right and wrong for the organization, thus distinguishing the acceptable from the unacceptable. It is helpful if the philosophy statement is sufficiently precise that performance in achieving it can be measured. At minimum, the statement of philosophy must be consistent with the law.

The statement of philosophy is different from the mission statement and should be developed separately. The philosophy statement provides a context for the mission statement; the mission statement is subordinate to it. Some organizations, however, include references to values in their mission statements. A mission statement that "the corporation owns and operates hospitals to provide care for the sick and injured" provides no information about the moral context of care. A mission statement that "the hospital provides care for the sick and injured in the context of humanitarian principles" is imprecise but provides a clearer values or moral context than the first.

Health services organizations with no specific, written philosophy nonetheless have an identifiable de facto or operational philosophy. The aggregate decisions and actions taken by the governing body and management reflect implicit, if ill-defined, philosophical bases. Management actions may be contradictory or inconsistent, and this suggests another negative aspect of not prospectively determining a comprehensive organizational philosophy. This lack of continuity and consistency will lead to incompatible, even contradictory, policies, procedures, and rules. The effect is diminished efficiency.

The importance of identified and shared values in organizations is now widely understood, if less frequently operationalized. In the early 1980s, however, it was a new concept, one that was synthesized by Peters and Waterman in their study of successful American corporations.[1] The quote attributed to IBM's former president, Thomas J. Watson, Jr., is instructive: "The basic philosophy of an organization has far more to do with its achievements than do technological or economic resources, organizational structure, innovation, and timing." That statement's context was the focus on customer service so important to IBM's reputation and financial success. If consumer and service are important to IBM, which has many characteristics of a products-based organization, consider the importance of customer and service in health care. The centrality of shared values is shown in Figure 5, the 7-S Framework, developed by McKinsey & Company.

Deal and Kennedy[2] also identified the characteristics of successful companies:

- They stand for something—that is, they have a clear and explicit philosophy about how they aim to conduct their business.

- Management pays a great deal of attention to shaping and fine-tuning these values to conform to the economic and business environment of the company and to communicating them to the organization.

- These values are known and shared by all the people who work for the company—from the production worker right through to the ranks of senior management.

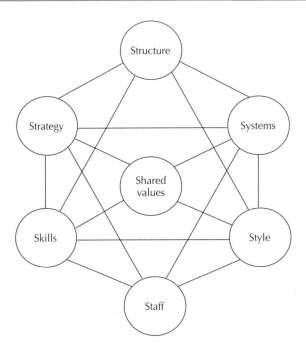

Figure 5.   The McKinsey 7-S Framework. (From McKinsey & Company, Inc. Reprinted by permission.)

Building on the importance of shared values or philosophy that make up a culture, Deal and Kennedy[3] identified the essential elements of a culture: 1) understanding and fitting into the business environment—the single greatest influence in shaping a corporate culture, 2) values—the basic concepts and beliefs of an organization, 3) heroes who personify the culture's values and are role models for employees, 4) rites and rituals that show employees the kind of behavior expected of them, 5) ceremonies that provide visible and potent examples of what the company stands for, and 6) the cultural network—the primary (but informal) means of communication within an organization that is the "carrier" of the corporate values and heroic mythology.

In further explaining corporate cultures Kennedy[4] noted the following:

> Culture isn't a single thing. It's not a budget; it's not a plan; it's not the shape of a building. It is an integrated pattern of all the things that go on in an organization on a day-to-day basis. Each company has its own unique culture, values, and standards communicated internally by style, dress, expectations, and assumptions.

New people in the workplace find out what is expected of them because their peers take them aside and say, "Look, don't wear jeans here. Come in to work on time, or you do this or that." They lay out some of the unwritten rules of behavior that are required for entrance into your workplace. That's how culture transmits itself to each new generation of persons. They don't come in and invent a whole new style of organization. They come in and learn from those around them what's going on in the organization and how they are expected to behave.

An organization's values are inextricably linked to its culture. To transform the organization so that its culture is a living reflection of values that facilitate the mission and vision, management must know which values are present in the culture. This presents somewhat of a chicken-and-egg situation. Regardless, management must biopsy the culture. This can be compared to a financial audit, except it is the organization's values that are being audited. Direct measures such as observation, staff surveys, exit interviews of department staff, and focus groups can be used. Proxy measures of culture include patient satisfaction surveys and service area surveys. In whatever ways it is done, however, management cannot effectively transform the organization's culture until its present content and course are known.

The barriers to establishing strong corporate cultures in any organization are a particular problem in health services organizations. For hospitals, barriers include:[5]

- Hospitals must serve diverse medical needs of heterogeneous populations.

- The number of external variables (forces outside the organization that affect it) is much greater for hospitals than it is in ordinary business enterprise.

- Hospital outcomes are difficult to define and to measure.

- It is difficult to nurture the keen proprietary sense of individual endeavors among leadership and management staff at all levels.

- Hospital board members are not active participants in its culture.

- Hospital physicians are a subculture, and peer acceptance and recognition, participation in professional activities, and stature based on professional contribution and expertise are more important than the rewards of belonging to a particular hospital.

- Elaborate peer reward systems in nursing are complicated by a deep search for professional identity.

- Support staff and especially allied medical personnel increasingly tend to have a professional identification independent of the hospital.

- Another special subculture in hospitals is the administrators who are caught between the role of facilitating the delivery of medical care and that of running a cost-effective "business" and, as a result, often isolate themselves from other subcultures.

Beyond these factors, and implicit in them, is the need for managers to view their relationships with staff and patients in a consistent fashion. Paying lip service to the organization's avowed goal of patient care but in fact focusing on economic or other nonpatient considerations is a contradiction that will not be lost on staff, who will respond to real incentives rather than platitudes. Not only must leader decisions and actions be consistent with organizational values, but staff must *perceive* that they are consistent, lest the leader be seen as a hypocrite. If values and how they are understood evolve over time, managers must solicit feedback to identify any disconnect between what they're saying and what employees are hearing.[6]

Management must know and understand the culture and values in its organization. Just as important, management must know how the culture and values mesh with or diverge from those the organization wishes to develop. The organization can mold a culture, but it can move neither faster than nor in directions that are opposed to or misunderstood by internal stakeholders. This congruence is critical. The organization's philosophy and derivative vision and mission statements are the primary points of reference for its corporate culture and subordinated activities. All efforts to develop excellence are a function of these statements.

A logic is evident in the link between the strength of a culture and organizational performance. The first piece of logic is that of goal alignment—a strong culture tends to cause staff to metaphorically march to the same drummer. Second, a strong culture aids in performance by creating an unusual level of motivation among staff—shared values and behaviors make staff feel good about working for an organization; the resulting commitment or loyalty makes them strive harder. Third, a strong culture aids in performance because it provides needed structure and controls without relying on a bureaucracy, which can diminish motivation and innovation.[7]

Closely linked to the concept of organizational philosophy and corporate culture is management's view of the organization's staff. McGregor's Theories X and Y, Maslow's hierarchy of needs, and the 14 points enumerated by W. Edwards Deming echo the importance of management's view of its employees, which is likely to be similar to how patients are viewed by a health services organization. Dysfunction is rife in an organization that treats employees as adversaries or as a means to an end and distrusts them while it urges staff to treat patients with dignity and respect. Employees see the hypocrisy and respond negatively. Peters and Waterman[8] sounded this theme, quoting Thomas J. Watson, Jr.: "IBM's philosophy is largely contained in three simple beliefs. I want to begin with what I think is the most important: our respect for the individual. This is a simple concept, but in IBM it occupies a major portion of management time."

Content of a Philosophy Statement

Organizational Content   The values and principles stated in an organization's philosophy establish a moral framework for its vision and mission. The philosophy provides a context and operative values—it gives delivery of health services a life, a meaning—and recognizes that these values are unique and represent more than delivering a product or rendering a service. Policies, procedures, and rules are derived from the mission statement and make the organization operational. The approaches taken by various types of health services organizations vary widely. Typically, those that are faith based have a greater focus on values and ethical principles. The commitment to values and ethical principles is not, however, exclusive to faith-based organizations. The Joint Commission on Accreditation of Healthcare Organizations (Joint Commission) recognizes the importance of an ethics framework; specific elements are identified.[9]

Sutter Health, a large West Coast multi-institutional system, has the classic trilogy of mission, vision, and values. Values include caring and compassion, excellence and quality, teamwork, honesty and integrity, and community.[10] Its statement of mission, vision, and values is reproduced in Appendix A. These values reflect some of the principles enunciated in Chapter 1, as well as some of the virtues.

Trinity Health is a faith-based multi-institutional health services organization that provides services across the continuum from acute care hospitals to long-term care and hospice. Its core values include respect, social justice, compassion, care of the poor and underserved, and excellence.[11]

Trinity Health's mission, core values, and vision statement are reproduced in Appendix A.

The George Washington University Medical Center includes a teaching hospital, schools of medicine and public health, and a physician group practice. Its vision is preeminence as a health institution; its mission includes teaching, research, clinical care, and improving health in general.[12] Virtues identified include altruism, compassion, integrity, and respect. Its statement is reproduced in Appendix A.

Sibley Memorial Hospital is a large nonsectarian East Coast community hospital. Including excellence, innovation, and continually improving care, teamwork, and job satisfaction in its values establishes both patient care and employment environments.[13] Sibley's mission, vision, and values statement is reproduced in Appendix A.

Mayo Clinic is a large multispecialty group practice that operates hospitals and a medical school, conducts research, and engages in postgraduate medical education. Its primary value is "The needs of the patient come first." Core principles include practice, education, research, mutual respect, commitment to quality, work atmosphere, societal commitment, and finances.[14] Its statement of mission, values, and principles is reproduced in Appendix A.

Sunrise Senior Living is a nonsectarian for-profit organization that provides a broad gamut of services to seniors. Its core values include passion, joy in service, stewardship, respect, and trust.[15] Its mission, foundational belief, core values, and principles of service are reproduced in Appendix A.

Relationship with Patients   It is difficult to imagine a health services organization that does not identify its role vis-à-vis patients in the context of respect for persons, beneficence, nonmaleficence, and justice, as well as the virtues identified in Chapter 1. These values mandate provision of medical services to patients with respect and in a manner that enhances human dignity. Staff members must know their responsibilities and duties toward patients in this regard. Patients are the reason why the organization exists, and all efforts are directed at meeting patient needs by safely delivering high-quality services.

Williams and Donnelly[16] asserted that accountability to the patient takes precedence over all other duties and relationships in health services organizations. Williams and Donnelly were pioneers when they had the temerity to assert that accountability to patients demanded that hospitals inform them if they had been harmed by medical misadventure. Their views are mainstream today; in fact, the expectation is much broader now. The Joint Commission requires that organizations provide information about unanticipated outcomes of care, treatment, and services to patients. The standards spell out how licensed independent practitioners (typically, these are physicians) or their designee are involved when unanticipated events occur.[17] This requirement continues to be controversial, if not as radical as in the 1980s. Informing patients and their families, as appropriate, of problems during treatment is the ethically (morally) right course. In addition, there is increasing evidence that telling patients and their families, as appropriate, about medical misadventures makes them less likely to seek legal redress because they believe the organization is being honest and that they are being treated fairly. However, this may not make believers of governing bodies, managers, and physicians. Intellectually, they may agree with the ethics of this level of accountability, but many will react with measured skepticism because the legal system demands an adversarial approach. This issue receives further attention in Chapter 8.

The economic hazards of implementing such a philosophy are significant, especially in organizations with a voluntary medical staff. Regrettably, the organization that becomes fully supportive of patients at the expense of its physicians risks alienating the physicians who are its economic livelihood. At the very least, the organization will have angry physicians. A desirable answer to this dilemma is to immerse physicians in the corporate culture, thus making its organizational philosophy part of their perspective. Hence, physicians will see substandard clinical treatment as endangering the corporate culture and will work with the organization—to the ultimate benefit of the patient.

The view expressed by Williams and Donnelly, and now by the Joint Commission, is consistent with the high degree of trust that the public places in health services organizations, and it is an appropriate measure of the duty organizations should meet in turn. The public has every right to expect that the organization and its managers will treat them with respect and dignity and will seek to right any wrongs. For many, this will result in a changed relationship with the organization.

Relationships with Staff   Like patients, employed and nonemployed (typically physicians) staff are entitled to be treated with respect and loyalty. Staff are the organization's most important asset because, ultimately, they determine the manner in which services are delivered. Like patients, staff must not be treated as a means to an end. The ethical aspects of these relations are most apparent in the organization's policies. Examples include reasonable and equitable performance appraisals and evaluation standards known in advance and fairly applied; forthright efforts to eliminate capriciousness, arbitrariness, and prejudice in human resources decision making; due process in grievances and disciplinary proceedings; and determination of the attributes and capabilities required for each position and matching staff with them.[18] These considerations of ethics in employee relations also make good management sense. Managers should note that employees who believe that they work in an ethical environment are six times more likely to be loyal to their employer than those who believe their employer is unethical. Employees need to have the organization's values communicated to them and to see that the actions of management fit with the stated values.[19]

Employees are in an unequal position of power with the organization and supervisors: The employment relationship limits their freedom of action. Consequently, for example, a manager who borrows money from employees acts unethically. Such an action jeopardizes management's credibility, but more important, it reflects a lack of respect for employees, who are being used as a means to an end. Employees are also used as a means to an end if they must undertake high-risk activities (e.g., caring for patients with highly infectious diseases) with poorly developed procedures and processes or inadequate training, supplies, and equipment. This example is a rare instance in which the duty of beneficence toward the patient is superseded by the virtues of loyalty and justice to staff and the principle of nonmaleficence, a decision supported by a utilitarian calculus.

Physicians are the economic life blood of health services organizations. In most instances, they are there at the organizations' sufferance, either as employees or independent contractors. In either relationship, the presence of these high-profile professionals complicates the organization's interactions with patients and other staff. If, for example, quality of care issues arise, the organization must meet its obligations to protect patients and further their interests by intervening, as necessary, in the physician–patient relationship. The resulting political and economic problems likely to arise for governance and management mean that intervention occurs only reluctantly and less often than it should.

Employees and medical staff should participate in developing the organization's philosophy and vision and mission statements. Increased congruence between the philosophies of organization and staff benefits all involved; most important, it benefits patients. Rapport between the organization and its staff is essential to developing a strong, positive corporate culture.

Relationship with the Community   In some geographic areas, community (service area) and patients or potential patients are synonymous. The organization's philosophy should specify its relationship to the community: What is its obligation to provide free or less-than-cost care to Medicaid patients or to those who cannot afford to pay? What is its obligation to provide controversial services such as abortion? Prospectively answering questions such as these causes the organization to consider important issues about itself and its role. This probing assists in honing an organizational philosophy and provides an opportunity for introspection and staff involvement in establishing and strengthening a corporate culture.

Going the Extra Mile[20]

The senior managers of a home health agency (HHA) serving five rural counties were indicted (and later convicted) of Medicare fraud. The HHA served more than 1,000 patients and had more than 225 employed staff and independent contractors. During initial criminal proceedings against the senior management, their further actions caused the HHA to go into bankruptcy. The payroll was weeks behind. By the end of the next 2-week pay period, the staff had not been paid for a month. Many were home health aides being paid less than $9.00 an hour. Most of the staff were parents.

A senior supervisor met with the staff and told them of the HHA's problems. As a group, they decided to continue caring for all the patients. Some managers loaned their staff money, even though it violated company policy. Within a few weeks, the bankruptcy judge released the payroll, and a semblance of normality returned. Continuity of patient care was maintained.

What a compelling case! The HHA staff had developed a strong culture of beneficence, nonmaleficence, loyalty, and honor—principles and virtues lacking among the corrupt senior management. Their actions reflect proudly on the highest traditions of the health services field. Loaning money to staff in violation of the company policy was morally justified, given the exigencies of the situation and the honorable purposes for which it was done. The staff and supervisor should be given kudos for their shared actions.

Relationship with Other Institutions   Revising the organizational philosophy is difficult but necessary as the external environment changes. The organization must deal forthrightly and honestly with other entities, even actual or potential competitors. This ethic fits with effective competition—it simply means the organization competes honestly, with no hint of fraud or deception. In the past, there were few incentives for health services organizations to cooperate, but significant changes in the delivery of health services and economic pressures will force them into networks or systems. Large differences in moral philosophies inhibit cooperative efforts, a problem that may be insurmountable when sectarian and nonsectarian organizations contemplate a merger or joint efforts.

Summary   The values that an organization reflects in its philosophy can be derived from religion, secular humanism, or a combination of these sources. Regardless of the source, organizations (and oftentimes individuals) will reflect values and virtues such as integrity, respect, altruism, compassion, honor, fidelity, courtesy, professionalism, sensitivity, and justice in their philosophies.

Moral considerations important to the organization must be addressed in its statement of philosophy or values. These may include the organization's position on specific clinical ethical issues. If, for example, its view of the sanctity of life prohibits delivery of certain services, this should be stated. The organization's view of its relationship with patients, staff (including nonemployed physicians), community, and other institutions should be described. Ideally, this statement is sufficiently detailed so that performance measures can be developed and applied.

Consistent with the moral philosophies and derivative principles and the virtues discussed in Chapter 1, the organization's philosophy must emphasize the importance of ensuring respect for persons and of benefiting patients and protecting them from untoward results. The principle of justice should be included in the philosophy statement. These values are inherent in the independent relationship between organization and patient and are not superseded by the relationship between physician and patient. Through its philosophy the organization also implicitly or explicitly states its accountability to the public, regardless of type of ownership.

DEVELOPING A MISSION STATEMENT

Vision statements are aspirational and inspirational. As such, they sketch what the organization would like to become. They set a direction for the organization and broadly state its role and activities.

Mission statements are the applied portions of the vision statement. They operationalize the means by which the vision is to be accomplished. The mission statement may originate in the articles of incorporation, the documents filed to establish the health services organization as a legal entity. The statement of objectives or the purposes for which the corporation was formed are useful in developing a mission statement. That the mission statement needs to be consistent with and reflect the organization's philosophy has been amply described. A simple mission statement is that a community hospital association will:

- Establish, operate, and maintain a hospital

- Engage in educational activities related to treating the sick and injured

- Engage in health promotion and disease prevention activities

- Promote and perform scientific research related to care of the sick and injured

- Engage in other activities designed to promote the general health of the community

More elaborate are the objectives (mission statement) of Sterling County Hospital,[21] in which elements of an organizational philosophy are included:

- To recognize man's unique composition of body and soul and man's basic right to life. Sterling County's concept of total care, therefore, embraces the physical, emotional, spiritual, social, and economic needs of each patient

- To affirm that the primary objective of our health services is to relieve suffering and to promote and restore health in a Christian manner that demands competence, mercy, and respect

- To generate and cultivate a source of allied health manpower by orienting and supporting personnel development in the areas of individual skills, knowledge, and attitudes

- To participate in the development of health services that are relevant to the total community needs by meaningful area-wide and regional planning and in a partnership for health concept

These mission statements show what the two organizations seek to accomplish. An important distinction is that the first has no values context, nor are its activities linked to a larger value system. The second statement has a more philosophical context.

Organizations state their missions differently. A pediatric medical center states that it will serve any child, regardless of ability to pay. Such a mission statement incorporates the philosophy that treating the child is primary; economics are secondary. Sectarian health services organizations cite their religious creeds; nonsectarian organizations typically link their activities to humanitarian motives. Publicly owned Sterling County Hospital is unique by having a religious reference in its mission statement. See Appendix A for other sample organizational philosophies and vision and mission statements.

RECONSIDERING THE ORGANIZATION'S PHILOSOPHY

A competitive environment will significantly affect the way many health services organizations born of eleemosynary (charitable) motives view themselves. Competition and reports of large profits will change how others, especially patients and communities, view them. Aggressive competition is at variance with the philosophy and historical mission of many organizations that serve the sick and injured and do so from a sense of duty and charity rather than from a desire to establish new product lines, increase their market share, or maximize net income over expense. The organization that does not possess the stamina, resources, or mind-set to reconsider its philosophy and mission may become uneconomic and cease to exist.

An Acceptable New Image?

Sebastian Hospital was founded by a Christian congregation in 1891. Its philosophy and mission statements include a strong commitment to care for the sick and injured regardless of ability to pay. This mission posed no problems during its first 90 years. Even after the hospital was purchased by the community in 1950, it continued to function in much the same fashion. Sebastian successfully weathered a controversy about abortion in 1973. The compromise solution limited where in the hospital abortions would be performed and how staff would be assigned.

Increasing cost pressures during the 1970s and diagnosis-related groups (DRGs) in the early 1980s caused substantial financial problems. A switch to all-payer prospective payment, which would prohibit cost shifting, was imminent. In addition, there was pressure for corporate reorganization. Planning consultants first recommended enterprises such as a physician office building, a parking facility, and a motel. Some of these suggestions complemented the primary mission. The trustees saw others suggestions as tangential. Another new type of enterprise was proposed: a joint venture with members of the medical staff.

The administrator was concerned that Sebastian's 100-year focus would change dramatically. It was one thing to manage a facility competently but quite another to be razzle-dazzle entrepreneurs. Would the caring reputation that Sebastian had achieved so successfully disappear in a blaze of marketing efforts and joint ventures? The administrator wondered whether Sebastian was hopelessly out of step with its environment.

This case illustrates the dilemma confronting many not-for-profit community hospitals. The same or similar problems affect most organizations in the sense that they must rapidly adapt to what seem to be revolutionary environmental changes. Interinstitutional competition is less problematic when a community has one of each type of institutional provider. Even in these cases, however, organizations are beginning to offer competing services. For example, hospitals often find themselves competing with members of their medical staff—most often for highly remunerative outpatient ancillary and diagnostic services. The loss of revenue to hospitals may mean the difference between economic life or death. Such economic tensions diminish the ability of not-for-profit organizations to carry out their historic missions.

Initially viewed with disdain by managers because it conjured up images of individuals with questionable parentage selling unneeded services of little value, marketing has become an accepted, even necessary, part of health services delivery. The preference is still to focus on health promotion and disease and accident prevention and treatment, but marketing is the buzzword; organizations that fail to heed it risk their survival.

Competition per se is not at variance with a charitable mission. The context has changed and the stakes have increased, but managers should view such changes as a challenge—an opportunity to do what they have been doing even more effectively. Successful corporate restructuring and effective marketing allow the organization to develop revenue streams that enable it to provide charitable services.

A more insidious problem, and one that is fraught with conflicts of interest, occurs in certain joint ventures between health services organizations, such as hospitals, and their medical staffs. Physicians who earn income by referring patients to providers in which they have an ownership interest or a profit-sharing arrangement have an ethical conflict of interest. States began to prohibit physician referral to such facilities or mandate disclosure to patients. Organized medicine took note of such conflicts of interest in 1985.[22] Since then, several federal laws have set limits on physician self-referral for federal program beneficiaries.

A different philosophical dilemma faced St. Joseph Hospital, which was established in 1870 and owned by various orders of Catholic sisters. In 1971, it was sold to the Creighton Regional Health Care Corporation, a not-for-profit corporation with a lay governing body, which operated St. Joseph as a Roman Catholic teaching hospital for Creighton University. In 1984, a contract was signed with American Medical International (AMI), a for-profit hospital system, under which AMI would acquire St. Joseph Hospital and operate it as a full-service Roman Catholic teaching hospital. Based on this transfer of ownership, the Catholic Health Association (CHA) terminated St. Joseph's membership because "the Hospital is not operated, supervised, or controlled by or in conjunction with the Roman Catholic Church in the United States."[23] The controversy surrounding the decision suggested that other important but unstated reasons were questions about the morality of the profit motive in health services and that other AMI hospitals performed abortions. Those challenging CHA's action argued that the profit motive was compatible with St. Joseph's mission and that the bondholders of St. Joseph's debt were paid several millions of dollars in interest—an action, it was argued, indistinguishable from that of paying dividends to stockholders. St. Joseph continues to be unaffiliated with CHA.[24]

What is important in this case is that CHA acted when a member hospital was no longer compatible with its philosophy and mission. Regardless of how one judges CHA, its decision was based on a specific philosophy—a crucial underpinning for any organization. The values issues arising from the merger of faith-based and nonsectarian health services organizations can be significant. This is especially true if there are limitations on types of medical services that can be provided (e.g., certain reproductive services in hospitals affiliated with the Roman Catholic Church). Put most starkly, the issue is whether the demands of nonadherents can trump the organization's philosophy (values). It is argued that in a pluralistic society, quasi-public organizations such as hospitals do not have the luxury of limiting services needed and demanded by the general public. Providing such services, however, necessarily causes the organization to violate its values or its institutional moral agency—that which for personal providers such as physicians would be called conscience. When a merger eliminates choice, the issue is often finessed by establishing a freestanding center for reproductive health that has limited, if any, connection with the faith-based organization.

UNDERSTANDING PATIENT BILLS OF RIGHTS

Patient bills of rights provide guidance about the appropriate ethical relationship between the patient and the organization and its staff. Titles vary, but bills of rights have been published by organizations including the American Hospital Association (AHA), the Joint Commission, the U.S. Department of Veterans Affairs (VA), and the American Civil Liberties Union (ACLU). In addition, health services organizations have developed their own statements. Bills of rights reflect the law on confidentiality and consent, for example, but no bill is legally binding. Philosophical differences are significant, however.

The AHA first adopted a Patient's Bill of Rights in 1973.[25] Before 1992, AHA's bill was more oriented to institutional than patient needs and included an element of paternalism (e.g., a provision that at times patients should not be fully informed of their medical conditions). Paternalism's deep roots in medical ethical tradition date to the Hippocratic oath and cause doing good (beneficence) to conflict with enhancing patient autonomy. The bill adopted in 1992 puts greater emphasis on patient rights. The institutional bias is muted but continues, and the implementation of some patient rights is limited (e.g., "The patient has the right to make decisions about the plan of care prior to and during the course of treatment and to refuse a recommended treatment or plan of care to the extent permitted by law *and hospital policy*" [emphasis added]). This example phrase suggests that hospital policy will prevail when the patient's wishes conflict with it. Patient responsibilities in the care process are also addressed.

The ACLU's patient bill of rights[26] was drafted as a model law with the intention that it would be enacted by the states. A demanding view of patients' rights distinguishes it philosophically from AHA's bill. The ACLU bill views the patient as an autonomous individual entitled to full involvement in the care process. For example, the bill mandates that each patient have a 24-hours-per-day patient rights advocate, who may act on behalf of the patient and, with the patient's consent, assert or protect the rights enumerated in the model bill. Patients also have a right to their medical records, upon request and payment of reasonable copying expenses. The ACLU bill details the information to be provided when consent for treatment is obtained. Gone, however, is a suggestion from the previous iteration that patients *have a duty* (emphasis added) to be fully involved in their care. The ACLU bill's stridency in protecting patient rights is unconventional, but its provisions are worth considering.

The Department of Veterans Affairs Patient Rights and Responsibilities[27] and the Joint Commission's Patient Rights and Organization Ethics

Standards[28] lie philosophically between the AHA's and ACLU's patient bills of rights. The VA's bill recognizes that some patients may have lengthy stays in nursing facilities or hospitals, and there are provisions on the rights to wear one's own clothes, keep personal items, and refuse visitors. Specifically mentioned are choosing whether to participate in research, participating in treatment decisions, and, it is important to note, access to the ethics committee. Advance directives are identified only by implication. In the 1990s, Joint Commission standards recognized the patient's responsibility to cooperate with caregivers. For 2004, its standards emphasize patient rights that organizations are expected to perfect, such as informed consent, providing information about caregivers, patient wishes relating to end-of-life decisions, a right to pain management, and a right to gain access to protective and advocacy services. Provisions address ethical issues in research and organ procurement. The Joint Commission's view of the organization's ethical obligation to patients is moving closer to the ACLU's.

Documents such as patient bills of rights set an ethical tone for relationships with patients and serve as a nonformal source of law should a dispute arise. The usefulness of such documents is limited by the organization's willingness to adopt one already available or to develop its own, and, more important, to implement the bill of rights by making its contents known to patients and monitoring processes that demonstrate its application.

STRATEGIC MANAGEMENT

The organization's philosophy also affects strategic management (planning). The philosophy must be articulated if objectives are to be consistent as well as set appropriately. The organization's view of its social responsibility should be reflected in its organizational philosophy and vision and mission statements. Only then should strategic management occur.

An organization's philosophy, vision, and mission state the ideal—ends thought to be unattainable in their idealized version but progress toward which is believed possible.[29] The mission statement must be usable to measure performance, define the organization's business, be unique to the organization, and be relevant to all stakeholders, and it should be exciting, challenging, and inspiring. In contrast, the vision is a verbal picture of what the organization's stakeholders want it to be.[30] In this respect, perhaps the most difficult aspect of developing an organization's strategy is

determining the balance between social responsibility and economic performance.[31] The perspective that the health services organization is a social
enterprise with an economic dimension may no longer apply; in fact, the
environment may have caused the obverse to be true. Resolving this
dilemma and the resulting problems will be increasingly difficult. Although
the governing body is primarily responsible for developing a philosophy
and vision and mission statements, senior management prepares and opera-
tionalizes the strategic plan. All participants must ensure that there is
consistency between the organization's philosophy and its specific policies,
procedures, and rules.

ACHIEVING CONGRUENCE OF PHILOSOPHIES

Several questions must be asked about the relationship between the manager's personal ethic and the organization's philosophy: To what extent must
organizational philosophy and the personal ethic of a manager mesh? If
the organization is to be a community of shared values, must all managers be
in full agreement with the philosophy? As a class, are managers sufficiently
professional to be effective in an organization when they may not agree
fully with its values? What degree of congruence is needed? A literal
interpretation of Deal and Kennedy's work suggests that philosophical
divergence is to be discouraged; all values must be shared by all employees,
including managers.

Some sectarian health services organizations require that managers
at mid-level and above be adherents to the religion of the sponsoring
group. Apparently, they judge their philosophy and mission so unique that
only co-religionists can effectively manage their organizations. Some moral
philosophies are unique, but this requirement seems largely unsupportable.
If this policy also breeds conformity and diminishes innovation, it becomes
counterproductive.

The organization's interview and preemployment processes should
explain its philosophy and determine the applicant's personal ethic about
health services and their delivery. This information permits both parties
to judge their philosophical congruence, which should occur whether or
not the applicant is a co-religionist, because even those of the same faith
often have divergent views. Similarly, nonsectarian organizations may not
want to employ individuals whose ethic constrains them from participating
in services such as electroconvulsive therapy. In such cases, this information
can and should be known prospectively.

It is key that persons may reach the same conclusions about an organization's activities and its relationship to patients using a moral philosophy that is independent of the organization's religious doctrine. These managers would be as effective in achieving the same goals as others in the organization because they share the same values, the same philosophy. The ultimate measure is the congruence between the organization's philosophy and the results of a manager's decision making, although there are other indications. Someone claiming to be morally neutral is potentially the most inimical to an organization seeking to implement a philosophy and strengthen its corporate culture.

CONCLUSION

This chapter examined the importance of a philosophy, or values, in determining and guiding an organization's vision and mission. From them are derived policies and procedures, the stuff from which the abstract and sometimes elusive aspects of an organization are operationalized. Developing a strong corporate culture is the result of shared values. Shared values are crucial in easing discontinuity and achieving corporate effectiveness. However, a school of behavioral science suggests that individuals who disagree must be willing to speak out, and it is problematic if the organization becomes an environment of "group think."

A variety of sources assists in developing an organization's philosophy, including religious affiliation or orientation and humanism or humanitarian motives. Employee and patient bills of rights are also important. Whatever sources an organization uses, the principles of respect for persons, beneficence, nonmaleficence, and justice, as well as complementary virtues, are essential.

NOTES

1. Thomas J. Peters & Robert H. Waterman, Jr. (1982, reissued 1997). *In search of excellence: Lessons from America's best run companies* (p. 15). New York: MacMillan Library Reference.
2. Terrence E. Deal & Allan A. Kennedy. (1982, reissued in paperback 2000). *Corporate cultures: The rites and rituals of corporate life* (p. 22). New York: Perseus Books Group.
3. *Ibid.*, pp. 13–15.
4. Allan A. Kennedy. (1985, October). Corporate values/corporate culture. In *Excellence in management: Lessons learned from other industries* (pp. 5–7). Report

from a special conference for the American College of Hospital Administrators Fellows.

5. Terrence E. Deal, Allan A. Kennedy, & Arthur H. Spiegel, III. (1983, January/February). How to create an outstanding hospital culture. *Hospital Forum*, *27*, pp. 21–28, 33–34.

6. Amy C. Edmondson & Sandra E. Cha. (2002, November). When company values backfire. *Harvard Business Review*, *80*(11), pp. 18–19.

7. John P. Kotter & James L. Heskett. (1992). *Corporate culture and performance* (p. 18). New York: The Free Press.

8. Peters & Waterman, pp. 15–16.

9. Joint Commission on Accreditation of Healthcare Organizations. (1998). Sample components of an organization ethics framework. In *Ethical issues and patient rights across the continuum of care* (p. 74). Oakbrook Terrace, IL: Author.

10. Sutter Health. (n.d.). *About us: Our mission*. Retrieved August 21, 2003, from http://www.sutterhealth.org/about/mission

11. Trinity Health. (2004). *Who we are*. Retrieved April 13, 2004, from http://www.trinity-health.org/who/mission.shtml

12. The George Washington University Medical Center. (2003). *GWUMC vision and mission*. Retrieved April 13, 2004, from http://www.gwumc.edu/mcinfo/aboutgwumc/vision.html

13. Sibley Memorial Hospital. (2002). *Employment at Sibley: Mission, vision, values*. Retrieved April 13, 2004, from http://www.SIBLEY.ORG/employment/emphil.tmpl

14. Mayo Clinic. (n.d.). *Mayo's mission*. Retrieved August 21, 2003, from http://www.mayoclinic.org/about/missionvalues.html

15. Sunrise Senior Living. (2003). *Principles of service and core values*. Retrieved April 13, 2004, from http://www.sunrise-al.com/difference/PrinciplesOfService.do

16. Kenneth J. Williams & Paul R. Donnelly. (1982). *Medical care quality and the public trust*. Santa Monica, CA: Bonus Books.

17. Joint Commission on Accreditation of Healthcare Organizations. (2004). Ethics, rights, and responsibilities. In *Accreditation manual for hospitals*. Oakbrook Terrace, IL: Author.

18. Bonnie J. Gray & Robert K. Landrum. (1983, July/September). Difficulties with being ethical. *Business*, *33*, pp. 28–33.

19. Study: Ethical climate closely linked to employee commitment. (2000, August 18). *ACHe-news*.

20. This case was developed from an incident related to the author by Dorothy H. Mitchell, R.N., M.S.H.A., Brunswick, GA, May 2003.

21. Ed D. Roach & Bobby G. Bizzell. (1990). Sterling County Hospital. In Jonathon S. Rakich, Beaufort B. Longest, Jr., & Kurt Darr, Eds. *Cases in health services management* (2nd ed., p. 144). Baltimore: Health Professions Press.

22. Editorial. (1985, September). Dealing with conflicts of interest. *The New England Journal of Medicine*, *313*, pp. 749–751.

23. Richard L. O'Brien & Michael J. Haller. (1985, July). Investor-owned or nonprofit? *The New England Journal of Medicine*, *313*, pp. 198–201.

24. Mary Jo Pearman, Membership Services, Catholic Health Association; personal communication, December 12, 2003.

25. American Hospital Association. (1992, October 21). *A patient's bill of rights.* Retrieved November 18, 2003, from http://www.hospitalconnect.com/aha/about/pbillofrights.html

26. George J. Annas. (1989). Appendix B. In *The rights of patients: The basic ACLU guide to patient rights* (2nd ed., pp. 283–291). Carbondale, IL: Southern Illinois University Press.

27. U.S. Department of Veterans Affairs. (2002, April). *Patient rights and responsibilities.* Retrieved November 22, 2003, from www1.va.gov/health_benefits/docs/Patient_Rights_and_Responsibilities.PDF

28. Joint Commission on Accreditation of Healthcare Organizations, 2004.

29. Russell L. Ackoff. (1981). *Creating the corporate future.* New York: John Wiley & Sons.

30. Russell L. Ackoff. (1999). *Re-creating the corporation: A design of organizations for the 21st century* (pp. 83–84, 87). New York: Oxford University Press.

31. James Webber. (1982, April 1). Planning. *Hospitals, 56,* pp. 69–70.

CHAPTER 4

CODES OF ETHICS IN HEALTH SERVICES

Many factors influence human behavior and interaction. Among the most basic are those arising from the individual's legal relationships with society—those increasingly pervasive laws, ordinances, regulations, and court decisions. Other formal sources of law, such as the bylaws of a corporation, apply only to a specific entity. The link between formal sources of law and ethics was described in the Introduction. In addition, there are nonformal sources of law, such as standards of justice, public policies, moral convictions, customary laws, and notions of individual equity. Both formal and nonformal sources of law are used by health services organizations. Codes of ethics adopted by professional associations are important because they state goals and aspirations, guide members, and serve as a reference point to discipline those who deviate from the norm.

In 1978, the U.S. Congress created the Office of Government Ethics (OGE) in the executive branch to prevent conflicts of interest on the part of government employees and to resolve those that occur.[1] The law requires financial disclosure and restricts activities after leaving government service; accepting gifts from outside sources; and outside earned income, honoraria, and employment. Remote or inconsequential financial interests are not thought to affect integrity and are exempt. OGE's primary source of information is the employee's annual financial disclosure statement. Similarly, states provide ethical and legal guidance for their employees.[2]

Self-regulation is a hallmark of the learned professions; historically, these professions were law, medicine, and the clergy. Their ethics are reflected in bar discipline, principles of medical ethics, and ecclesiastic law. As law and medicine, as well as newer professions, sought regulation (economic protection) through legislation or as regulation was forced on them, many of their ethical principles were incorporated into statutes or regulations or, for lawyers, court-adopted rules of professional conduct.

Groups seeking professional status adopt codes of ethics. Codes are common in health services, and managerial, clinical, and technical groups have them. Their language is usually general, and performance standards are typically so vague as to make fair enforcement impossible. In the latter regard, the profession of law is a notable exception. A wag would say that this is as it should be because lawyers seem plagued by ethics problems. The American Bar Association (ABA) is a private association that has developed Model Rules of Professional Conduct. These model rules, as well as codes of conduct developed by state bar associations, reflect the profession's ethics. These statements of professional ethics take on the weight of judicial sanction because a state's highest court uses them to develop its rules of professional conduct for lawyers licensed in the state. These rules are used to sanction errant lawyers. For example, as officers of the court, lawyers have a duty to inform the appropriate professional authority if they know that another lawyer has violated the rules of professional conduct in a way that raises a substantial question as to the lawyer's honesty, trustworthiness, or fitness as a lawyer in other respects.[3] The state's highest court typically appoints a board of professional responsibility to enforce its rules and to review and investigate complaints, which are heard by a special panel of judges. Adverse action by this panel results in penalties ranging from admonition or probation to suspension or revocation of the lawyer's license.

It is clear, however, that even with reasonably stringent enforcement, a code of ethics can only guide the behavior and decisions of individuals who want to do the right thing but need help determining what that is. Individuals trying to get away with something are always on the fringe of a profession, and principles of ethical conduct (and legal requirements) only encourage them to become more devious to avoid being caught. Even in the absence of a code, some actions inevitably raise questions of character.

Mr. B

Mr. B sought a job as a health services consultant. He contacted two firms and was interviewed by both. One offered him a position. Mr. B verbally accepted the offer, even though it meant moving his family. Several days later, as a courtesy, he called the second firm to tell them he had taken a position. The managing partner said, "Gee, that's really too bad. I was going to offer you a job in your area and pay you $5,000 more than you got from the other firm."

Mr. B faces an ethical problem. There is no written agreement, but he verbally accepted the first offer—he gave his word. Were Mr. B to call the first firm and explain what happened, they would likely release him. After all, who wants a disgruntled employee? This action does not affect his ethical obligation to take the job he accepted, however. Having given his word, he made a commitment. Mr. B is morally bound to meet it. The virtue of promise keeping applies here. Only if Mr. B can show morally overriding considerations, such as great hardship to his family, can he avoid his commitment.

CODES FOR MANAGERS

In addition to what is considered minimally acceptable, codes also state the vision of the profession. The goals stated in the vision may be unachievable. The profession must work toward them, nonetheless, because progress is possible. These aspects of codes of ethics are similar to the philosophy and vision statements developed by organizations.

In the sister field of business, the corporate scandals of the late 20th and early 21st centuries highlighted the importance of business ethics. These scandals caused educators to reconsider the place of teaching ethics in graduate business programs and to give their graduates a better grounding in the values that will prevent similar problems in the future. Like any business skill, the importance of reinforcing application of appropriate values in business has long been known, and experts agree that ethics can be taught *and* learned and that moral development takes place in everyone.[4] The implications? Classroom and continuing education in ethics for health services managers are essential, despite the skepticism of some.[5]

Health Services Executives

First among health services management professional associations is the American College of Healthcare Executives (ACHE), known prior to mid-1985 as the American College of Hospital Administrators (ACHA). In 2004, the ACHE had about 30,000 members. The ACHE has had a Code of Ethics since 1939, 6 years after its founding. Initially, it was linked to the code of ethics for hospitals developed by the American Hospital Association (AHA). Ensuing iterations made the ACHE's code distinct; it also became more explicit than the AHA's code. A major revision of the code occurred in 1987; significant changes were made in 2003.

The preamble establishes a context for the 2003 code and continues the concept introduced in 1987 that health services managers are moral advocates (the term *agents* was used in 1987) who must evaluate the possible outcomes of their decisions. It is suggested but not explicitly stated that health care executives are morally responsible for their decisions. Noteworthy is the executive's obligation to act in ways that will merit the trust, confidence, and respect of health care professionals and the general public, and that, therefore, they "should lead lives that embody an exemplary system of values and ethics." This code expectation substantially melds the public and private lives of health care executives and is reinforced by a code provision that directs health care executives to refrain from participating in any activity that demeans the profession's credibility and dignity.

The 2003 iteration has five sections that detail the health care executive's responsibilities to the profession, to patients or others served, to the organization, to employees, and to the community and society. The final section charges affiliates who have reasonable grounds to believe that another affiliate has violated the code with a positive duty to communicate such facts to the committee on ethics. The lengthy section on conflicts of interest in the previous iteration has been replaced by a modest and largely inadequate "Avoid financial and other conflicts of interest."

In 2003, the section on the executive's responsibilities to the organization was substantially expanded. Added were the need to report negative information, prevent fraud and abuse and aggressive accounting that may result in disputable financial reports, act to minimize clinical and management errors and disclose them when they occur, implement an organizational code of ethics and monitor compliance, and provide ethics resources to staff to address organizational and clinical issues. All are important additions.

Arguably, the code pays too little attention to the role of managers in resolving biomedical ethical issues. It does, however, include the need to establish processes that resolve values conflicts between patients and staff and that ensure patient autonomy and self-determination. A continuing lapse is attention to the independent moral duty that health care executives owe to patients. For example, the code has yet to define the limits of loyalty (fidelity) to the organization and the point at which it is superseded by an ethical duty to the patient. This is a vital facet of the manager as moral agent (advocate) and an essential element of the code as a living document that builds professional self-respect and esprit de corps.

Disciplinary actions under the code are highly structured and emphasize fairness. The ethics committee receives complaints alleging unethical conduct. The process includes the committee chair's screening the complaint, informing the respondent (the affiliate) of the allegations, investigating the allegations, and making a recommendation to the board of governors. The respondent may appeal the committee's adverse findings and recommendations through a process that ends with the ACHE's board of governors. All information developed in the process is privileged.

The lengthy grievance process is consistent with the expectation of procedural and substantive due process in private associations. Respondents can seek judicial review of these decisions, but courts intervene in the actions of private associations only reluctantly. Expulsion is the maximum disciplinary action available to the ACHE or any other private association. Because affiliation is not linked to licensure, expulsion is significant only if colleagues and potential employers consider it important. If they do, the former affiliate's employment and career opportunities become more limited. Enforcement has the attribute of making codes of ethics vital, living documents that offer greater usefulness to members as they confront ethical issues and work to solve them.

The ACHE supplements the code by issuing Ethical Policy Statements that suggest a standard of behavior and offer specific guidance for members. They have addressed issues such as an ethical environment for employees, decisions near the end of life, impaired health care executives, and health information confidentiality.[6] The 2003 ACHE Code of Ethics is reproduced in Appendix B.

Nursing Facility Administrators

The American College of Health Care Administrators (ACHCA) has approximately 4,500 members who are primarily managers of long-term care facilities. Its 2003 code is reproduced in Appendix B.

Members are obliged to meet four "expectations," which are divided into prescriptions and proscriptions.[7] The expectations state that members shall: 1) hold paramount the welfare of persons for whom care is provided; 2) maintain high standards of professional competence; 3) strive, in all matters relating to their professional functions, to maintain a professional posture that places paramount the interests of the facility and its residents; and 4) honor their responsibilities to the public, their profession, and relationships with colleagues and members of related professions. The prescriptions and proscriptions are analogues. Examples of issues presented include addressing the quality of services; maintaining confidentiality of information about recipients of care; providing continuing education; handling conflicts of interest; and fostering increased knowledge, supporting research, and sharing expertise.

Like the ACHE, the ACHCA expects members to provide information to its standards and ethics committee of actual or potential code violations and to cooperate with inquiries into matters of professional conduct related to the code of ethics. The latter requirement suggests a disciplinary dimension, but neither enforcement nor appeals processes are included. The code's preamble states that the ultimate responsibility for applying standards and ethics falls to the individual. The ACHCA code pays even less attention to biomedical ethical issues than does the ACHE code—an important lapse for both groups.

CODES FOR CAREGIVERS

Physicians

Codes of ethics in medicine date from the 18th century B.C. and the Code of Hammurabi, which established fee schedules for physicians and veterinarians. Harsh punishments could result if patients were harmed because of treatment, including loss of a physician's hands if treatment resulted in the loss of a patient's eye or life.

A very different code developed from the teaching and work of Hippocrates (circa 460–370 B.C.). The Code of Hammurabi was imposed by a ruler, but the Hippocratic philosophy governing relationships among physicians and between physicians and patients was developed by Greek physicians, one of whom may have been Hippocrates, for their own use. The Hippocratic oath has never received public sanction or force of law. It established standards of conduct, some of which are found in contemporary codes of medical ethics, as well as in state licensing and regulation of physicians.

The Hippocratic oath contains a largely obsolete section describing expected relationships between physicians and their teachers and students. Other provisions no longer used include restrictions on performing surgery, assisting in abortion, and only applying dietetic measures in healing. Hippocratic prohibitions on assisting in suicide and refraining from sexual misconduct with patients and others in the household, as well as broad restrictions on confidentiality of information learned during treatment, are found in contemporary codes, explicitly or implicitly.

The American Medical Association (AMA) was founded in 1847. Its first code of medical ethics was based on the work of Sir Thomas Percival, English physician, philosopher, and writer. Revisions of the AMA's code, Principles of Medical Ethics, occurred in 1912, 1957, 1980, and 2001.[8] The revision of the 1980 principles added precision to professional ethics for physicians. The changes were not as dramatic as those between the 1957 and 1980 versions, however. The 1980 version eliminated proscriptions on advertising and voluntarily associating with practitioners who have no scientific basis for treatment. In addition, the 1957 principles had a strong element of paternalism—physicians were expected to act in ways that *they considered to be in the patient's best interests* (emphasis added). Eliminating that provision reflected a major philosophical shift for the AMA. In commenting on the changes between the 1957 and 1980 versions of the principles, Veatch[9] observed, "It is the first document in the history of professional medical ethics in which a group of physicians is willing to use the language of responsibilities and rights," rather than that of benefits and harms.

The 2001 iteration (reproduced in Appendix B) continues to emphasize providing competent medical care, honesty in all professional interactions, and safeguarding patient confidences. Changes from the 1980 version include adding *rights*, with the expectation that physicians will provide medical care with "respect for human dignity and rights," will "maintain a commitment to medical education," and will participate in activities contributing to "the betterment of public health." New principles VIII and IX state that "A physician shall, while caring for a patient, regard responsibility to the patient as paramount" and that "A physician shall support access to medical care for all people," respectively. Principle II has been reworded to state that AMA members "shall . . . strive to report physicians deficient in character or competence, or engaging in fraud or deception, to appropriate entities."[10] Critics of organized medicine argue that this continuing duty has been widely ignored.

The AMA's Council on Ethical and Judicial Affairs assists members in interpreting the principles by publishing opinions on issues such as experimentation, genetic engineering, abortion, and terminal illness. These opinions usefully supplement the Principles of Medical Ethics. The Council's 1994 statement, "Fundamental Elements of the Patient–Physician Relationship," complements the AMA's principles by focusing on the rights of patients (see Appendix B).

Just as it is clear that health services managers and their organizations benefit from increased attention to ethics, there is also evidence that physicians (and their patients) can benefit from education in ethics, professionalism, and moral reasoning: "[Orthopaedists] with higher moral reasoning and levels of professionalism . . . perform better clinically [and] also have fewer malpractice claims."[11]

Nurses

The American Nurses Association (ANA) code of ethics was first formally adopted in 1950, although precursors date from the "Nightingale Pledge" of 1893.[12] The preface to the 2001 iteration of the Code of Ethics for Nurses (reproduced in Appendix B) states that the code includes humanist, feminist, and social ethics; adherence to ethical principles; and the cultivation of virtues. It also asserts that

> The ethical tradition of nursing is self-reflective, enduring, and distinctive . . . [and that] The Code of Ethics with Interpretive Statements provides a framework for nurses to use in ethical analysis and decision making. The Code of Ethics establishes the ethical standard for the profession. It is not negotiable in any setting nor is it subject to revision or amendment except by . . . the ANA.[13]

Noted in a description of the code's evolution are doing no harm (nonmaleficence), benefiting others (beneficence), loyalty, truthfulness, social justice, and the autonomy of patient and nurse.[14]

Code expectations run a gamut that includes principles to guide practice, primary commitment to the patient, individual accountability, duties to self and others, improving health care, advancing the profession, collaboration, and obligations to the profession. Many of the code's nine provisions are specific. An interpretive statement follows each. Like physicians, nurses are obligated to counter or expose problematic practice: "The nurse promotes, advocates for, and strives to protect the health, safety, and rights of the patient." The interpretive statement discusses these obligations in the context of privacy, confidentiality, research, standards and review, and questionable and impaired practice.[15] Apparently, the nursing field has the American public's confidence. In four of the five times nurses were included in national surveys, they were perceived as the most honest and ethical professional group; in 2003, they outpolled physicians 83% to 68%.[16]

CODES FOR ORGANIZATIONS

Hospitals

The AHA is the most important trade association for hospitals. AHA last revised its guidelines for ethical conduct in 1992.[17] The guidelines are divided into community role, patient's care, and organizational conduct. Members are expected to improve community health status and deliver high-quality, comprehensive services efficiently. The importance of coordinating with other health services organizations is emphasized. Some provisions are specific: the need for informed consent; confidentiality; and mechanisms to resolve conflicting values and ethical dilemmas among patients and families, medical staff, employees, the organization, and the community. Members should try to accommodate the religious and social beliefs and customs of patients whenever possible. The guidelines identify the expectations regarding employee policies and practices and the accommodation of religious and moral values held by employees and medical staff. Conflicts of interest are defined. Neither disciplinary nor grievance proceedings are included.

Long-Term Care Facilities

The American Health Care Association (AHCA) is the national association of state associations of long-term care facilities, primarily nursing facilities. Its code of ethics was developed for use by the AHCA as an organization, but it is intended to serve as a model for its state members and, in turn, their facility members. The AHCA's organizational values, as identified in the preamble, include concern for individuals in need, quality service, service to the community, integrity and honesty, fairness, accountability, respect for employees, and stewardship. Topics in the body of the code include moral responsibility, good business practices, making difficult choices, acting responsibly, the obligation to provide quality service, dealing with conflicting values, the use of information, responsible advocacy, potential conflicts of interest, respect for others, and fairness in competition.[18] AHCA's code is not a tool for certification and has no sanctions for failing to meet its standards. Some states require nursing facilities receiving Medicaid funds to follow a patient bill of rights based on that of the AHCA.

The American Association of Homes and Services for the Aging (AAHSA) is the national association that represents not-for-profit or government-sponsored organizations that provide housing, health, community, and related services to meet the needs of older adults. AAHSA's ethics are reflected in its "Membership Creed," which was first adopted in 1991. Its current creed, which was adopted in 2001, includes a set of beliefs and a set of values, both of which are accompanied by brief explanations. The beliefs focus on the relationships that AAHSA members establish with the people they serve, personal responsibility with shared burdens, voluntary association, meeting unmet needs, the role of caregivers, and stewardship of resources and the environment. Values include concern for those served, the wise use of resources, honesty, justice in access and compensation, respect, and accountability. The creed includes no reporting or disciplinary process.

PHILOSOPHICAL BASES FOR CODES OF ETHICS

Codes of ethics for the health professions blend various moral philosophies and ethical theories. To varying extents, the principles of respect for persons, beneficence, nonmaleficence, and justice, as well as various of the virtues, are found in all codes.

The ACHE and ACHCA codes blend consequentialism (teleology), deontology, and virtue ethics but emphasize the latter two. Respect for persons and beneficence predominate. The statements on confidential information, for example, are grounded in deontology and virtue ethics, not in consequences. As noted, the duty to report violations was added to the ACHE code in 1987. In 2003, it required that "An affiliate of ACHE who has reasonable grounds to believe another affiliate has violated this *Code* has a duty to communicate such facts to the Ethics Committee."[19] In 2003, the ACHCA code contained a similar provision.

The preamble of the 2001 Principles of Medical Ethics of the AMA provides the context of its amended view of physician duty and respect for patients: "A physician must recognize responsibility to patients first and foremost, as well as to society, to other health professionals, and to self."[20] This philosophy is absent in the Hippocratic oath and the 1957 AMA principles, which emphasized paternalism. This change carries important implications for resource allocation by suggesting that physicians must consider the societal effects of individual treatment costs. This admonition is based on justice rather than beneficence, which focuses on patients, and adds a dimension of utilitarianism—to consider the greatest good for the greatest number.

As noted, the underpinnings of the ANA's Code of Ethics for Nurses include several moral philosophies. The code remains grounded in deontology, however, which is duty based. Within this philosophical context, respect for persons, nonmaleficence, beneficence, and justice undergird relationships with patients. Self-improvement, collaboration, and integrity are stressed.

APPLYING CODES OF ETHICS

Use and Enforcement

As noted, codes of ethics must be living documents that are used and applied by an association's members. General education about code provisions is the obvious first step. In addition, the professions must provide members with regular information about the code's interpretation, application, and enforcement. However, more attention should be given to making health services administrative or institutional codes living documents that are useful in guiding decisions. Encouraging and responding to this interest remain important challenges to the professional associations. It is encouraging that the majority of managers in leadership positions have used the ACHE code to teach others about expected behaviors and to counsel colleagues.[21]

Educating, counseling, and propagating professionalism among members are vital uses for codes. They assume even greater importance and usefulness when they are enforced. Unenforced, they are platitudes, seemingly intended primarily for public consumption. Enforceable codes are precise and include interpretations of provisions. Absent sufficient detail to guide members, enforcement results in arbitrary decision making and a lack of fairness. As noted, private associations are unlikely to be held to constitutional requirements of due process, but it is nonetheless fair (just) that they meet such a standard. This theme should underlie an association's relationships with members. Enforcement with feedback to members provides additional knowledge and understanding for the profession and makes the code a living document. This crucial attribute uses casuistry in building a body of cases and experience.

When health services professionals are licensed, disciplinary actions are usually a matter of public record. Reports of disciplinary actions against the licenses of physicians and other caregivers appear occasionally in the press. Among health services managers, only nursing home administrators are licensed—the result of historical problems in nursing facilities. Scandals elsewhere in the field of health services could lead to demands for licensure of other managers, an approach that is less desirable and probably no more effective than self-regulation. This scenario highlights the importance of the profession's voluntary efforts and the need to enforce usable, living codes of ethics.

Separating Private and Public Actions

Health services managers are quasi-public figures; the public's interest in them and their organizations is a function of the latter's prominence in the community. A manager's public role is greater in small communities, in which the organization, especially an acute care hospital, is economically, politically, and socially very significant. This prominence means that health services managers are community leaders ex officio. They are in a fishbowl whether or not they desire it. Managers of major health services organizations in urban areas are also community leaders by reason of their appointment. Health services managers must be prepared to accept this trust and to use the public's confidence to improve the community's health. However, such a role demands exceptional performance in all respects.

Community leaders are entitled to some claim of privacy, but greater prominence invariably diminishes privacy. Younger, less experienced managers have difficulty understanding that persons in positions of prominence cannot escape public scrutiny. Younger managers jealously guard their privacy, and most consider what happens in their personal lives as irrelevant to their performance as managers. Would that this were so, but their role in the organization and the public's expectations deny them this luxury.

Three elements affect the dynamic between public and private lives: 1) the corrupt moral standard that the right or wrong of an action is unimportant—the question is whether one is caught; 2) the organization's culture and the community standard of behavior and morality; and 3) administrative effectiveness. "It's okay if you don't get caught" or "It's okay, everybody's doing it" are unacceptable bromides for health services managers. The following simple examples highlight the effect of such views. Most employees would be embarrassed to be seen photocopying personal papers at their place of employment or to have their superiors note personal long-distance telephone calls made at the organization's expense. Wasted time, personal use of office supplies and equipment, and personal telephone calls will neither result in disciplinary action by a professional association nor by the organization (except in extreme cases). Such actions must be regulated by the individual's personal ethic. Members of the profession must consider that small infractions are governed by the principles developed in Chapter 1, as well as by their personal ethic.

The organization's philosophy and the community standard of morality are important because they affect managers' views of what is acceptable, thus tempering the manager's personal ethic. The microcommunity that is the organization develops a corporate culture whose mores and standards are unique, demanding, and ignored at one's peril.

Organizational Culture

It Just Isn't Done!

Several university faculty were invited to have lunch with 20 middle- and senior-level managers of a data processing firm. The group was enthusiastic and highly motivated, and most members were younger than age 40. Lunch was a break in a long day of seminars and meetings. When the waiter asked for drink orders, no one from the firm ordered an alcoholic beverage. Instead, they ordered milk or soda. One of the faculty remarked about this unusual behavior and was told there was an unwritten company policy that no member of the staff should go back to work after having an alcoholic beverage.

This attitude may seem straitlaced, and it is certainly different from the "two-martini lunch" once described as the norm in business. Yet this "rule" reflected the group's self-view (culture), and substantial peer pressure would likely be directed at anyone who disregarded it. On both a macro- and a microlevel, this is the type of peer pressure health services managers exercise for the good of patient and profession.

Administrative effectiveness is a question for the manager's manager, who determines whether problems have fatally flawed someone's ability to lead. Managers with badly tarnished reputations lose their effectiveness. Managers who are ridiculed, whose character deficits are blatant and widely known, or for whom respect is eroded or gone must be dismissed.

An example of private behavior considered unacceptable in a health services manager is driving while intoxicated (DWI). Regardless of the view held by professional associations, governing bodies are intolerant of managers charged with DWI, even though such behavior for a housekeeper would go unnoticed. Problems such as DWI run counter to the organization's view of the manager qua leader and its philosophy, which will be unwritten for problems such as alcohol and drug abuse, illicit sexual activity, and spouse abuse. Illegal activities are unethical per se. They are not explicitly prohibited because they are so obviously unacceptable.

A further reason such behavior is unacceptable is that the governing body has no wish to be embarrassed by an errant manager. An organization faced with scandal will separate itself from the source. This reaction reflects the instinct for organizational survival as well as indignation and moral revulsion. Instilling an awareness of the importance of ethical behavior in others is a continuing challenge.

It may seem unfair that managers are held to a higher standard than the larger community. Employees and the public expect more of leaders than of followers. The health services management profession correctly expects its members to avoid the temptations and problems affecting those outside it.

This a Laughing Matter?

One afternoon, Joan Zimmerman, the chief operating officer of a large hospital, encountered two younger members of her management staff conversing in hushed tones. As she approached unnoticed, they burst into laughter. One of the two blushed and turned his eyes downward as Zimmerman greeted them and asked lightheartedly about the source of their amusement. Neither spoke. Sensing there was something she should know, Zimmerman pressed for an answer. The awkward situation was interrupted by Zimmerman's pager, which asked her to call the operator immediately. Later, one of the two managers asked to see Zimmerman. He related an amazing story about the female director of a support department with a high turnover rate. In routine exit interviews conducted by human resources, several young male employees said they were leaving because they could no longer endure the sexual harassment by the department's director, who insisted that the young men have sex with her. Employees who refused were given the worst schedules and treated badly in other ways.

Zimmerman was told that the problem had existed for some time and was an open secret in the hospital. She was shocked and distressed that she had not been told.

This case has several dimensions. First, sexual harassment is against the law. Second, sexual harassment breaches the principle of respect for persons. Third, the unfair treatment of staff by the department head breaches the principle of justice. Finally, the department director has failed to meet the virtues of self-control, temperance, and integrity.

The immediate problem is to investigate the allegations against the department director and take disciplinary action, if appropriate. Also of concern is that younger managers were amused, not outraged. Their reaction may show immaturity rather than approval; regardless, it is a problem that needs attention. Managers lead by words and actions; actions are far more important.

Two other issues must be addressed. The first is that Zimmerman was unaware of the problem. The second is the lack of action taken by staff who knew of the allegations, which, if true, cast a shadow over the organization. Zimmerman must make clear to all staff that such behavior is intolerable. It breaches the trust reposed in managers, breaches their fiduciary duty to the staff and the organization, and is inconsistent with any organizational philosophy worthy of the name. If the allegations are true, the actions of the support department director diminish the regard in which all managers in the organization are held and, ultimately, diminish organizational effectiveness. Cynicism can become a cancer that slowly destroys the organization.

CONCLUSION

Most codes of ethics provide only general guidelines. Even specific provisions require interpretation and the courage to apply them. Interpretation is crucial, because even great detail cannot address the nuances and intricacies of all circumstances. A highly detailed code would be excessively legalistic; applying it would be impractical and nightmarish.

Of the professional groups in health services management, the ACHE has the most detailed code. This detail enhances its usefulness to guide health services managers, whether or not they are ACHE members. In most respects, however, the code is too general to provide performance standards.

Codes in the health services field carry only the sanctions available to the professional association, of which expulsion is the maximum disciplinary action. This limitation is unlikely to affect the individual's legal right to engage in the profession.

In addition to the expectations of ethical codes, most clinicians are regulated by state law. Licensure statutes—or *practice acts*, as they are often called—incorporate ethical principles similar to their private associations, and licensing boards are usually composed of individuals from the profession being regulated. This composition tends to give the group's ethical precepts the force of law; breaching them could lead to license suspension or revocation. It is noteworthy that the proceedings of public regulators are distinct from those of private associations or professional groups. A license is a condition of membership in the professional association, but membership in the association is not required for licensure—an appropriate distinction between private and public action.

For groups such as hospital managers, the lack of licensure increases the importance of self-regulation. The public looks to such professionals as important in safeguarding health services delivery. Unless self-regulation is effective and maintains the public's confidence, licensing or another form of governmental regulation will result.

Another pragmatic consideration is what contributes to managers' success. Historically, integrity was identified as the personality trait most important for success and more important than any skill or other trait or factor.[22] Integrity's importance undoubtedly continues. This additional stimulus to be ethical and above reproach in all aspects of their lives should cause health services managers to be vigilant about themselves and their colleagues. These are significant reasons for maintaining the public's trust in health services managers and their organizations.

More important than pragmatism to encourage ethical behavior is that it is the right thing to do—it is a principle for life and the profession. The slightest hint of impropriety in personal behavior must be avoided. What a tragedy for the late Hyman G. Rickover, father of the nuclear submarine fleet and a retired U.S. Navy admiral, with an astounding 64 years on active duty, to be forced to admit that be took gifts from defense contractors. Rickover claimed that the gifts were trinkets and that taking them did not affect his judgment. The Secretary of the Navy insisted that the gifts were worth tens of thousands of dollars. Whatever the facts, these revelations badly, and sadly, tarnished a distinguished career. It is just such situations that health services managers must assiduously avoid. Failing this, managers damage the public trust, risk their careers and reputations, and violate the principles of any personal ethic worthy of the name.

NOTES

1. Office of Government Ethics (OGE). (n.d.). *About OGE: Background and mission.* Retrieved November 4, 2003, http://www.usoge.gov/pages/about_oge/backgrnd_mission.html
2. Anita Cava, Jonathan West, & Evan Berman. (1995, Spring). Ethical decision-making in business and government: An analysis of formal and informal strategies. *Spectrum, 68*(2), pp. 34–35.
3. American Bar Association. (n.d.). *Rule 8.3: Reporting professional misconduct.* Retrieved April 14, 2004, from http://www.abanet.org/cpr/mrpc/rule 8 3.html
4. Peter Arlow & Thomas A. Ulrich. (1983, Spring). Can ethics be taught to business students? *Collegiate Forum,* p. 17; Archie B. Carroll. (2003, February 17). Can ethics be taught? *UGA News Service.* Retrieved November 14, 2003, from http://www.uga.edu/columns/030217/news12.html; Ameet Sachdev. (2003, February 14). Ethics moves to head of class. *Chicago Tribune On Line.* Retrieved November 14, 2003, from www.chicagotribune.com/business/chi-0302140374feb14,0,623998.story?coll=chi-business-hed
5. Dan Seligman. (2002, October 28). Oxymoron 101. *Forbes,* pp. 160, 162, 164.
6. American College of Healthcare Executives (ACHE). (2003). *ACHE professional and public policy statements.* Retrieved October 31, 2003, from http://www.ache.org/policy/index.cfm
7. American College of Health Care Administrators. (n.d.). *Advocacy: Code.* Retrieved April 14, 2003, from http://www.achca.org/achca.asp?DP=content&FN=code_of_ethics.asp

8. Tanya Albert. (n.d.). AMA's Principles of Medical Ethics may be infused with new "lofty ideas." *American Medical News* [On line]. Retrieved August 18, 2003, from http://www.ama-assn.org/amednews/2001/01/01/prsa0101.htm

9. Robert M. Veatch. (1980, June). Professional ethics: New principles for physicians? *Hastings Center Report, 10,* p. 17.

10. American Medical Association. (2003). *Newly adopted principles of medical ethics, June 2001.* Retrieved March 12, 2004, from http://www.ama-assn.org/ama/pub/category/4256.html

11. DeWitt C. Baldwin, Jr., & Wilton H. Bunch. (2000, September). Moral reasoning, professionalism, and the teaching of ethics to orthopaedic surgeons. *Clinical Orthopaedics and Related Research, 378,* pp. 97–103.

12. From American Nurses Association. (2001). *Code of ethics for nurses with interpretive statements* (p. 27). Washington, DC: Author.

13. *Ibid.,* pp. 5–6; extract reprinted by permission.

14. *Ibid.,* p. 27.

15. *Ibid.,* pp. 12–16.

16. Joseph Carroll. (2003, December 1). Public rates nursing as most honest and ethical profession. In *Gallup Poll: Poll analyses* Retrieved December 3, 2003, from http://www.gallup.com/content/login.aspx?ci=9823

17. American Hospital Association. (1992). *Hospital management advisory: Ethical conduct for health care institutions.* Chicago: Author.

18. American Health Care Association. (2003). *Code of ethics.* Retrieved November 23, 2003, from http://www.ahca.org/quality/qf_ethics.htm

19. American College of Healthcare Executives. (2003). *Code of ethics.* Retrieved October 31, 2003, from http://www.ache.org/abt_ache/code.cfm

20. American Medical Association. (2003, July 15). *E-principles of medical ethics.* Retrieved January 14, 2004, from http://www.ama-assn.org/ama/pub/category/8292.html

21. William A. Nelson & Paula P. Schnurr. (2003, November/December). Affiliates comment on code of ethics. *Healthcare Executive, 18*(6), pp. 54–55.

22. Walter J. Wentz & Terence F. Moore. (1981). Administrative success: Key ingredients [Special issue]. *Hospital & Health Services Administration, 2,* pp. 85–93.

CHAPTER 5

ORGANIZATIONAL RESPONSES
TO ETHICAL PROBLEMS

Thus far, little has been said about how organizations can be organized to solve administrative and biomedical ethical problems. The starting point in such efforts is the organization's philosophy, which reflects its values and establishes moral direction and a framework for the vision and mission statements. The organization's philosophy is subject to the minimum standard set by external constraints such as criminal and civil laws and their derivative regulations and court cases. For example, federal guidelines to protect human subjects are a starting point for the organization's relationship with patients participating in federally funded clinical research.

The personal ethic of the manager, as employee and leader, influences the organizational philosophy and is influenced by it. In addition, the manager organizes the organization and allocates resources to prevent and solve ethical problems. Such problem solving occurs in the context of the organizational philosophy but is affected by the manager's personal ethic, which should be more specific and comprehensive than the organizational philosophy. This dynamic reinforces the importance of the personal ethic, lest the manager lose an essential attribute of leadership—clear moral direction.

Since the 1970s health services organizations have established various means to solve ethical problems; most prominent are institutional ethics committees (IECs), institutional review boards (IRBs), and infant care review committees (ICRCs). IECs can provide a broad range of assistance on administrative and biomedical ethical issues. IRBs are specialized IECs that focus on research ethics. They are more helpful in preventing and solving problems in biomedical ethics than administrative ethics. ICRCs review care for infants with disabilities.

INSTITUTIONAL ETHICS COMMITTEES

The progenitors to IECs were abortion selection committees—which determined, prior to *Roe v. Wade*—whether a pregnant woman's health or life was at sufficient risk to justify an abortion, and medical morals committees in Roman Catholic hospitals, which assessed certain treatment decisions in light of Church teachings.[1] Later, in the 1960s, committees selected recipients of renal dialysis at a time when there were many more medically suitable patients than machines.

The 1976 court decision regarding Karen Ann Quinlan directed establishment of an "ethics" committee that was to review her prognosis. Such committees confirmed prognoses and helped determine whether to continue life-sustaining treatment. Prognosis committees were often called "God squads" because they determined when treatment would be withdrawn so the patient died from the underlying disease process(es).

The role of IECs in the 21st century is much broader. An early source of information about IECs was a national survey completed for the President's Commission for the Study of Ethical Problems in Medicine and Biomedical and Behavioral Research, which was published in 1983.[2] Smaller hospitals did not have an IEC, and IECs were not ubiquitous in large hospitals. Hospitals with teaching programs were most likely to have IECs. It was estimated that there were fewer than 100 IECs nationwide. The Quinlan case had encouraged hospitals to establish IECs.

The number of IECs grew rapidly in the early 1980s. By 1985, surveys done by the National Society of Patient Representatives found that 59% had them. The Baby Doe controversies in the early 1980s caused many hospitals to establish specialized IECs to solve the ethical problems accompanying newborns with profound disabilities. The growth in numbers of new IECs slowed in the late 1980s, however.[3] This lack of growth was confirmed by 1993 estimates that nationally, approximately 60% of hospitals had IECs; state and regional ethics networks put the number at 65%–85%.[4] By contrast, a 1993 survey by the Catholic Health Association found that 92% of members responding had an IEC.[5] A Hastings Center report suggested that hospital ethics committees have matured and must reconsider their roles to determine whether they should be involved in new ways and in other aspects of organizations.[6] In the 1990s, IEC involvement in case consultation seemed to decline; IECs were more likely to be involved in issues of appropriateness of technology, patients' rights, relationships among health care providers, and conflicts of social values.[7]

Nonacute health services are moving from hospitals to other types of settings. Growth in the need for and use of IECs will be greatest in nursing facilities, health maintenance and managed care organizations, and integrated delivery networks. A survey by the American Association of Homes and Services for the Aging found that the numbers of ethics committees among its members had increased from 29% in 1990 to 45% in

1995 and that many others were in the planning stage. The committees review cases and consult, make and review policy recommendations, and educate and advise staff and administration. Of organizations with committees, 86% surveyed found them useful.[8]

IECs in nonacute care organizations are likely to develop differently, in ways consistent with their unique activities and roles. It has been suggested that unlike physicians on IECs in hospitals, physicians on IECs in nursing facilities play a minor role and that administrative staff are much more important. Staff education levels in nursing facilities are lower, which may exacerbate cultural and class differences between staff and patients. In addition, because nursing facilities are heavily regulated, it is also likely that considerable focus will fall on legal rather than on ethical issues.[9] An important context for the use of ethics committees (or a similar mechanism) is the requirement of the Joint Commission on Accreditation of Healthcare Organizations (Joint Commission) that hospitals have a mechanism to resolve ethics issues, a requirement usually met by establishing an IEC.[10]

Organization

Complex health services organizations, especially acute care hospitals, should establish an ethics committee with at least two subcommittees, each of which addresses different types of ethical issues. An alternative is to have two ethics committees, one for administrative ethical issues and one for biomedical ethical issues. Specialization is necessary because a committee prepared to address biomedical ethics problems is likely to be inadequately prepared to address administrative ethics problems. Greater specialization is needed within the broad categories of administrative and biomedical ethics (e.g., ICRCs). Committee proliferation or overlap must be avoided, but the various types of ethical problems must be addressed effectively. Because of the need to solve general, organizationwide problems and specific, sometimes very technical, problems, the committee with subcommittees model should be considered.

Veatch[11] argued that the different ethical tasks undertaken by IECs are mutually exclusive because they emphasize different ethical principles. He recommended the ethics committees be organized using the following models:

1. *An autonomy model*—implements decisions of competent patients whose wishes are known

2. *A social justice model*—grapples with broad issues such as organizational health care policy, resource allocation, and cost effectiveness

3. *A patient benefit model*—makes decisions for patients unable to make decisions for themselves

Ethics committees that use autonomy models are accountable to the patient, whereas ethics committees that use a social justice model must be accountable to the organization (or the community). The first and third models emphasize biomedical ethical issues. The second model could address administrative as well as biomedical issues, if it were determined desirable to address the two types in one committee.

Purpose and Role

Since their early, focused beginnings, IECs have broadened their activities considerably. Administrative and biomedical IECs undertake generic activities such as policy development, education, case review, and guidance for individuals upon request. Specific activities for administrative IECs could include developing consent forms and procedures, considering criteria for macro resource allocation, and providing guidance on issues related to whistleblowing. Specific activities for biomedical IECs could include developing do-not-resuscitate (DNR) and patient consent policies, addressing involuntary discharge, addressing patient safety, and advising on withholding or withdrawing life support.

IECs play two roles of general importance. One is to assist in developing or reconsidering the organizational philosophy (to move the organization toward a more desired culture) and the derivative vision and mission statements. The experience and range of its interdisciplinary membership are likely to produce better reasoned and more thorough results. Education is the second role. The IEC's composition and its members' experience make it a reservoir of knowledge and expertise, and the typical case-based approach reflects casuistry. These resources should be made available to the governing body and staff. Such attributes add a level of sophistication to the organization and improve the quality of clinical and administrative decision making.

Before considering ethical problems, an IEC must develop a statement of its ethic, the framework for which is the organizational philosophy. The IEC's ethic is not a determination of how to solve each type of problem but is a statement of general principles that guide deliberations and determine its recommendations. This exercise is essential to the effectiveness of the IEC because it identifies and minimizes differences in members' personal ethics. Only by understanding and enunciating its own ethic can the IEC, for example, appreciate how its values differ from those of a patient, an understanding that is essential if patient autonomy is to be respected.

In terms of biomedical ethics, the principal benefits of IECs that have been identified since the late 1970s include facilitating decision making by clarifying important issues, shaping consistent policies about life support, and providing opportunities for professionals to air disagreements. IECs appear not to have been effective at increasing the ability of patients' families to influence decisions or at educating professionals about issues relevant to life support decisions. IECs focus almost exclusively on biomedical ethical problems and devote little time to administrative ethical issues, such as conflicts of interest, or to consulting on policy formulation and macro allocation decisions.

In the early 1980s, the President's Commission found that IECs were involved in few cases and were dominated by medical professionals to the exclusion of patients and, frequently, family members.[12] After a spurt of involvement in the mid-1980s and early 1990s, case consultation appears to have declined. Yet, the problem of patient representation, control, and attendance has continued.

The problem of attendance by patients and family raises significant questions of patient autonomy, especially in terms of resource allocation and consent. Among organizations with culturally diverse stakeholders, IEC members must be sensitized to the views that various cultures hold about medical services and especially about significant events such as death and the process of dying.

Last Wishes

A Native American was admitted to Memorial Hospital's emergency department in grave condition. His cardiac insufficiency was terminal. He was able to communicate his wishes, verified by his friend, that extreme measures not be used and that he be allowed to die naturally and peacefully. Death was expected within hours or a few days. His friend explained to nursing staff that in their religion a dying person's spirit could only enjoy eternal bliss if the person died in the open and the spirit could go to the sky, unfettered by the walls and ceilings of a building. Nursing staff wanted to meet the dying man's wishes but were uncertain what to do. They could not take the patient outdoors until he was in the final moments of the dying process. They monitored him closely. When they determined that he had died—even though a doctor had not pronounced him dead—they put him on a gurney, covered him, and took him outside through the service entrance. After a few moments away from the building, they returned his body to the nursing unit. His friend came back to the hospital a short time later. He thanked the staff for letting the dead man's spirit "go to the sky."

Nursing staff were able to accommodate the patient's wishes without compromising his care or that of other patients. They acted appropriately, if outside traditional bounds of the nurse–patient relationship. Meeting patients' spiritual needs, generally, has been identified as important to faster response to treatment and reduced likelihood of depression. Failure to meet them increases risk of death and poor mental health and reduces quality of life. Yet, clinicians receive little or no training in the subject.[13]

Membership

The President's Commission found that biomedical IECs were interdisciplinary. Physicians were the most common type of member, averaging 5.25 members per committee. Committees averaged one member of the clergy. Other members found on fewer than half the committees were attorneys, laypersons, social workers, and physicians in graduate education programs (residents). Administrators served on only about half of the committees. The commission found no strong community link, something that governing body members and individuals from the organization's service area could provide. Community members would bring an important perspective to decision making.[14] That managers were underrepresented may reflect limited interest in clinical matters—a problem managers must remedy. It was suggested in the early 1990s that nurses are also underrepresented in terms of both their number in health services organizations and the number of biomedical ethical problems they encounter.[15]

An administrative IEC will include fewer clinical personnel and more governing body members and managers. Yet, clinical staff should be included. The ample evidence that health services organizations are most effective when they involve clinicians in management decisions will certainly apply to solving administrative ethics problems.

Relationships

The IEC's relationships vary depending on its activities (role), which may be general or specific. General activities span the organization and can be divided into administrative and biomedical ethics. General levels include refining the organizational philosophy, ethics education, macroallocation decision making, and policy development (e.g., a conflict of interest policy).

Common specific-level activities are case and microallocation consultations and situational analyses. An example of a specific activity is whether a particular decision is consistent with the organizational philosophy.

The IEC should be proactive in developing and revising the organizational philosophy and in considering the ethical implications of macroallocation of resources. Similarly, the IEC should take the initiative in reviewing the consent process. However, the committee may choose a more passive role and wait to be consulted in specific instances of conflicts of interest and misuse of confidential information (for an administrative IEC) or in specific clinical matters (for a biomedical IEC).

It stands to reason that IECs are most effective when they wait to be consulted rather than when they interpose themselves in clinical or administrative decision making. As a consulting body, the committees only make recommendations to decision makers. IEC participation in biomedical and administrative decision making may be optional or mandatory. Whether the advice given by an IEC need be followed may be optional or mandatory, as well. Table 1 shows the combinations.

Physicians are unlikely to accept mandatory–mandatory involvement by a biomedical IEC. Furthermore, this type of involvement is not desirable for situations in which the physician is willing to develop alternatives and communicate them to the patient and others concerned. Even if the physician is unwilling to share decision making with an ethics committee, there are benefits to making its analysis and recommendation available to decision makers.

Important to an IEC's functioning is its location in the organization. Various options have been used and include making the IEC a standing committee of the governing body, medical staff, or administration. Concerns that IECs will be dominated by physicians causes some experts to suggest that they should be a governing body or administration committee. Members should be chosen for their ability to analyze ethical issues in an unbiased manner and not as the representative of a group.

Table 1.   Matrix of possible roles for institutional ethics committees (IECs)

Involvement of committee in decision making	Acceptance and use of advice provided by IEC
Optional	Optional
Optional	Mandatory
Mandatory	Optional
Mandatory	Mandatory

The Administrative Institutional Ethics Committee

The chief executive officer (CEO) of Community Health Plan (CHP) had been approached by a group from "north of the river." This area of the city was economically depressed and over the previous decade had lost many of its health services delivery organizations and physicians to the suburbs. It seemed to be in a downward spiral, with no end in sight. Decreasing numbers of insured patients meant that organizations were increasingly unable to serve the area. The city-owned hospital had made several ill-fated attempts to serve the area north of the river with a clinic system, but its efforts were scandal ridden. The clinic system became a political football with little credibility in the community.

The representatives from north of the river were community leaders, none of whom appeared to have political ambitions. They seemed genuinely willing to do whatever they could to assist in securing high-quality health services for their community. They proposed that CHP establish and staff three storefront clinics in the area. The community leaders stated that they would find volunteers to remodel the facilities and work in clerical jobs.

The CEO presented the proposed initiative to the administrative IEC, which included members of the governing body, managers, and physicians and other caregivers. In making the presentation, the CEO stressed the health plan's historical role in providing services to those in need, its not-for-profit status, and its continuing modest surplus. The members listened patiently, but the minute the CEO finished, all of them seemed to speak at once. Several members opposed the proposal and made the following points about the suggested venture:

1. The area north of the river was the city's responsibility. Providing care to the needy is not something a small not-for-profit health plan like CHP should attempt.

2. The organization's primary obligation was to enhance benefits for its enrollees and not to become involved in new schemes. New services had been requested by several of their physicians and many plan members.

3. The modest surplus the plan had accumulated over several years could be easily consumed by the proposed venture. The chief financial officer noted that an increase in reinsurance premiums was expected in the next quarter.

4. If the plan pulled the city's political chestnuts out of the fire by providing even stopgap assistance, the city would never get its house in order and develop the system needed north of the river.

Several members spoke in favor of working with the community north of the river and made the following points:

1. Helping the north-of-the-river community was the right thing to do. The people living there deserved health care services. Someone noted that the plan's own start came about when several physicians in the community fought the prevailing attitude among their peers about the prepaid practice of medicine.

2. Those opposing the proposal were putting dollars ahead of people's health. They must be willing to assist those who were less fortunate.

3. Plan members would support such an initiative if it were properly explained to them.

4. The positive publicity could further the plan's interests by increasing the number of enrollees.

It seemed to the CEO that this was a no-win situation. The organizational philosophy was not well developed and the proposal was a major step. Should something be done to help the north-of-the-river community? The IEC members had raised valid points that merited further discussion.

This case describes issues arising from decisions about the macroallocation of resources. The problems were more complex because CHP was being asked to volunteer assistance and to do so from its own meager surplus. Relevant theories of justice in allocating resources include retribution or compensatory justice (distributing resources so as to make up for past wrongs); just desserts (help would go to those who had not earned it and CHP's leadership had no right to risk the plan's solvency, which was something the membership paid to achieve); egalitarianism in access to health services and whether it was government's responsibility to provide it to the community north of the river; and utility as a prospectively determined element of beneficence.

A significant problem for CHP was that it did not consider this aspect of its relationship with unique subsets of the community in formulating its organizational philosophy and vision and mission statements. It would do well to develop these prospectively in a comprehensive fashion rather than address them ad hoc. Resource allocation receives further attention in Chapter 13.

Summary

IECs are useful in many ways. Overall, their effects will improve clinical and administrative decision making. However, one cannot assume that the mere presence of an IEC preordains its success. As with all undertakings, IECs should be evaluated so that performance can be improved.[16]

IECs present significant potential problems. Organizational concerns, especially legal ramifications and the avoidance of public embarrassment, can easily overwhelm concerns about patient goals.[17] At the extreme, it has been suggested that because IECs represent organizations, they cannot be objective; as a result, when a dispute arises, they will take management's side to avoid risk and thus fail in their vital role as patient advocates.[18] Management must ensure that IECs are not subverted in this manner.

INSTITUTIONAL REVIEW BOARDS

Health services managers may think research and experimentation are exclusive to academic health centers, in which rigorous protection and standards of review are applied. Many health services organizations, however, engage in research, some of which may not even be known to nonclinical managers.

Ethical Principles in Research

Contemporary codes of research ethics emphasize the subject's voluntary, informed consent. The modern emphasis on consent in research began in 1900 when a Prussian government commission identified unambiguous consent as essential.[19] The research subject's mental competence receives less attention than does consent. A provision in the Nuremberg Code (1949) states that subjects should be able to halt the experiment if they no longer wish to continue. This proviso places a heavy burden on the subject, who may become incapacitated by the experiment itself or by an unrelated medical problem or who may be intimidated by the setting or individuals involved. Subjects also usually lack the technical expertise to understand when their safety is threatened. This weakness was partially corrected in the Declaration of Helsinki (1964, revised 1975 and 1989), which recommends establishing an independent committee to review and approve the experimental protocol.

In 1978, the National Commission for the Protection of Human Subjects of Biomedical and Behavioral Research issued the *Belmont Report: Ethical Principles and Guidelines for the Protection of Human Subjects of Research*, which identified the ethical principles and guidelines for research involving human subjects. Its most influential contribution was the enunciation of three basic ethical principles: 1) respect for persons (met through an informed consent process), 2) beneficence (weighing risks and benefits), and 3) justice (fair selection of subjects). The Belmont Report provided important guidance on the boundaries between research and clinical medicine.[20] Its principles and guidelines are reflected in the type of committee required by the U.S. Department of Health and Human Services (DHHS).

All research codes and guidelines permit nontherapeutic research and recognize that volunteers for whom the experimental treatment offers no potential diagnostic or therapeutic benefit are needed for certain research. The utilitarian language present in all codes balances the risk to the subject (in nontherapeutic research) with the benefit to society. Conversely, emphases on voluntary and informed consent suggest a Kantian philosophy and reflect the principles of respect for persons and nonmaleficence, as well as the virtues of fairness, honesty, and trustworthiness. This view is found in the DHHS regulations ("Protection of Human Subjects"; Public Welfare, 45 C.F.R., 2001).

A primary problem with research codes other than federal regulations is that they inadequately separate the physician's roles as healer and researcher. The ethical burden on physicians is heavy because the duality of interests of physician-researchers puts them at high risk of encountering an actual conflict of interest. What is good for the research subject as patient may diminish the integrity of the experimental design. This problem is exacerbated in nontherapeutic research because the risk to the subject is not balanced by potential benefits. American Medical Association (AMA) guidelines recognize the dilemma and stress adequate safeguards for the welfare, safety, and comfort of the subject and written consent after full disclosure.[21]

Establishing Institutional Review Boards

To protect human subjects, health services organizations conducting research should establish an IRB, which is an independent committee comprised of scientific and nonscientific members that meets the requirements of federal law.[22] IRBs conduct initial and continued review of research involving human subjects. Committees with similar activities are considered IRBs, as well.

In the health services field, the DHHS and the Food and Drug Administration (FDA) are the most important federal entities that require an IRB to review, approve, and maintain oversight of research studies. The DHHS requirements for IRBs and protection of human subjects are applicable to research funded (i.e., supported or conducted by and regulated under a specific research statute) by 17 federal agencies and departments that have adopted the "common rule" or "federal policy" for the protection of human subjects.[23] Examples of federal agencies that use DHHS requirements are the Department of Defense, the Department of Veterans Affairs, the Environmental Protection Agency, the National Science Foundation, and the Consumer Product Safety Commission.

Research that involves human subjects and is wholly or partly federally funded must be reviewed by an IRB with a process that meets DHHS criteria. Although technically not required, research funding applications typically include assurances that the organization will comply with DHHS IRB requirements for human subjects (and other DHHS requirements for the protection of human subjects) for *all* of its research, federally funded or not.[24]

The FDA regulates the interstate sale of drugs, biologicals (i.e., vaccines), and medical devices and has the same requirements as DHHS. Unlike the DHHS, however, compliance with the FDA's guidelines, including the use of IRBs, is necessary regardless of funding source. A few states (e.g., New York) regulate medical research, but in most cases, health-related research is regulated by either the DHHS or FDA.

The FDA does not regulate surgical experimentation. For example, the FDA did not judge that coronary artery bypass surgery or radial keratotomy (ophthalmic surgery) were safe and efficacious or that they should be generally available. Neither does the FDA regulate innovative clinical care, which is defined as new uses of existing treatments, drugs, biologicals, and devices. Innovative care is distinguished from standard clinical activity, and its use requires more than the review and consent procedures for standard therapies. Absent government regulation, the organization's managers and clinical staff are essential in monitoring the activities of clinicians who develop innovative uses of drugs or treatments or who attempt new surgical procedures.

It is not easy for hospitals, most of which have no ongoing research programs, to define experimentation and innovative therapy. Nonetheless, definitions are important, not only because they determine whether there is a need to meet legal requirements or to form an IRB but also because the organization must ensure that its own, presumably more rigorous, procedures for consent and protection of the patient are followed. The following case illustrates the problem.

This Is Experimenting?!

An internal auditor conducted an audit of supplies used in biopsies. The data for kidney biopsies revealed significant discrepancies: The use of biopsy packs exceeded the number of procedures by 50%. The auditor was puzzled, but double-checking requisitions and utilization data showed them to be correct. Theft was unlikely.

The auditor made informal inquiries and spoke to technicians in the cytology laboratory. One agreed to speak confidentially about the additional kidney biopsies. The technician told the auditor that one of the nephrology fellows was using a second biopsy pack to take additional tissue during kidney biopsies. The tissue was sent to cytology for special studies ordered by the fellow. The technician said the fellow was testing a new theory about treating end-stage renal disease.

Is this research? Yes, because the nephrology fellow's activities meet the definition of research as systematic investigation designed to develop or contribute to generalizable knowledge. Taking additional tissue or using part of the specimen in the manner described is experimentation, although the act of obtaining it is not experimental. By trying to prove or disprove a theory, the nephrology fellow is performing research. However, taking the additional tissue requires consent separate from that for the routine, initial biopsy. There is no evidence a second consent was obtained. Taking more tissue or performing a second biopsy puts the patient at additional risk, without any actual or potential diagnostic or therapeutic benefit. The organization and its managers have an absolute duty to prevent unauthorized research, and policies and procedures regarding it are essential. Innovative treatments, too, must be closely monitored. With innovative treatment, the level of concern increases with the degree of risk. Adequate consent is essential for both experimentation and innovative therapy.

Ethical considerations also exist in the economics of this case. The second study adds to the laboratory's workload. If the charges (or costs) are paid by third-party payers who are told they are part of a patient's diagnosis or treatment, the organization is acting dishonestly toward the payer.

Organizational policies must distinguish standard clinical care from experimental procedures. Obtaining a few extra milliliters of amniotic fluid during amniocentesis causes moderate additional risk. Taking unused urine routinely collected for other purposes or performing analyses on the expelled placenta pose no risk to the patient but require consent nonetheless. Minor or nonexistent risks do not justify ignoring patients' rights and the duties owed to them. DHHS and FDA regulations recognize minimal research risk and permit special review procedures. Protocols for research in these categories can receive expedited review and approval from the IRB.

Defined as attempting new means, methods, and techniques, medicine has always engaged in research; without it medical knowledge would stagnate. Protecting the rights and welfare of human subject remains problematic, however.

Fever All Through the Night

Vice President for Administration Beverley Atchison finished reading the minutes of the utilization review committee. Atchison noted that a lengthy discussion had occurred with regard to the seemingly overlong stay of a pediatric patient. In fact, the attending pediatrician had appeared before the committee to explain the length of stay and her unique treatment regimen.

The case involved a child with a fever of unknown etiology. Routine tests after hospitalization showed no pathology. The physician explained that she had read about fever therapy in the literature and was impressed with its possibilities. Therefore, she decided to determine its appropriateness in cases of fever of unknown etiology. She ordered Tylenol if the fever went above 102.5 degrees Fahrenheit. Otherwise, there was to be no intervention.

The pediatrician stated that the efficaciousness of fever therapy was proven because after 3 days the child made a full recovery. The regimen raised numerous questions among the committee members, however.

This regimen is innovative; it could even be classified as experimental. The case raises two ethical issues: Did the child's parents receive information about the treatment adequate to give informed consent? This question bears directly on how the hospital determines that informed consent is obtained in such cases. At the very least, the therapy was innovative; special consent and review procedures should have been used. If fever therapy is determined to be experimental rather than innovative, the second issue is whether the research was therapeutic or nontherapeutic. Experimental treatment that may benefit the subject is therapeutic—the subject is also a patient. Nontherapeutic research involves healthy subjects or patients with medical problems other than those that might benefit from the experimental treatment. Nontherapeutic research must receive closer attention because the subject will not benefit and may also be at increased risk.

Had this innovative (perhaps experimental) therapy been presented to an IRB for review and approval, additional safeguards would have been required. An IRB reviewing pediatric research must be persuaded of the justification for the therapy's risks and benefits. The IRB must find that the activity falls into one of four categories: 1) research not involving greater than minimal risk; 2) research involving greater than minimal risk but presenting the prospect of direct benefit to the individual subjects; 3) research involving greater than minimal risk and having no prospect of direct benefit to the individual subjects but likely to yield generalizable knowledge about the subject's disorder or condition; or 4) research not otherwise approved but that represents an opportunity to understand, prevent, or alleviate a serious problem affecting the health or welfare of children.[25]

Notable in the fever therapy case is the nursing staff's apparent lack of concern about the unusual orders. Nursing's code of ethics emphasizes protecting the patient and requires the nurse to intervene if the patient is unnecessarily placed at risk. Timely reporting should have been accomplished through the nursing hierarchy. This part of the case suggests a much more widespread problem in terms of protecting patients and furthering their interests.

Membership and Purpose

Institutions may choose their own IRB members, but federal regulations (and perhaps state law) govern composition of the membership, the nature of the review that is conducted, and conflicts of interest of IRB members.[26] IRBs review research proposals for conformity with the law, standards of professional conduct and practice, and institutional commitment and regulations. IRBs acceptable to the DHHS have a minimum of five members with varying backgrounds (must have at least one whose professional interests are scientific and one whose interests are nonscientific) and who are capable of reviewing research proposals and activities of the type commonly performed by the organization.[27]

An IRB that is acceptable to the DHHS must apply the following requirements in reviewing research activities:[28]

- Minimize risks to subjects.

- Determine that risks to subjects are reasonable relative to anticipated benefits, if any.

- Select research subjects equitably.

- Obtain informed consent from each prospective subject or each subject's legally authorized representative.

- Appropriately document informed consent.

- Monitor the data collected to ensure the safety of subjects.

- Protect the privacy of subjects and maintain the confidentiality of data.

Additional safeguards must be in place when some or all of the subjects are likely to be vulnerable to coercion or undue influence. Examples include children, prisoners, pregnant women, persons with mental retardation, or those who are economically or educationally disadvantaged. Several provisions identify the information needed for informed consent.

The FDA uses the same basic elements of consent as the DHHS but applies special provisions when the subject is in a life-threatening situation that necessitates use of the test article and when the subject cannot provide legally effective consent, when time is insufficient to obtain consent from the subject's legal representative, and when no alternative method of generally recognized therapy that provides an equal or greater likelihood of saving the subject's life is available.

Requirements

Regulations issued in 1981 eliminated the requirement that any organization receiving DHHS funding had to use DHHS guidelines in *all* research, regardless of funding source. This marked a shift in the role of the federal government in protecting human subjects and in research, generally. The change also magnified the responsibilities of managers and researchers and put greater reliance on the organization's policies and procedures and on managers' personal ethic in judging the research. Problems such as those in the Willowbrook case, which is discussed in subsequent paragraphs, are likely to increase state regulation of research.

As a practical matter, organizations with multiple research funding sources, one of which is the federal DHHS, are likely to use the same DHHS-qualified IRB for all research protocols. It is easy to slip, however, and managers must be alert to potential ethical problems in formal research programs as well as in isolated innovative therapy or surgical experimentation.

A mix of moral philosophies and values is found in the DHHS regulations. Beneficence and its subsidiary, cost–benefit analysis, determine the benefits of research. Conversely, a Kantian (deontological) perspective and principles of respect for persons and nonmaleficence underlie the requirements for consent, privacy, and confidentiality. The virtues of honesty, trustworthiness, and integrity are appropriate here, too.

It has been argued that nondiagnostic and nontherapeutic research on children and adults who are considered legally incompetent should be prohibited.[29] Congress *has not* given the FDA authority to require extensive testing on children. The ethical, economic, political, legal, and scientific problems of research involving children are so daunting that researchers have been reluctant to undertake it. Despite efforts by Congress and the FDA to encourage testing of pharmaceuticals and biologicals on children, little research involving children is done, and most prescriptions for children are based on physician trial and error.[30] It is estimated that 50%–75% of drugs used in pediatric medicine have not been studied adequately to provide appropriate labeling information.[31] Nontherapeutic research on children is permitted, however. A risk–benefit ratio is applied, and no child can be placed in unnecessary jeopardy. Assent from the child and consent from parents or legally authorized representatives are required.

Hepatitis for Children with Mental Retardation?[32]

Willowbrook State Hospital, an institution for the care of people with mental retardation in Staten Island, New York, housed more than 5,000 residents in 1971.

Dr. Saul Krugman was a consultant in pediatrics and infectious diseases. When he began work at Willowbrook in the early 1950s, he discovered that major infectious diseases, including hepatitis, measles, shigellosis, parasitic infections, and respiratory infections, were prevalent. Conditions at Willowbrook were like those found at similar facilities elsewhere in the United States. Dr. Krugman and his colleagues undertook a study of these diseases, including research on a measles vaccine and hepatitis.

In 1956, Dr. Krugman, Dr. Joan Giles, and Dr. Jack Hammond began studies on hepatitis. The final phase of the research (1965–1970) involved 68 children ages 3–10. The researchers injected an infected serum to cause hepatitis in the residents of their research unit. The objective was to gain a better understanding of hepatitis and possibly develop methods of immunizing against it. The research was approved by the Armed Forces Epidemiological Board, one of the funders of the research; the executive faculty and the Committee on Human Experimentation of New York University, where Dr. Krugman held a faculty position; and the New York State Department of Mental Hygiene.

The researchers defended their decision to expose the children to strains of hepatitis on the following grounds:

- They were exposed to the same strains that were endemic to the facility.

- The were admitted to a special, well-equipped, and well-staffed unit and were isolated from exposure to other infectious diseases prevalent in the institution. The health risk was thus lower for those in the experiment than for those in the hospital at large, in which multiple infections occurred.

- They were likely to have a subclinical infection followed by immunity to the particular hepatitis virus.

The researchers also emphasized that only children whose parents gave informed consent participated in the experiment.

A storm of adverse publicity arose when the experiment was made public in 1967 by a New York state senator, who charged that children were being used as human guinea pigs. Nevertheless, the research continued. In 1971, the group's work produced spectacular results, when Dr. Krugman and co-workers were able to immunize a small group of children against serum hepatitis (hepatitis B [HBV]). The preliminary results were hailed as a scientific breakthrough. In defending the research, Dr. Krugman reported that the injections that induced hepatitis in the research group were given only after employing great thought and professional discretion and only with the informed consent of the parents. He stated that the doses were small and that the inoculations usually produced the infections without making the children sick. (After 12 years of legal and regulatory controversy, Willowbrook State Hospital closed at the end of 1987, when a federal court approved a final settlement.)

Although Dr. Krugman and his colleagues made a convincing case for undertaking and continuing the research, the Willowbrook case illustrates several ethical problems. The consent obtained from parents or surrogates was given under duress—they almost certainly believed that children who were part of the group purposely infected with HBV would fare better than children living among the population at large, in which conditions were much worse. Such considerations make it difficult to apply the principles of beneficence and nonmaleficence.

The general benefit of being in the special unit is an argument that should receive some credence. The children were somewhat protected from other diseases prevalent at Willowbrook and received treatment for the sequelae of HBV. In addition, it can be argued that this research is therapeutic; even though the children did not have HBV, they were almost certain to become infected with it. Children in the unit were also likely to be less harmed in other ways than would children in Willowbrook, thereby generally meeting the principle of nonmaleficence. The real problem, however, is that the children were being used as a means to an end, despite a potential for great social benefit if the research were successful.

The protocol for the studies had been approved by prominent and appropriate review bodies and the research continued for 16 years (1956–1971). Assuming effective consent from parents or legally authorized representatives, federal guidelines would have permitted this nontherapeutic research. At the same time, however, the organizational philosophy through its managers could have applied a more demanding standard—using the virtues of justice, compassion, and integrity—to the point of prohibiting the research. In fact, research that is not clearly therapeutic for children and others unable to give voluntary and competent consent is so fraught with ethical problems that it is rarely undertaken. Regrettably, this conundrum has resulted in a dearth of certain types of clinical knowledge, especially that of the therapeutic effects of drugs and biologicals on children, which, as noted, is ultimately to their detriment.

A question of justice in allocating state funds is raised by the horrific conditions at Willowbrook. Is it fair that human beings are treated so? Failing to increase state appropriations, however, the principles of respect for persons, beneficence, and nonmaleficence must be applied within financial limits.

The research conducted on children at Willowbrook seems to be from another era—an era with far less attention to protecting human subjects, especially children. Yet, three decades later an even more unacceptable example of research involving children occurred in Baltimore, Maryland, and involved the Kennedy Krieger Institute, an affiliate of The Johns Hopkins University. The Environmental Protection Agency–funded study, with state and city governmental sponsors and collaborators, sought to find inexpensive alternatives for reducing or eliminating the risks of lead paint from homes. A large number of families with healthy young children were placed in rental housing with various levels of lead risk abatement. Parents were not told of the full extent of the risk; upon discovering it, they sued.[33] Maryland's highest court faulted The Johns Hopkins Hospital IRB and ruled that "in Maryland a parent . . . cannot consent to the participation of a child or other person under legal disability in nontherapeutic research or studies in which there is any risk of injury or damage to the health of the subject."[34]

Exempt Research and Research Warranting Expedited Review

Six categories of research are exempt from DHHS requirements. Examples are research conducted in established or normally accepted educational settings involving normal educational practices; research involving use of educational tests, survey and interview procedures, or observation of public behavior; and research involving the collection or study of existing data, documents, records, and pathological or diagnostic specimens. Limits are specified.[35]

DHHS regulations identify research warranting expedited review as a category to which different provisions apply. Expedited review allows special procedures for approval of certain types of research that pose no more than minimal risk to human subjects. The review is conducted by the IRB chair or by one or more experienced reviewers designated by the chair. In reviewing the research, the reviewer exercises all authority of the IRB. Research may be disapproved only in accordance with the nonexpedited procedure.[36] Subject to limitations, research categories appropriate to expedited review include clinical studies of drugs and medical devices; collection of blood samples; collection of biological specimens such as hair and nail clippings and deciduous teeth; collection of data through noninvasive procedures; research using materials collected for other purposes; collection of data from various types of recordings; research on individual or group characteristics or behavior; and continuing review of research previously approved by the IRB.[37] Expedited review greatly facilitates several kinds of research.

Falsification of Research Data

A unique dimension to problems in research occurred in the late 1970s and early 1980s.[38] John Darsee, a fellow in cardiology at Emory University and Harvard University and a brilliant physician of unusual talent, perpetrated an amazing fraud. Darsee was found to have falsified large quantities of research data on the genetic and biochemical factors affecting heart disease. Some of these data had been published in leading medical journals. Other data were being used for papers in process. Many of the articles listed prominent physician-researchers as coauthors, some of whom later asserted they had no knowledge that they had been identified as such.

Darsee's champions supported him until evidence of his deception proved overwhelming. Darsee's detractors argued that his supporters were too easily charmed by his personality and talents. When researchers and administrators at Emory and Harvard learned of the fraud, they withdrew his papers and abstracts that had been submitted for publication. The only course for articles already published was to urge readers to disregard them. It is claimed that no patients were harmed because of Darsee's clinical work, a claim verifiable only by reviewing medical records. Much more potential harm, however, lies in the fact that Darsee's list of publications includes more than 100 articles and abstracts. Readers unaware of the fraud cannot know which publications contain false data.

The organizations involved acted forthrightly when the problems were discovered. What happened violated both the ethics of research and proscriptions imposed by funding organizations, such as the National Institutes of Health. The most pointed questions, however, concern the adequacy of surveillance, not only of Darsee but also of all physicians in training who engage in research and collect research data. Subsequent self-assessment at Emory led to new safeguards in reviewing the work of physicians in training and in monitoring the use of names of teaching staff as coauthors. Research findings are also reviewed much more extensively since the Darsee affair. Despite the safeguards, some people argued that "[they] won't prevent the generation of fraudulent data, but under this system someone like Darsee couldn't send out articles at the rate of one a week without raising suspicions."[39]

Summary

Regulations such as those imposed by the DHHS focus responsibility on the organization and its IRB. Irrespective of legal requirements, the organization's managers are charged with independent duties under the principles of respect for persons, beneficence, nonmaleficence, and even justice (e.g., equitable selection of research subjects) in order to protect the patient. The virtues of honesty, integrity, and trustworthiness are applicable, as well. Managers must establish and maintain systems and procedures to prevent unauthorized research and to provide the necessary extra protection when innovative treatment or surgical research are proposed or undertaken. The Darsee affair raises a unique set of potential problems in teaching and research institutions. Most important are staff awareness about the parameters of acceptable practice and the courage to act.

INFANT CARE REVIEW COMMITTEES

ICRCs are another type of specialized IEC. They focus on the biomedical ethical problems of infants with life-threatening conditions. The Child Abuse Amendments of 1984 (PL 98-457) directed the DHHS to encourage establishment of ICRCs in health facilities, especially those with tertiary-level neonatal units. The DHHS identified the following guidelines for ICRCs:

> (1) educate hospital personnel and families of disabled infants with life-threatening conditions; (2) recommend institutional policies and guidelines concerning the withholding of medically indicated treatment from infants with life-threatening conditions; and (3) offer counsel and review in cases involving infants with life-threatening conditions.[40]

The guidelines make it clear that the DHHS considers it prudent to establish an ICRC but that the organization decides whether to do so. Chapter 10 provides the background for the original Baby Doe regulations and the Child Abuse Amendments.

Certain aspects of the ICRC's membership and administration recommended in the guidelines are notable. Members should include individuals from varied disciplines and perspectives because a multidisciplinary approach provides the expertise to supply and evaluate pertinent information. The committee should be large enough to represent diverse viewpoints but not so large as to hinder its effectiveness. Recommended membership includes a practicing physician (e.g., pediatrician, neonatologist, pediatric surgeon), practicing nurse, hospital administrator, social worker, representative of a disability group, lay community member, and a member of the facility's medical staff, who is the chairperson.[41] The recommendation to include a representative of a disability group in the ICRC runs counter to the principle that members of such committees should not represent specific groups.

The DHHS suggested that the ICRC have adequate staff support, including legal counsel; that the ICRC recommend procedures to ensure that both hospital personnel and patient or resident families are informed of its existence, functions, and 24-hour availability; that the ICRC self-educate about pertinent legal requirements and procedures, including state law requiring reports of known or suspected medical neglect; and that the ICRC maintain records of deliberations and summary descriptions of cases considered and their disposition.[42]

Many groups, including the AMA, the American Hospital Association (AHA), and various medical specialty associations, objected vociferously to the original Baby Doe regulations and sought to block implementation. The Child Abuse Amendments and regulations, however, were supported by health services trade associations, which ran the gamut from institutional and personal providers to specialized groups. In fact, the associations were instrumental in developing the law and regulations. The new law was enthusiastically backed by the AHA, and few hospitals will have philosophical problems complying with it.[43]

SPECIALIZED ASSISTANCE

This section outlines assistance for organizations and their managers and clinical staffs in solving administrative and biomedical ethical problems. Analogues to IECs and specialized committees such as IRBs and ICRCs that can assist managers to identify and solve administrative ethical problems are not as well developed but should be given further nurturing and attention.

Ethics Consultation Service

An Ethics Consultation Service (ECS) is one way that health services organizations can provide specialized personnel to advise and assist in solving biomedical ethics problems. Doing so is similar to establishing a clinical service. The ECS is staffed by ethicists with graduate degrees in philosophy, often at the doctoral level, and by clinical personnel who may be physicians or other caregivers. The clinicians have a special interest and/or preparation in ethics and provide a bridge between the ethicist and clinical staff attending the patient. They also are a resource for the ethicists. In this model, an ethicist is on call, and the clinical member of the ECS is involved as needed. The ECS reports to the hospital IEC, which develops and recommends policy to the governing body. The IEC also serves as a sounding board for problems that develop during ethics consultation. A variant uses a primary consultant who is assisted by other members of the ECS. The primary consultants and those assisting them come from various backgrounds, but all have intensive and specialized training in ethics and all participate in case reviews, ethics instruction, and regular meetings of the ECS staff.[44]

Ethicists

A less formal approach than the ECS is common in larger hospitals but should not be limited to them: Large hospitals are likely to employ full- or part-time ethicists. As in an ECS, the ethicists are often doctorally qualified philosophers who may be faculty members at a university or medical school and who consult with clinical staff on biomedical ethical issues.

Organizations needing the assistance of an ethicist can look beyond universities and medical schools and consider anyone with specialized preparation in ethics and its application in health services delivery. In this case, as with the ECS, an ethicist is the clinically oriented, problem-solving extension of an IEC.

Dispute Resolution

Treatment options and decisions regarding them often cause disputes among stakeholders, such as clinicians, patients, and families. The various types of ethics committees (e.g., IECs, IRBs, ICRCs) may be able to resolve disputes, but their connection to the organization raises concerns among some stakeholders as to their objectivity. Arbitration and mediation should be considered to resolve such disputes. Arbitration involves a neutral person to whom the parties to the dispute have given the authority to make a decision that all have agreed to accept. Mediators are neutral individuals who work with the parties to reach a result that is acceptable to them; mediators have no authority to make a decision. Competent neutrals can minimize the power imbalances present in health services settings, especially when nonclinicians are involved in the dispute.[45] One objective of improved dispute resolution is to weld a multidisciplinary group into a cohesive and mutually supportive team so that they can resolve their differences and maintain the quality of patient care. Formal dispute resolution could also assist the various types of ethics committees, because it seems overly optimistic to think that the act of establishing an interdisciplinary ethics committee means that it will be successful.

CONCLUSION

This chapter examined committees established to address ethical issues. These committees include the general type, which the chapter called IECs, and IRBs and ICRCs, which are specialized ethics committees. In addition to hospitals, ethics committees can provide assistance in a wide range of health services organizations, including nursing facilities, managed care organizations (MCOs), and hospices, all of which experience ethical problems similar to those found in hospitals. The greatest growth is likely in nonhospital settings. Hospice and nursing facilities, for example, confront issues related to dying and death; MCOs have issues of resource allocation and physician incentive plans. Ethics committees in all settings will be involved in solving complex ethics issues, some of which (e.g., organizational philosophy) may come under mandatory review.

ECSs and ethicists can be involved on a more discretionary basis to assist in identifying and analyzing the moral obligations, rights, responsibilities, and considerations of justice that bear on a general issue or on the ethical issues in a specific clinical case.[46] They can assist physicians and are more likely to be used than are biomedical ethics committees, which physicians may view as cost ineffective. Beyond considerations of efficiency, it may be more palatable for physicians to consult with a single ethicist than to seek guidance from a committee. Ethicists can serve a similar function for managers by assisting them in identifying and solving administrative ethics problems and working with an administrative IEC.

Economic pressures resulting from cost cutting by third-party payers—especially government—and new competitive pressures are affecting all health services organizations, especially acute care hospitals. Managers may be tempted to use economic justification for decisions that implicitly, or even explicitly, affect quality of care negatively. The conflict between economic interests and quality considerations lies near the surface in most relationships with patients. The technical nature of health services and the average consumer's limited ability to judge results make it imperative that individuals associated with health care delivery expend every effort to further the quality of care and protect the interests of patients.

NOTES

1. Judith Wilson Ross, John W. Glaser, Dorothy Rasinski-Gregory, Joan McIver Gibson, & Corrine Bayley. (1993). *Health care ethics committees: The next generation* (p. 1). Chicago: American Hospital Publishing.
2. President's Commission for the Study of Ethical Problems in Medicine and Biomedical and Behavioral Research. (1983). *Deciding to forego life-sustaining treatment: A report on the ethical, medical, and legal issues in treatment decisions* (p. 443). Washington, DC: U.S. Government Printing Office.
3. Right-to die: An executive report. (1989, November 20). *Hospitals*, p. 34.
4. Ross et al., p. ix.
5. Joanne Lappetito & Paula Thompson. (1993, November). Today's ethics committees face varied issues. *Health Progress*, p. 34.
6. Cynthia B. Cohen, Ed. (1990, March/April). Ethics committees. *The Hastings Center Report, 20*, pp. 29–34.
7. Lappetito & Thompson, p. 34.
8. American Association of Homes and Services for the Aging. (1995, July). *Summary report: Survey on ethics involvement in aging services.* Washington, DC: Author.
9. Ross et al., p. 8.
10. Joint Commission on Accreditation of Healthcare Organizations. (2004). Ethics, rights, and responsibilities. In *Hospital accreditation standards* (pp. 99–116). Oakbrook Terrace, IL: Author.
11. Robert M. Veatch. (1983, July). Ethics committees proliferation in hospitals predicted. *Hospitals, 57*(13), pp. 48–49.
12. President's Commission, p. 448.
13. Harold G. Koenig. (2003, July/August). Meeting the spiritual needs of patients. *The Satisfaction Monitor.* Retrieved October 17, 2003, from http://www.pressganey.org/products_services/readings_findings/satmon/article.php?article_id=94
14. Marilyn M. Mannisto. (1985, April). Orchestrating an ethics committee: Who should be on it, where does it best fit? *Trustee, 38*(4), pp. 18–19.
15. Ross et al., p. 5.
16. Linda S. Scheirton. (1993). Measuring hospital ethics committee success. *Cambridge Quarterly of Healthcare Ethics, 2*, pp. 495–504.

17. Mannisto, pp. 17–20.

18. Amy Haddad & George Annas. (1994, July). George Annas quoted in "Do ethics committees work?" *Trustee, 47*(7), p. 17.

19. Abbey S. Meyers. (2000, January 30). A lot of rules, too many exceptions. *The Washington Post,* p. B3.

20. PricewaterhouseCoopers. (2001). *PricewaterhouseCoopers IRB reference book* (p. 13).

21. American Medical Association. (Updated June 1994 and June 1999). *Clinical investigation.* Retrieved January 2, 2004, from http://www.ama-assn.org/ama/pub/category/print/8422.html

22. Public Welfare, C.F.R. 45, Part 46, and Food and Drugs, C.F.R. 21, Part 56.

23. Mark Barnes & Sara Krauss. (2000, August 31). Conflicts of interest in human research: Risks and pitfalls of "easy money" in research funding. *BNA's Health Law Reporter, 9*(35), p. 1383.

24. *Ibid.*

25. PricewaterhouseCoopers, pp. 199–200.

26. Barnes & Kraus, p. 1382.

27. Public Welfare, 45 C.F.R. § 46.107 (2001).

28. Public Welfare, 45 C.F.R. § 46.111 (2001).

29. Paul Ramsey. (1970). Research involving children or incompetents. *The patient as person* (p. 252). New Haven, CT: Yale University Press.

30. Peter B. Budetti. (2003, August 20). Ensuring safe and effective medications for children. *Journal of the American Medical Association, 290*(7), pp. 950–951.

31. Rosemary Roberts, William Rodriguez, Dianne Murphy, & Terie Crescenzi. (2003, August 20). Pediatric drug labeling: Improving the safety and efficacy of pediatric therapies. *Journal of the American Medical Association, 290*(7), pp. 905–911.

32. Articles from several issues of *The New York Times* were used to prepare the Willowbrook case and background information: January 11, 12, and 13, 1967; March 24, 1971; April 18, 1971; January 11, 1972; May 25, 1981; January 8, 1984; April 19, 1985; and March 3, 1987.

33. Manuel Roig-Franzia & Rick Weiss. (2001, August 21). Md. appeals court slams researchers. *The Washington Post,* p. B1; Manuel Roig-Franzia. (2001, August 25). My kids were used as guinea pigs. *The Washington Post,* p A1.

34. Grimes v. Kennedy Krieger Institute, 366 Md. 29, 782 A.2d 807 (2001).

35. Office for Protection from Research Risks. (1997, December 23). *Summary of basic protections for human subjects.* Retrieved August 17, 2003, from p. 2 of http://ohrp.osophs.dhhs.gov/humansubjects/guidance/basics.htm

36. Public Welfare, 45 C.F.R. § 46.110 (2001).

37. Office for Human Research Protections. (1998, November 9). *Categories of research that may be reviewed by the institutional review board (IRB) through an expedited review.* Retrieved August 17, 2003, from http://ohrp.osophs.dhhs.gov/humansubjects/guidance/expedited98.htm

38. *Emory Magazine.* (1983, December), pp. 6–15.

39. *Ibid.,* p. 15.

40. Final Rule, Child Abuse and Neglect Prevention and Treatment Program, 45 C.F.R. §1340 (1985).

41. Services and Treatment for Disabled Infants; Model Guidelines for Health Care Providers to Establish Infant Care Review Committees, 50 Fed. Reg. 14893(1985).
42. *Ibid.*
43. *Summary: Survey of infant care review committees.* (1984). Paper presented at the Annual Meeting of the American Academy of Pediatrics, Chicago.
44. John C. Fletcher, Margo L. White, & Philip J. Foubert. (1990). Biomedical ethics and an ethics consultation service at the University of Virginia. *HEC Forum, 2*(2), pp. 89–99.
45. Jerry P. Roscoe & Deirdre McCarthy Gallagher. (2003, Spring). Mediating bioethical disputes: Time to check the patient's pulse? *Dispute Resolution Magazine 9*(3), pp. 21–23.
46. John C. Fletcher, Norman Quist, & Albert R. Jonsen (1989). *Ethics consultation in health care.* Chicago: Health Administration Press.

ADMINISTRATIVE ETHICAL ISSUES

Virtually all administrative problems that arise in managing health services organizations and programs have ethical dimensions. These ethical problems are qualitatively distinct from those encountered in the business world.

Business ethics literature burgeoned in the 1980s, and courses in business policy and ethics are now common in graduate and undergraduate business programs. Little tradition exists in business of an independent duty or obligation beyond that established by law; emphasis is correctly on profitability and *caveat emptor* (let the buyer beware). Business ethics literature examines concepts such as honesty, integrity, and benevolence; duties of employees to each other and the organization; and duties of organizations to employees. These aspects are similar to those that health services managers apply. Absent, however, is the concept of respect for persons, which emphasizes autonomy, fidelity, and confidentiality. Neither is beneficence a focus in business ethics. The principle of justice is found only at its periphery. The differences between business and health services are cited not to criticize business but to distinguish the two fields of endeavor, whose foci and purposes are, simply put, quite different.

The public's view and that of the health services field have been that health services managers have a higher calling, one that goes well beyond the financial bottom line. Codes of ethics in health services assist in defining this calling and the intrinsic duties of managers. This definition stems from the link with medical and nursing professionals and the not-for-profit status common to the health services field. For acute care hospitals, historic links with religious orders and Samaritan motivation created a special set of relationships. The totality of this higher calling emphasizes the caring as well as the curing aspects of health services delivery. It reflects society's sense of the sick as a unique group, one with special status that needs protection and is not to be exploited. Despite occasional, harsh criticism, especially of financial management and the quality of care, the Samaritan image of health services organizations is largely intact.

The administrative ethics issues confronting health services managers run a gamut from conflicts of interest to governing body and medical staff relations to independent duty to the patient. Such problems can be subtle and appear in many guises, but they are identifiable and solvable by alert, conscientious managers. The ethical issues and concerns of managers in their relationships with the organization, staff, patients, and community are considered in Chapters 7 and 8. Also included is the effect of acquired immunodeficiency syndrome/human immunodeficiency virus (AIDS/HIV) on these relationships and the special duties and responsibilities that are raised.

Section III identifies and examines administrative ethical issues. By and large, they are distinct from the biomedical ethical issues considered in Section IV. Differences between administrative and biomedical ethical issues are important, but the two often blur in practice. Patient consent provides an example of these differences. Administrative ethics of consent likely affect patients as groups rather than individuals and affects managers' relationships with the organization, peers, profession, and community. Biomedical ethics of consent usually affect patients as individuals or as specific types of patients. The two merge in the ethical duty of the organization to assure itself that patients have freely given informed consent to clinicians for treatment. Administrative and biomedical ethical problems actually or potentially affect one another. The primary focus of each type of ethical problem is different, however.

CHAPTER 6

CONFLICTS OF INTEREST
AND FIDUCIARY DUTY

onflict of interest is the most commonly reported administrative ethical problem confronting health services organizations. Trade associations, such as the American Hospital Association (AHA), have issued policy statements about conflicts of interest. Conflicts of interest arise from differing interests and exist when duties are owed to two or more persons or organizations and meeting the duty to one makes it impossible to meet the duty to the other. The classic case occurs when a decision maker (a director [trustee] or a manager) is also a decision maker for an organization with which the health services organization does business. The manager cannot meet the duties owed to both organizations—the duties conflict. Conflicts of interest also arise for clinicians. Conflicts between duties owed to different patients by the same physician, for example, are an important reason to separate the organ transplant team from the physician treating the potential donor. Other conflicts of interest arise when the differing duties owed to the organization by a physician are in conflict with those owed to patients or colleagues or when patients with the same diagnosis and physician but in different payment categories receive different care in the same organization.

Conflicts of interest are insidious; one can slip into them almost without realizing it. There is sometimes a fine line between acceptable and unacceptable behavior, a pragmatic view recognizing that the relationships of normal business often create differing interests, which may result in actual conflicts of interest.

The manager's relationships with the organization and interactions with the health system and other organizations in it can cause conflicts of interest. In addition to potentially affecting the manager's relationship with the organization, conflicts of interest can affect managers' relationships with the profession and their personal development.

Conflicts of interest are often subtle and can affect all managerial activities. Has the manager who uses a position of influence and authority

123

to gain titles, stature, and income at the expense of the organization or patient care acted ethically? Is the manager who is lax in developing and implementing an effective patient consent policy and process acting ethically? Is it ethical for a manager to review and cleanse negative information from reports to the governing body? Is it ethical for a manager who has reason to believe that quality of care problems may exist in a clinical department to do nothing to prove or disprove their presence? Is it ethical for managers who have serious concerns about their abilities to continue managing? To the complexity of such questions from an ethical perspective must be added the legal implications. Regardless, managers must first be concerned about their independent, positive duty to the patient.

There is significant evidence that many conflicts of interest are not consciously understood by persons making decisions—they honestly believe that what they are doing is truly in the best interests of the organization or individuals involved. Incentives in compensation programs unconsciously drive decision making that leads to conflicts of interest.[1]

Yet, managers must avoid any hint of wrongdoing, especially the suggestion of divided loyalties. A bad odor emanates from a situation in which a hospital's chief executive officer (CEO) owns stock in a corporation that contracts for the hospital's data processing business and in which the principal stockholder and CEO is the hospital's comptroller. This odor lingers regardless of discounted price or other advantages the hospital may gain. Outside observers cannot help but think that the relationships have hidden aspects that are detrimental to the organization or its patients and that managers are reaping a personal advantage. Attempts to convince the public otherwise probably reinforce the perception of wrongdoing. The only course of action is to avoid arrangements or entanglements that contain any hint of duality of interests that could lead to conflicts of interests. The problem is well put by Harlan Cleveland in *The Future Executive*: "If this action is held up to public scrutiny, will I still feel that it is what I should have done, and how I should have done it?"[2]

FIDUCIARY DUTY

Fiduciary is an ethical and legal concept arising from Roman jurisprudence. A fiduciary relationship exists whenever confidence and trust on one side result in superior position and influence on the other. Superiority and influence raise duties of loyalty and responsibility. The definition suggests that numerous fiduciary relationships exist in health services. Governing body members, for example, are fiduciaries. Their duty of loyalty prevents them from using their position for personal gain, and they must act only in the organization's best interests. This definition has been interpreted to mean that no secret profits can be made in dealings with the organization and that the governing body member may not accept bribes or compete with the organization. The duty of responsibility requires governing body members to exercise reasonable care, skill, and diligence, as demanded by the circumstances.[3] Members of governing bodies have a duty to avoid errors of omission and errors of commission. Breaching these duties could result in personal liability, whether or not the corporation is organized for profit.

Trusts are common in the health services field. Many not-for-profit health services organizations engaging in charitable activities were established because of a gift or bequest that directed the establishment of a trust; trustees manage the assets of the trust. Examples are trusts to defray the costs of a patient unit or specific clinical activity in a hospital. Other uses include funding schools of nursing or providing scholarships to educate health services personnel.

The term *trustee* is commonly used to describe governing body members of not-for-profit corporations in the health services field, even though there is no trust and they are not true trustees. Technically, the legally correct term is *director* or *corporate director*. The title *trustee* is preferred in the not-for-profit sector, however, perhaps because governing body members want to be distinguished from governing body members in for-profit organizations, in which *director* is used.

The legal standard for true trustees is much more stringent than is that applied to directors of corporations or to individuals responsible for monies or properties not held in trust. True trustees actually hold title to property or the corpus of the trust and manage it for the beneficiary. True trustees must act in good faith and practice undivided loyalty in administering the trust. All situations and relations that interfere with discharging these duties must be avoided. Breaching these standards results in personal liability.

In many jurisdictions, the standard of care required of directors of not-for-profit corporations who are not true trustees is higher than that required of other corporate directors. The usual standard for directors who are not true trustees is that they are liable for ordinary negligence, errors in judgment. The minority rule is that to be legally liable, directors must have committed an act of gross negligence, usually defined as an intentional failure to perform a manifest duty with reckless disregard of the consequences.

Sibley Memorial Hospital

An important court case involving governing body members of a health services organization is *Stern et al. v. Lucy Webb Hayes National Training*

School of Deaconesses and Missionaries et al. (1974).[4] The members of the governing body of Sibley Memorial Hospital, a not-for-profit hospital in Washington, D.C., were called "trustees" even though they were not true trustees. David M. Stern brought a class action suit against Sibley Memorial Hospital on behalf of his minor son and other patients, alleging that patients had overpaid for care because several governing body members had engaged in mismanagement, nonmanagement, and self-dealing (succumbing to self-interest). The suit alleged that the acts of omission and commission resulted from a conspiracy between those trustees and various financial institutions with which several trustees were affiliated. The court found no evidence of a conspiracy. In considering the other allegations, however, it determined that:

> The charitable corporation is a relatively new legal entity which does not fit neatly into the established common law categories of corporation and trust . . . the modern trend is to apply corporate rather than trust principles in determining the liability of the directors of a charitable corporation, because their functions are virtually indistinguishable from those of their "pure" corporate counterparts.[5]

This ruling meant that defendant trustees were held to a less stringent standard of care.

The court found that the trustees had violated their duties as fiduciaries, even when held to the lesser standard. Mismanagement occurred because the trustees ignored the investment sections of yearly audits, failed to acquire enough information to vote intelligently on opening new bank accounts, and generally failed to exercise even cursory supervision over hospital funds. Nonmanagement was evidenced by the same failure to exercise supervision and was most starkly demonstrated because although certain trustees were repeatedly elected to the investment committee, they did not object when the committee failed to meet in more than 10 years. The allegation of self-dealing was substantiated by the following: A number of trustees were officers of banks in which Sibley kept hundreds of thousands of dollars in noninterest-bearing checking accounts and in which interest-bearing accounts paid less than market conditions would have permitted, and one trustee advised approval of and voted to approve a contract for investment services with a corporation of which he was president.

The court did not find evidence of personal gain by the trustees, although in several instances they had been associated with organizations that had benefited from the transactions. That there was no evidence of a conspiracy seems significant to the ruling.

The court did not order any trustees removed from the governing body, and no personal liability was attached to their wrongdoing. To prevent similar problems in the future, the court ordered the governing body to adopt a written investment policy, review relevant committees to determine whether hospital assets conformed to the policy, and establish a regular process of disclosure of governing body members' business affiliations. Before the case was decided, the governing body adopted the AHA's guidelines on conflicts of interest. This action occurred long after the fact but was thought to demonstrate the governing body's good faith. The conflict of interest statement suggested by the AHA is shown in Figure 6. It reflects the less stringent corporate director standard.

The decision in Sibley was handed down by a federal trial court and therefore has limited legal significance as a precedent. Nevertheless, it is one of the few cases that considers the standard of care for governing body members (directors) of not-for-profit organizations. Fiduciary duty requires that governing body members exercise reasonable care, skill, and diligence; under a negligence theory, they are liable for acts of commission or omission that violate this standard. *Reasonable care* is the care an ordinary, prudent director would exercise under the same or similar circumstances. The rule enunciated in Sibley is that governing body members (directors) of a not-for-profit corporation who are not true trustees may be liable for ordinary negligence as well as gross negligence or willful misconduct. This standard is usually imposed on the board of directors of a business enterprise.

CEOs and other managers are not fiduciaries in the same sense as directors, but they are held to a similar standard: a duty to exercise reasonable care, skill, and diligence, or the care that an ordinary, prudent manager would exercise in the same or similar circumstances. Many states' laws provide immunity from liability for governing body members of not-for-profit organizations. Often, however, the statutes contain limitations and exclusions from immunity, loopholes, and vague language, thus providing little real protection for directors and officers against liability.[6]

ETHICAL OBLIGATIONS OF TRUSTEES AND DIRECTORS

Legal standards represent a minimum standard of performance. What are the ethical obligations of trustees and directors? The AHA guidelines in

Disclosure of Certain Interests of Governing Board Members

WHEREAS, The proper governance of the nation's health care institutions depends on governing board members who give of their time for the benefit of their health communities; and,

WHEREAS, The giving of this service, because of the varied interests and backgrounds of the governing board members, may result in situations involving a dual interest that might be interpreted as conflict of interest; and,

WHEREAS, This service should not be rendered impossible solely by reason of duality of interest or possible conflict of interest; and,

WHEREAS, This service nevertheless carries with it a requirement of loyalty and fidelity to the institution served, it being the responsibility of the members of the board to govern the institution's affairs honestly and economically, exercising their best care, skill, and judgment for the benefit of the institution; and

WHEREAS, The matter of any duality of interest or possible conflict of interest can best be handled through full disclosure of any such interest, together with noninvolvement in any vote wherein the interest is involved:

NOW, THEREFORE, BE IT RESOLVED: That the following policy of duality and conflict of interest is hereby adopted:

1. Any duality of interest or possible conflict of interest on the part of any governing board member should be disclosed to the other members of the board and made a matter of record, either through an annual procedure or when the interest becomes a matter of board action.

2. Any governing board member having a duality of interest or possible conflict of interest on any matter should not vote or use his personal influence on the matter, and he should not be counted in determining the quorum for the meeting, even where permitted by law. The minutes of the meeting should reflect that a disclosure was made, the abstention from voting, and the quorum situation.

3. The foregoing requirements should not be construed as preventing the governing board member from briefly stating his position in the matter, nor from answering pertinent questions of other board members since his knowledge may be of great assistance.

BE IT FURTHER RESOLVED: That this policy be reviewed annually for the information and guidance of governing board members, and that any new member be advised of the policy upon entering on the duties of his office.

Figure 6.   Conflict of interest statement of the American Hospital Association (AHA). (Reprinted with permission of the American Hospital Association; copyright © 1990.)

Figure 6 assist governing body members to avoid conflicts of interest. They emphasize disclosure—putting other governing body members on notice about potential or actual conflicts. In the Sibley case, it is uncertain that disclosure would have made a difference. The trustees almost certainly knew about their colleagues' outside affiliations and activities. Adopting the AHA guidelines and knowing their content might have alerted them to the ethical problems of self-dealing and mismanagement. A conflict of interest statement probably would have made no difference as to nonmanagement because the trustees did not take seriously their fiduciary duty to invest hospital funds prudently.

Health services managers possess the characteristics of fiduciaries. They are also moral agents, and an important part of their work is assisting the organization, through the governing body, to meet its ethical and legal obligations. Concomitant with this effort, managers have a duty to help the governing body avoid conflicts of interest and problems of nonmanagement. Managers are the conscience of the organization; they recognize potential administrative and biomedical ethical problems and act to avoid them or minimize their effect.

Hermann Hospital

A scandal uncovered in early 1985 involved activities of both administrators and trustees of the Hermann Hospital, an 800-bed facility, and the Hermann Hospital Estate, a trust established in 1914 to provide charity care to the poor of Houston, Texas. An investigation of the two entities showed evidence of theft, kickbacks, insider stock deals, lavish perquisites and expenditures, and costly trips taken by trust and hospital executives and employees at the trust's expense. Among the allegations were that the former executive director of Hermann Hospital paid money to his mistress for work that was never done and that he received kickbacks from overcharges paid by Hermann Hospital to a company of which he was president. The trust sued the former hospital executive director, asking that he repay $100,000 in kickbacks, $500,000 that he allegedly paid his pregnant mistress, and other funds he allegedly laundered. The suit also alleged that he took improper trips that, with related expenses, cost the hospital $250,000. In addition, it alleged that he used Hermann Hospital's name, credit, and money to create an interior decorating firm for his mistress, most or all of whose income came from the hospital.

The Hermann Hospital Estate's former executive director was alleged to have stolen more than $300,000. Allegations against a trust employee stated that a luxury automobile was traded in at less than 20% of its market value for a new automobile paid for by the trust. The undervalued automobile was then purchased by the employee at the grossly understated price. In addition, there was evidence that trustees and employees had entertained lavishly at trust expense. Newspaper accounts stated that the

Hermann Hospital Estate actually spent less than 3% of its funds on financially disadvantaged patients.

As a result of the investigation, two trustees and eight high-ranking trust and hospital executives resigned. Three individuals connected with the estate, including a trustee, were indicted on criminal charges.[7]

Many of the activities at the Hermann Hospital Estate and Hermann Hospital were unethical because they violated the law. The misconduct involved in this case goes well beyond a breach of that minimum standard. The trustees violated their fiduciary duty to protect trust assets by squandering funds that should have been spent treating patients. True trustees and directors alike must avoid anything that could be considered a conflict of interest and/or an improper benefit from their association with an organization. Similarly, hospital managers must be above reproach in all that they do. They act unethically when there is self-dealing or when organization assets are diverted, whether or not these are criminal offenses.

Cedars of Lebanon Hospital

Unlike Sibley Memorial Hospital but like Hermann Hospital, circumstances at the Cedars of Lebanon Hospital involved a hospital CEO who engaged in both unethical and criminal behavior. The latter resulted in a prison term for the CEO. As noted, criminal behavior is in itself unethical. In addition to conflict of interest, the case contains instances of self-dealing, bribery, and failure to obey federal laws:

- The CEO owned a consulting firm in the Caribbean with which the hospital contracted for architectural consulting services that were never performed.

- The CEO falsified governing body minutes to cover the fraudulent contract with his own consulting firm.

- The CEO received more 2,500 shares of stock with a market value of $75,000 in a computer company from which the hospital had purchased a $1.8 million diagnostic computer to be used for multiphasic screening; later underutilization of the equipment caused a loss of more than $2,000 per day.

- The CEO bribed public officials to obtain approval for construction and loans for an unnecessary addition to the hospital.

- The CEO attempted to ease the hospital's desperate cash flow situation by not paying federal withholding on employees' salaries.[8]

Other violations of ethical principles occurred, but these five are illustrative. The CEO's activities forced the hospital into receivership; he was later convicted and sent to prison. Important in the Cedars of Lebanon case is that the governing body paid grossly insufficient attention to the CEO's activities and did not meet their duties as fiduciaries.

CODES OF ETHICS AND CONFLICTS OF INTEREST

As noted, conflict of interest may be only a matter of degree—certain behavior, if limited, is unlikely to cause, or is presumed not to cause, a problem. Exaggerated, the same behavior is likely to have the appearance of a conflict of interest, if not an actual conflict. Gratuities are an example in applying this criterion. Few would say that a conflict of interest arises when a manager is treated to lunch in the cafeteria by a sales representative. A 2-week, all-expenses-paid vacation suggests something very different. Extravagant gratuities, benefits, or kickbacks can be reasonably assumed to encourage or reward certain behavior. Nevertheless, the appearance of a conflict of interest results by accepting *any* gratuity from those with whom business is done—even to the extent of a small gift or inexpensive lunch.

Health care executives are expected to conduct themselves personally and professionally so that all decisions are in the best interests of the organization and those it serves. They are expected to disclose to the appropriate authority direct or indirect personal or financial interests that pose potential or actual conflicts of interests, as well as to inform the appropriate authority of appointments or elections to governing body or committees inside or outside the executive's organization that pose a potential or actual conflict of interest. Gifts or benefits are not to be accepted if offered with the express or implied expectation of influencing management decision making.

These guidelines rely on the judgment of managers. Only they possess the knowledge about personal activities and those of the organization that will permit them to determine when there are potential or actual conflicts, when a solution is required, or when certain facts should be disclosed or brought to the attention of the appropriate authority. As noted, conflicts of interest are often subtle and insidious—avoiding them or minimizing their effect once they occur requires constant vigilance.

The Code of Ethics of the American College of Health Care Administrators (ACHCA) assists managers in preventing and solving conflicts of interest. It states that the health care administrator shall

Disclose to the governing body or other authority as may be appropriate, any actual or potential circumstance concerning him or her that might reasonably be thought to create a conflict of interest or have a substantial adverse impact on the facility or its residents. [Furthermore, he or she shall not] participate in activities that reasonably may be thought to create a conflict of interest or have the potential to have a substantial adverse impact on the facility or its residents.[9]

ACCEPTING GRATUITIES AND BENEFITS

Health services organizations must help staff avoid conflicts of interest by adopting policies to guide their decision making in the acceptance (or nonacceptance) of gratuities and benefits. Failing to receive guidance, staff and managers will act in ways that they believe are consistent with the organization's culture.

Bits and Pieces

John Henry Williams liked his new job in the radiology department of Affiliated Nursing Homes and Rehabilitation Center. He had been appointed acting head when his predecessor, Mary Beth Jacobson, asked for a 6-month maternity leave. John Henry would be responsible for two and one half technicians, an appointments clerk, and $350,000 in equipment. He would have the authority to purchase radiographic supplies, the annual value of which was approximately $110,000. Most supplies were obtained from three vendors, companies from which the Center had bought for years.

As Mary Beth oriented John Henry, she emphasized how much she liked the meetings with sales representatives from the three vendors. Over the years, one had become a close personal friend. She told John Henry that most meetings were held at the nice restaurant near the Center. Some were held in her office and, if so, the reps always brought along "a little something." When John Henry asked what she meant, Mary Beth gave some examples: perfume, a bottle of brandy, and a pen set in a leather case. John Henry remembered thinking that his wife would like the perfume, but he was more interested in the lunches. It would be a chance to get away from the dreary cafeteria as well as his boring sandwich from home. Mary Beth said the lunches were nothing fancy. She estimated the cost to the sales rep to be similar to that of the small gifts—in the $40–$50 range.

John Henry asked Mary Beth whether there was a policy about accepting gifts from vendors. Mary Beth was upset by the question, which implied something might be wrong with what she was doing. She responded curtly that the Center trusted its managers and allowed them discretion in such matters. John Henry then asked if accepting gratuities might suggest to other staff that her decisions were influenced by the pecuniary relationship with the sales reps. Mary Beth's anger flashed: "I know you think that what I'm doing doesn't look right. That's not fair! I work long hours as a manager and get paid very little extra. It takes effort and time to order and maintain proper inventory. If things go wrong, it's my neck in a noose. The lunches and small gifts make me feel better about my efforts. My work has been exemplary. I'd be happy to talk to anyone who thinks otherwise!"

This case illustrates a common problem in many health services organizations. Several facts support Mary Beth's position: Taking clients to lunch and providing small gratuities is common in business relationships. The organization incurs no direct cost because everything is paid by the sales representatives, who use their expense accounts. At least one sales representative has become a personal friend. Taken individually, it seems unlikely that Mary Beth's judgment could be influenced by the modest value of the lunches and gratuities, but a long-term pattern could result in a different interpretation. It must be asked, however, whether other potential vendors are being ignored because of what have become "cozy" relationships with vendors.

Apparently, there is no organizational policy to guide John Henry. Neither the American College of Healthcare Executives (ACHE) code nor the ACHCA codes address the more subtle aspects of conflicts of interest. Although it is impossible to judge the giver's true motivation, vendors try to develop good relationships with buyers, and gifts are one way this is done. External evidence, including what is offered and accepted, must be used to infer that a conflict of interest exists.

Decision makers may gain or potentially gain from conflicts of interest in many ways. Often ignored are situations in which the parties understand that the decision maker will be considered favorably for employment or other benefits in the future. A promise or suggestion of future benefit necessarily creates a duality of interests that can lead to actual conflicts of interest and should be prohibited in professional codes of ethics. Classic nonhealth-sector examples of these circumstances are common. Active-duty military personnel interact with contractors and suppliers; on retirement, they accept employment with the same organizations. Former members of Congress and staff of federal agencies find lucrative employment as lobbyists or employees of organizations they formerly affected. Federal law limits how soon such contacts can occur, but advising those who actually make contact is permitted—a very large loophole. Former health services executives are employed by consulting firms with which their organizations have done business. Such problems in the health services field are more than theoretical, and their likelihood increases as health care becomes more politicized and as large aggregations of health services organizations become more common.

Anyone who takes something of value knowing the giver intends to influence the recipient acts unethically. Bribery is obvious: The recipient knows what is being done and what (or who) is being bought. Typically, however, the relationship of giver and recipient is more subtle. What does the pharmacy director do about the proffered lunch from the drug retailer? Does the CEO stop a dietitian from accepting a basket of holiday fruits, nuts, and sweets from the greengrocer? What about a modest gift from the equipment salesperson who was the successful bidder during the renovation program completed 3 years ago? Or 10 years ago? Such transactions suggest potential conflicts of interest. The gift might be given to receive special consideration in the future, or it might be payment for past decisions.

Such situations become even more complex because it is difficult to distinguish the conflict-fraught activities of managers and staff from normal interactions. People develop relationships and friendships, whether as buyer and seller or as professional colleagues. As friends or professional colleagues, however, one should expect the buyer to be equally generous in making gifts to the seller.

Health services organizations must establish a policy on gratuities and benefits. There are three basic options. One is to prohibit staff from accepting any gratuity or benefit offered in the course of business. Such a policy is simple—there is no need to try to judge the giver's intent. This clear, unequivocal rule can be used by staff to refuse gratuities and benefits that may make them feel uncomfortable, thus adding to its usefulness. Declining gratuities of trivial value may make some staff feel awkward, but this is not a significant negative aspect. Most important, such a policy eliminates the need to judge whether there is an expectation of influencing management decision making. Option one is the position of the Association for Healthcare Resource & Materials Management. Its Personal Ethics states: "Never enter into any transactions that would result in personal benefit or a conflict of interest."[10]

The second option is pragmatic but more complex because judgment and difficult decisions are occasionally required. A criterion of reasonableness is applied to the first option. This allows for various circumstances and recognizes that staff have friends and relationships. What must be assiduously avoided, however, is any hint of wrongdoing or suggestion that there is a conflict of interest present in decision making. As noted, such a balancing is achieved only with difficulty. The test should be what the reasonable person objectively viewing the situation would conclude about the intent of the giver and the effect of the gratuity or benefit on the decision maker.

A third option is a hybrid of the first two and is a compromise for organizations that prefer not to enforce an absolute prohibition but want to minimize conflicts of interest and provide staff with a rule for a reference point. This policy considers all gratuities and benefits as coming to and belonging to the organization. They are made available for its use by sending them to the materials manager, either for redistribution to staff or other corporate uses. If given to the organization or widely shared with staff, the potential for a personal conflict of interest ceases to exist, even though a conflict between the organization and patient care may continue.

Option three is similar to a health services organization that receives gratuities and benefits from businesses. Suppliers of goods and services commonly make cash or in-kind contributions to not-for-profit organizations. Accepting them is not a conflict of interest. The contribution benefits the organization directly and as a whole, just as would a price cut or a discount. This option makes it difficult to accept consumable gratuities or benefits such as meals and paid travel, but even here accommodations can be made. Free travel, for example, can be raffled to staff or used to reward someone for a significant success. The gratuity or benefit does not accrue to one person, even though the reflected glory of such contributions may enhance the reputations of those who manage the organization. In addition to enhancing management's reputation, it raises the question of future favorable treatment for vendors because of gifts made previously.

Only a Matter of Degree

Stimson received four Super Bowl tickets in the mail. Attached was a note from the local sales rep for a major equipment manufacturing company, which read: "Thought you might be able to use these." The nursing facility of which Stimson is CEO recently decided to build an addition for a rehabilitation unit. The sales rep's company manufactures equipment that could be used in the unit. Stimson had called the manufacturer several months earlier to discuss equipment that might be available in order to make the specifications for the bidding process more precise.

Stimson is in a difficult situation. Super Bowl tickets are expensive, difficult to obtain, and generally highly prized. However, their intrinsic value is subjective; some recipients would place little value on them. Absent a personal relationship, such as a long-standing friendship, the proffered tickets seem intended to influence the CEO's decision. Important to discussing this conflict is whether Stimson is the sole owner of the organization. If so, Stimson's interests and the organization's are one—there is no economic conflict of interest. Nevertheless, the owner's financial interests may conflict with the interests of facility residents, a different type of conflict.

APPROVAL OF SELF-DIRECTED EXPENDITURES

More subtle questions of conflict of interest can be self-induced. It seems a safe assumption that health services managers usually identify a personal obligation to put patient interests before their own. How much, then, should be spent to refurbish the CEO's office? What type of automobile should be leased for senior management? Answers to such questions vary by type of organization and ownership.

Patient or Self?

Anderson is the CEO of Community Hospital, a not-for-profit organization. Anderson has assembled an effective administrative staff. Because Anderson's results have been good year after year, the governing body pays little attention to internal operations and focuses on fund-raising and community relations. Anderson has a large discretionary fund available. In the past it has been used for entertainment, gifts, and staff education.

At the urging of several governing body members and managers, Anderson redecorated the administrative suite. Rosewood and leather sofas were ordered, elegant carpet and drapes were installed, a burled oak desk was delivered, and several original oil paintings were purchased through the interior decorator. The project's cost totaled $50,000.

When the cost was criticized, even by the more financially successful members of the medical staff, Anderson reacted defensively. Anderson's primary argument to justify the expenditure was that the CEO of a multimillion-dollar enterprise needed the accoutrements of his office to be effective. Few critics were placated.

Whether such expenditures are appropriate varies by context and setting. A big private hospital with a large endowment, in which the CEO's office is expected to reflect success and sophistication, will view this case differently from a public hospital, in which each nickel is spent reluctantly.

Organizations at either extreme, however, could fund worthwhile administrative and clinical projects with $50,000. No one expects a CEO to sit on a lawn chair or use brick and board bookshelves, but the criterion should be good judgment tempered by reason. Again, it is useful to view such actions as would an informed, objective outsider.

CONFLICT OF INTEREST WITH NO DIRECT PERSONAL GAIN

The case of Miriam Hospital is similar to that of Hermann Hospital.[11] Both cases lie between those of Sibley Memorial Hospital and Cedars of Lebanon Hospital. This case has an element of conflict of interest; other aspects make it unique.

Miriam Hospital

Before 1980, routine blood tests at Miriam Hospital were performed by a 6-channel analyzer. In 1980, the hospital purchased and put into operation a 12-channel analyzer. Because of a computer programming error, patients continued to be charged for both sets of tests, even though only the 12-channel machine was used.

A year later, Blue Cross raised questions about the unusually high laboratory charges at Miriam as compared with other hospitals. The explanation was that doctors at Miriam simply ordered more laboratory tests. In 1982, a professional standards review organization audit clerk uncovered the double billing. The manager of information systems was ordered by his immediate superior to eliminate the programming error. Shortly thereafter, however, he was told by top officials at Miriam to reinstate the programming error.

Later in 1982, a Blue Cross auditor uncovered the same problem and asked for a copy of the program. The manager of data processing was told to erase any evidence in the program that showed that the original error had been reintroduced. Blue Cross received the sanitized program.

A short time later, two data processing personnel were accused of allowing an outside company to use Miriam's computer in contravention of hospital policy. Each was offered the opportunity to resign. Fearing he would be made a scapegoat, one data processor told his story to Blue Cross, who went to the state's attorney general. Six months later, a grand jury brought indictments against the hospital and several senior managers. The charges included obtaining money under false pretenses, conspiracy, and filing false documents. The alleged overbilling totaled almost $2.8 million.

The hospital's and managers' defense was based on their interpretation of the rules under which reimbursement was made. They argued that the rules required hospitals to continue using the same accounting methods for the entire fiscal year, even though there were errors such as those found in this case. An end-of-fiscal-year audit would determine what financial adjustments were needed.

Unlike Cedars of Lebanon Hospital and Hermann Hospital, there is no evidence that managers at Miriam gained personally from their decisions. Miriam Hospital was the only direct beneficiary of the double-billing procedure. This explanation does not excuse the action, ethically or legally, but does put it in a different light. Unlike the Sibley case, these executives did not benefit other organizations to the hospital's detriment. Regardless, to the extent that the double billing improved Miriam's financial situation, the managers enhanced their positions. Thus, they benefited through continued employment, enhanced status and reputation, and, perhaps, proffered financial rewards from the organization. Miriam's financial position was unclear; some sources stated it could not afford to refund the overcharges, even though management stated that doing so posed no problem. Saving a financially troubled organization at personal risk is altruistic and self-sacrificing; however, such efforts also benefit managers. Nevertheless, selfless or self-sacrificing activities cannot take precedence over moral values and ethical codes. The end cannot be used to justify the means. These managers ignored the virtues of honesty, integrity, and trustworthiness.

SYSTEMS CONFLICTS

Health services managers typically serve on governing bodies of health-related organizations. Examples of such organizations include health planning agencies, charities, insurance companies, Blue Cross plans, managed care organizations, and hospital associations. Increasingly, the duality of interests caused by such service has great potential for conflicts of interest. Conflicts of interest can be prevented by disclosing to the governing body (and other parties) the potential for them because of service on governing bodies or committees outside the manager's organization. Such information puts the organization on notice and allows it to judge the extent of the potential conflict of interest. If an actual conflict occurs, the manager must withdraw. However, changes in the health services environment may have rendered these precautions inadequate.

The dilemma begins with the manager's civic obligation and professional responsibility based on a general duty of beneficence to assist the community in meeting its health needs. These efforts are reinforced by codes of ethics and the stimulus of governing bodies. Health services managers should be encouraged to apply their professional expertise to improving community health services, but the potential for conflicts of interest is apparent and can be present even if other health services providers are not discussed. If a health services manager is a governing body member of an insurer, for example, there are potential conflicts of interest as to rates, programs, and covered services. Furthermore, some insurers are becoming competitors of traditional health services organizations by developing service delivery capability. Even if managers abstain from debating or voting on matters directly affecting their organizations, it is impossible to avoid being privy to corporate thinking and strategies for other activities that in general and specific ways affect the managers' health services organizations. Once known, this knowledge cannot be ignored.

Increased competitiveness in the field of health services makes all information about one's competitors important in order to meet threats to market share or to blunt unfriendly initiatives. In fact, the virtues of loyalty and conscientiousness require a manager to preserve or expand the organization's market share. If managers minimize the problem of conflict through disclosure and withdrawal when necessary, they diminish their effectiveness as a governing body member of the organization and potentially violate their fiduciary duty. Furthermore, they risk charges of impropriety simply by participating in other organizations.

How is this problem solved? How does a health services organization obtain important expertise without exposing itself and manager-directors to charges of impropriety and conflicts of interest? One option is to permit service only by individuals from noncompeting organizations. This solution has the disadvantage of potentially excluding individuals with operational experience in that geographic area. However, over time, out-of-area directors will develop expertise. This solution is complicated by the growing number of integrated delivery systems, which replace the traditional, locally based organization with one that is regional or national.

A second option is that health services organizations use full-time governing body members—persons who are governing body members of noncompeting organizations and who are not employed elsewhere. Full-time directors are common in business enterprise but rare in health services, especially in the not-for-profit sector. These individuals are usually paid, an expenditure that should pose no problem for health services organizations, especially the larger ones. Organizations that are unable to bear the cost should consider option three.

The third option uses professionally prepared and experienced individuals not actively managing health services organizations. Examples include retired health services managers and health services administration educators. Physicians and well-informed members of the public could also serve effectively. This option possesses most of the advantages of option two. Here, some payment is desirable because it will produce higher levels of commitment and higher-quality involvement.

Managers working to improve community health services through cooperative efforts face an increasingly competitive environment. This challenge makes some types of cooperation difficult or impossible. Other types, such as sharing services and participating in joint ventures, are stimulated. Survival is a primary corporate goal for health services organizations, and new ethical guidelines are needed to address these problems.

CONCLUSION

Avoiding conflicts of interest requires constant vigilance. Managers of government-owned facilities risk fines and criminal charges if they are involved in conflicts of interest. The likelihood of legal penalties is less in the private sector. This does not obviate the ethical problem, however. Disclosure to eliminate or minimize the problem is stressed by the ACHCA and AHA. Disclosure presumes that one recognizes duality of interests that could lead to potential conflicts of interests. Failure to recognize conflicts means that managers may be well into a conflict situation before they realize it. Conflicts of interest can be subtle, and continual questioning and self-analysis are needed to identify them. Their potential and actual effect will increase as competition intensifies.

In addition to disclosure, conflicts of interest may be avoided or eliminated in other ways, including divesting a potentially conflicting outside interest, seeking guidance from the governing body, and not participating in or attempting to influence matters in which conflicts may exist. Such steps eliminate the conflict or put the governing body on notice. Both are important, but managers must remember their moral agency and must prevent conflicts of interest or work to minimize their negative effects once they are present.

Systems conflicts will cause unique problems as well as opportunities in competitive environments. To avoid conflicts of interest, managers must be alert and may need to withdraw from all involvement in governing and advising competing or potentially competing health services organizations.

Nontraditional means will be required to maximize the assistance that individuals experienced in health services can offer while minimizing the potential for systems conflicts.

NOTES

1. Mahzarin R. Banaji, Max H. Bazermand, & Dolly Chugh. (2003, December). How (un)ethical are you? *Harvard Business Review 81*(7), p. 61.

2. Harlan Cleveland. (1972). *The future executive* (p. 104). New York: Harper & Row.

3. Arthur E. Southwick. (1988). *The law of hospital and health care administration* (2nd ed., pp. 123–126). Chicago: Health Administration Press.

4. Stern et al. v. Lucy Webb Hayes National Training School of Deaconesses and Missionaries et al., 381 E Supp. 1003 (1974).

5. *Ibid.*, p. 1013.

6. James E. Orlikoff. (1990, January). What every trustee should know about D & O liability. *Trustee, 43*, pp. 8–9.

7. *The Houston Post*, articles dated March 5, 9, 10, 12, 13, 16, and 19, 1985, and *The Washington Post*, article dated March 21, 1985.

8. Summarized from a case study written by the late Milton C. Devolites, Professor Emeritus, Department of Health Services Administration, The George Washington University, Washington, D.C. The case was prepared from various issues of *The Miami Herald* and *The Miami News* published in 1974.

9. American College of Health Care Administrators. (2003). *Advocacy: Code.* Alexandria, VA: Author.

10. Association for Healthcare Resources & Materials Management. (2003, August 27). *Code of ethics and professional conduct.* Chicago: Author.

11. *Providence Journal-Bulletin*, articles dated September 22, 1983; October 2, 5, and 6, 1983; and May 16, 1984.

CHAPTER 7

ETHICAL ISSUES REGARDING ORGANIZATION AND STAFF

A wide variety of administrative ethical issues arise as health services managers do their jobs. Issues linked to employee performance appraisal, for example, are a function of formal relationships. Other issues, such as working with independent practitioners of the medical staff, often result from less organizational formal relationships. Managers have an ethical and legal fiduciary relationship with the organization as represented by the governing body. In an ethical sense, managers are fiduciaries for all staff in the organization, and this relationship raises special obligations. Self-dealing was examined briefly in Chapter 6 but is addressed further in this chapter.

In the course of their duties, health services managers are privy to copious confidential and insider information. Much is sensitive; almost all is proprietary. Administrative information is distinguished from that collected, used, and maintained for patient care. Using and safeguarding both types of confidential information is a major ethical concern in health services organizations, but it receives little attention.

ORGANIZATIONAL CONTEXT OF RELATIONSHIPS

Managers are employed to carry out the organization's mission in the context of its philosophy. The governing body selects and evaluates the chief executive officer (CEO). In turn, the CEO selects and evaluates subordinate managers, perhaps down to the middle management level. Regardless of organizational level, managers are moral agents who are ethically accountable for the effects of nonfeasance, misfeasance, and malfeasance on patients, staff, and organization. Their decisions are not excused because they are employees or because they were following orders. The law may hold individuals who are not prime actors or decision makers to a different standard, but managers remain morally accountable.

As an employee, the manager has a duty of loyalty to the organization and its staff. In terms of the organization, this duty means that the manager supports the employer's goals and activities and keeps confidential what is learned. Disagreements about policy and its implementation are neither broadcast nor otherwise shared with individuals who have no "need to know." The duty of loyalty has special importance in light of a common malady, backbiting the employer. Backbiting is not the grumbling or complaining usually considered normal, perhaps even healthy behavior. Although employees may have a legitimate reason to complain about their treatment (even the best employer does not get it right every time), rabid, negative comments are problematic. Employees who persistently speak ill of their employer act in an unacceptable fashion and should find new employment, voluntarily or involuntarily.

Managers must achieve the difficult balance between loyalty to the organization and fidelity to their personal ethic and professional integrity. Where does the manager draw the line? How far should a manager go in following the crowd or in standing alone? A clear and well-considered personal ethic is needed to answer questions such as these. Professional codes of ethics play a role but provide only general guidance and are unlikely to be useful in helping a manager decide what to do in specific cases. At the extreme, the limits of loyalty are part of whistleblowing, which is examined in Chapter 8.

As posited previously, the manager has an independent duty and responsibility to the patient; at minimum, this means that managers protect patients from unnecessary risk and further their interests. What follows from that duty is the need for integrity and the courage to speak out and act to make that responsibility a reality. What happens, however, when the duty to protect the interests of patients conflicts with the duty of loyalty in achieving part of the organization's mission?

She Only Had to Ask

Richard Weidner experienced angina on mild exercise. His internist referred him to a cardiologist at University Hospital for a cardiac catheterization. After the cardiologist examined Weidner, she explained the procedure and obtained his consent. As the cardiologist turned to leave, Weidner asked her, "You'll be taking care of me, won't you, doc?" The doctor replied, "I'll see you in the cardiac cath room." Weidner was reassured and especially pleased that he had had such a long, friendly visit with his cardiologist.

That afternoon, Weidner was lying on the table waiting for the catheteriza-tion to begin. He had a clear view of the television monitor, and as the procedure began he saw the catheter moving from his groin toward his heart. At one point he asked a question and was startled when his cardiologist appeared near his head and described what was happening. When Weidner asked who was threading the catheter, she told him it was a resident in cardiology.

Later, Weidner was in the recovery area waiting to be discharged. He was quite agitated that a resident had performed the procedure, especially because he thought he had an understanding with his cardiologist. He described what had happened to the nurse and demanded an explanation. The nurse tried to calm him. "You know," she said, "this is a teaching hospital—we train residents so they can perform these procedures to help other people." Weidner was not placated. He said, "Had I been asked, I probably would have agreed to have the resident participate. But they didn't ask me, and I'm damned angry about it. Please tell a manager to see me immediately. I want some answers!"

Weidner was not harmed physically, but he was emotionally distraught. He believed that he was misled and that a promise was broken. Weidner was concerned about who would perform the procedure and sought reassurance from the cardiologist, whom he trusted. Her answer was evasive. She purposefully or negligently misled him and thus breached her obligation to tell the truth. In sum, Weidner was deceived and treated disrespectfully. What happened does not seem to be the result of maliciousness; all involved would likely be distressed to learn of Weidner's anger about his treatment. Weidner's expectations and understanding were unmet, however.

What should the manager of cardiology do when Weidner relates his story? Except to reassure and placate, little can be done for Weidner. Perhaps a promise to Weidner that it will not happen again will be helpful. More important is what should be done to prevent similar problems. The manager of cardiology should be the force for staff education and necessary process changes. The personal ethic of this manager's peers and the organi-zational philosophy should demand this level of attention to the principle of respect for persons and the virtues of trustworthiness and integrity.

To become fully qualified, physicians in residencies need specialized training, which can only be gained by treating patients. Far less acceptable, of course, is the assumption that all patients are willing to participate in medical education. Being used as a means to an end is a crude summary of utilitarianism and one incompatible with the principle of respect for persons; specifically, the elements of autonomy and truth telling were violated in this case.

The forms used to admit patients to teaching hospitals disclose their involvement in medical education. Few patients, however, read or understand the implications of that disclosure. Judged by legal standards of informed consent, the act of signing such a form has questionable validity. More important than the law, however, is the organization's ethical obligation to inform patients of what being a teaching institution means in terms of their care. Even if the form has been read and understood, minimum ethical conduct demands that patients be informed when teaching activities are to occur and that permission is again obtained. Medical education and consent are covered more fully in Chapter 9.

ORGANIZATIONAL INFORMATION

In addition to some types of clinical information, the manager is privy to confidential information about the organization, much of it proprietary. As with patient information, a basic criterion for other confidential information is need to know. Examples of confidential organizational information include decisions about capital equipment, medical staff recruitment and development, business and marketing strategies, and financial and human resources programs. Equally important, but less commonly included, are general information concerning the staff and organization and specific information such as the strengths, weaknesses, and peculiarities of individual managers or governing body members.

In a competitive environment, "loose lips" will result in significant adverse consequences. It is unethical to deliberately or negligently make confidential information available to unauthorized organizations or individuals. This is true whether the manager's organization is put at risk or actually experiences a loss or the manager disclosing the proprietary information gains personally.

The 2003 American College of Healthcare Executives (ACHE) code directs the health care executive to "respect professional confidences." This wording provides little guidance about confidential information in the organization. Managers, governing body members, and staff must ensure that confidential information is safeguarded. Physicians who are independent contractors—a typical arrangement in hospitals—have limited loyalty to the organization; this makes sharing proprietary information with them problematic. In a competitive environment, health services organizations increasingly provide confidential information to physicians only on a need-to-know basis.

Self-Dealing

Narrowly defined, self-dealing occurs only when a person with access to confidential information uses it for advantages such as monetary gain, unfair personal advantage, or self-aggrandizement. Misuse of confidential information that does not involve self-dealing is simply a breach of confidentiality. Examples of misusing insider information include the following: a manager, knowing that the organization will establish a surgi-center in a specific location, purchases the property through a straw man (an agent), who then resells it to the organization at a profit that the two share; a manager discloses information about organizational decision making that gives acquaintances an advantage in doing business with it (misuse of confidential information); and a manager seeking revenge for perceived insult discloses market strategies to competitors, with no resulting personal gain. Strictly speaking, only the first scenario illustrates self-dealing. If the manager in this example is decision maker for both the sale and the purchase, there is also a conflict of interest.

What's a Manager to Do?

S.L. Rine joined the management staff of a large health services provider after working at a similar organization for several years. Rine is a member of ACHE and wants to build the best set of credentials in the shortest time. His goal is to become a CEO.

Rine is responsible for several support departments as well as the administrative aspects of some clinical areas. Shortly after beginning employment, Rine realized that the organization is very political. Much of what happens at the senior level is the result of personal relationships and obligations.

Maintenance is one of Rine's departments; it is responsible for all of the grounds. Rine learned that grounds crews were being sent to the homes of senior members of the governing body to maintain their lawns, shrubs, and trees. Rine asked the maintenance director to explain and was told that the practice had a long history and should be left alone. When Rine asked the director for a cost estimate of the grounds work being done at the private homes, the director refused, saying that he feared the wrath of the governing body members who were benefiting. Rine pondered what to do.

Soon after talking to the maintenance director, Rine had lunch with the laboratory director. Without discussing specifics, Rine described the problem in maintenance. The laboratory director exclaimed, "That's nothing!" and went on to describe how two governing body members were selling reagents and supplies to the laboratory at higher-than-market prices. Rine asked the laboratory director why she had not done anything about the situation. She replied that her predecessor had tried to stop the practice and was fired. Again, Rine pondered what to do.

This case has two dimensions, one involving governing body members, the other involving managers. Governing body members whose yards are maintained by the organization or who sell to the laboratory at inflated prices are explicitly or implicitly using their authority for personal benefit. Selling overpriced reagents and supplies to the laboratory seems more unethical than receiving free grounds maintenance; in principle, however, the two acts are indistinguishable. Both improperly divert (steal) organizational resources. Most destructive for the organization's moral health is that the governing body members are setting bad examples, which at best make the staff cynical and at worst encourage them to also use their authority improperly.

The second dimension is the role of managers. Knowing about improper (i.e., unethical or illegal) behavior but not acting (nonfeasance) is no better than committing an unethical act (malfeasance). Codes of administrative ethics are of limited help. Rine and the laboratory manager agree that the behavior is unacceptable. Their problem is to identify their ethical obligations and act on them.

By confronting those involved, Rine will achieve little more than embarrassing them, and Rine may be fired. Managers can and should take any available steps, however. One is to question generic unethical activities at every opportunity and to encourage colleagues to speak out. If several managers agree that certain behavior is unethical, they draw strength from one another. They can implement or can try to implement a policy of competitive bidding for all purchases, including the laboratory. They can develop and propose an organizationwide policy on self-dealing and abuse of authority. In short, they must take whatever steps they can to end unethical practices. As moral agents, they cannot close their eyes to such problems. Nonfeasance is not an option.

Misuse of Insider Information

Persons in an organization with access to information not available to the public are known as insiders. Ethical problems arise when managers use such information in a manner that is inconsistent with their fiduciary duty, the obligation to be trustworthy. Benefiting oneself or one's associates are examples. Some misuse of confidential information has a salutary effect and must be distinguished. An example is whistleblowing that occurs when internal efforts at reform fail and the manager's moral agency demands external disclosure of information about practices that may affect the safety of patients or the public. The protection of such groups takes precedence over a duty of loyalty (fidelity) to the organization, even if the manager becomes subject to civil or criminal sanctions.

A common misuse of confidential (nonpublic) information occurs when employees (insiders) use it to make advantageous stock market transactions. Historically, health services organizations were largely unaffected because relatively few were publicly traded for-profit stock corporations. This status has changed dramatically since the late 1960s. Regulation by the Securities and Exchange Commission or state counterparts does not diminish the seriousness of the unethical conduct inherent in misusing insider information. Again, the law is a minimum that does not necessarily set an appropriate level of ethical behavior.

Just Part Owner

Jane Abernathy is the CEO of a large urban not-for-profit nursing facility. She is a voting member of all governing body committees. Following a retreat, the governing body's planning committee recommended that rehabilitation become a significant new initiative. For the past several months, the capital expenditures committee has considered the purchase of equipment to increase the nursing facility's capacity in rehabilitation. The part-time physician-director of rehabilitation wants to become a full-time employee.

Following an uncle's death 2 years ago, Abernathy inherited 1,000 shares of INCO, Inc., stock. She submits an annual statement of her investments and holdings as part of the governing body's conflict of interest disclosure requirement. The next report is due in 8 months. INCO's last annual report stated that 10 million shares of common stock are publicly held. INCO manufactures rehabilitation equipment similar to that which Abernathy's facility may buy.

The capital expenditures committee's draft report includes purchase of INCO equipment. Abernathy dislikes making private information available to the governing body and is distressed about this apparent need for special disclosure.

In theory, Abernathy faces a duality of interests that could lead to a conflict of interest. Also, there is a potential to misuse confidential information to engage in self-dealing if Abernathy recommends purchasing equipment from a manufacturer in which she owns stock. Abernathy's ownership interest is remote, however—a mere .01% of the company's stock. Thus, the personal gain is so small that it is unlikely Abernathy's decision could be influenced by her stock ownership or, if it were, that she would have any measurable benefit. Abernathy's objectivity becomes more suspect as her ownership interest increases. Nevertheless, Abernathy should disclose her holdings in INCO, even though she finds doing so distasteful.

RELATIONSHIPS WITH THE GOVERNING BODY

The CEO is the governing body's agent in achieving the organization's mission. In turn, the CEO selects, hires, evaluates, and retains subordinate managers. The CEO and other managers and staff are moral agents, not just the organization's morally neutral arms and legs.

As previously noted, some sectarian health services organizations require that mid- and senior-level managers be adherents to the religion of the sponsoring organization. This requirement is too restrictive; co-religionists often hold different views about various doctrines or the rigor of their application. An effective corporate culture is built on managers (and other staff) who understand and accept the organization's philosophy. Nonsectarian philosophies and aspects of secular humanism often have values like those of organized religion. Culling for values occurs in recruiting and selecting staff, and it is here that ethical compatibility should be determined. Applicants, too, should assess their fit with the organization's culture during the interview.[1] Focusing on congruence of values widens the field from which to recruit competent managers; such diversity inevitably benefits the organization.

The governing body and the CEO and senior management (shown in Figure 7 as "Administration") must define the scope of their respective functions. Figure 7 also suggests the need to distinguish senior and middle management. Governance, administration, and management must understand their respective activities or they will interfere in one another's spheres, with resulting inefficiency and frustration of organizational goals. The diagram is not intended to depict relationships and spheres as isolated. It must include permeability of ideas and communications, but separateness as well as jointness must be clear.

Early leaders in hospital administration asserted that the risk of conflicts of interest that existed when the CEO or members of the medical

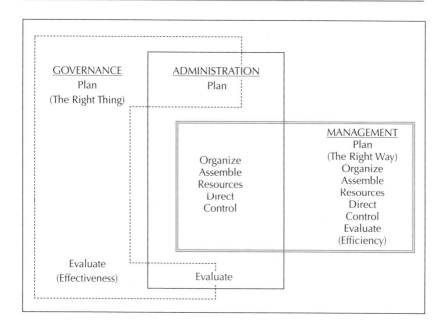

Figure 7.   A model of hospital governance, administration, and management. (Reprinted from *Trustee*, *34*, p. 6, by permission, June 1981. Copyright © 1981, American Hospital Publishing, Inc.)

staff were on the governing body far outweighed any benefit to be derived.[2] The environment has changed dramatically, however. The current thinking is that the disclosure of duality of interests or potential conflicts of interest prevents or minimizes their actual occurrence. In 1989, 42% of hospital CEOs were full voting members of the governing body, an increase from 38% in 1985.[3] This study found that an average of two physicians with medical privileges at a hospital were members of its governing body.[4] The trend toward greater participation of CEOs and medical staff members on the governing body has continued, and as of 2004, it is believed essential that these types of professionals fully participate in the governing body.

Anecdotal evidence suggests a trend toward a greater proportion of internal governing body members (senior managers employed by the organization) relative to external members. Internal members are desirable because of their general and organization-specific expertise. This duality of interests necessarily increases the potential for conflicts of interest, however.

Regardless of governing body membership, the CEO and senior managers link governance to the operating components of the organization.

As the governing body's agents, they provide it with the information and recommendations upon which macrodecisions are made. This enables senior managers to filter or sanitize data and make themselves look good or to mislead, as occurred in the Cedars of Lebanon case (see Chapter 6). A key issue is how much and what types of information the governing body should receive. The governing body makes this determination. The CEO and senior managers should make recommendations, but governing body members must be sufficiently informed to know which data it needs and how to interpret them. Level of involvement and expertise are special problems in organizations that rely on voluntary governing body members.

It is natural that managers want their performance to be viewed in a good light. Pressures in the external environment may tempt managers to engage in "creative reporting" about their performance. However, managers are obliged to be truthful in governing body interactions, an ethical duty arising from virtues such as courage, trustworthiness, veracity, and candor. Deception is antithetical to these virtues. This does not mean staff must emphasize unfavorable information; a balanced picture is prudent and desirable. It does mean that the governing body must be informed of problems honestly and in a timely manner. Managers must be alert to understated or misrepresented problems from their subordinates as well. Truthfulness is linked to whistleblowing, which is discussed in Chapter 8. Standardized and routinized reporting minimizes the potential to manipulate the system or the data.

I Wonder If They Even Care?

Stu White had just returned to his office from a monthly governing body meeting. His assistant, Barbara Jones, noticed that he was agitated and asked, "How was It?" White responded by describing the governing body's chronic problem, something Jones had heard before. He said, "I think I could tell them that the moon is made of green cheese and they would believe it! They don't seem to know, or care, what happens in this nursing home!" White described how he did all of the thinking for the governing body. He also described how there was no reporting system until he had established one. He emphasized that the organization had been lucky to have honest managers because, as he put it, "anybody else could have been hauling it [money] out of here by the carload."

The information flow problem White faces results from governing body members' lack of awareness or their unwillingness to be fully involved and accountable for the organization, duties that are unquestionably theirs. White is in a powerful position. He works with a governing body that takes little interest in understanding the organization's affairs, and he determines what information it receives. This problem is not uncommon, even if not as extreme as described here. CEOs and other senior managers possess knowledge superior to the governing body's in at least two respects. They are expert about health services generally and they intimately understand the organization's activities and functioning. Managers' fiduciary relationship requires them to be certain that they provide information the governing body needs. They act ethically when they present and interpret information that accurately portrays the organization. White must educate the governing body as to its responsibilities. Next, he must help them identify the data and reports they need to meet those responsibilities. Failing to change the governing body's culture sets a scenario with significant potential to harm the organization. Someone less scrupulous than White would be in a position to delay or withhold negative information, thus preventing timely action and increasing the probability of damage.[5]

RELATIONSHIPS WITH THE MEDICAL STAFF

Relations between physicians and the organization and its managers raise several ethical issues that are present whether the organization is designed as a matrix or is organized along the lines of the traditional functional hierarchy. Schulz and Johnson[6] suggested that the CEO's role has evolved from business manager to coordinator to corporate chief to management team leader, the predominant role at this writing. As a management team leader, the CEO is a partner with physicians in their joint efforts to provide the best possible care. This evolution causes the green-eyeshade mentality of health services managers to become no more than an historical curiosity. In collegial relationships, peers identify and solve problems of mutual concern. Regardless of the role and degree of collegiality the CEO has duties and responsibilities that inevitably cause disagreements with physicians.

Managers are ethically (and legally) expected to be aware of the quality of clinical practice and to intervene as necessary. This expectation reflects their important ethical responsibilities to protect the interests of patients. This managerial role has positive and negative aspects. Although they are not competent to judge the quality of clinical practice, managers act through experts who are. This situation is similar to that of a manager responsible for pharmacy or dietetics. Here, too, the manager relies on technical expertise to assess performance and make decisions. Some physicians react negatively to the slightest hint of such involvement, which they see as interference in clinical decision making. In fact, managerial involvement also serves the physician's best interests because it helps to ensure high-quality medicine is practiced. Anecdotal evidence suggests that the more competent physicians are less likely to object to a review of their work. It must be stressed that the manager is not judging quality of care directly but only in cooperation with those clinically competent to do so. Conflicts of duties, perhaps even conflicts of interest, arise because managers must maintain harmonious relationships with physicians while ensuring patients' interests. As moral agents, physicians are expected to meet the principles of respect for persons, beneficence, and nonmaleficence, as well as the virtues of courage, compassion, and caring. Lapses do occur, however.

The manager must be attentive to the needs and activities of physicians because they are essential to patient care. Their clinical service to and relationships with patients are the reason the organization exists. Conflicts with the medical staff result from enforcing medical staff bylaws, resource allocation decisions, and relationships between physicians and staff. Other important responsibilities of senior management are to help the medical staff keep its bylaws and rules and regulations current and to assist in enforcing their administrative provisions. A typical example of the latter responsibility occurs when a hospital CEO or medical director applies the medical staff bylaws and its rules and regulations to suspend a physician's admitting privileges. This action occurs most often because of tardy completion of medical records. Absent dire circumstances in which summarily suspending a physician's privileges is warranted, disciplinary actions use established procedures and are not taken single-handedly. Because of the independent duty owed to patients, even exclusively clinical problems cannot be ignored by managers. Clinical and nonclinical managers must act as the need arises. Sometimes mistakes occur, as in the following case.

Oops!

Dr. M is a graduate of a foreign medical school who has been a successful cardiologist on the staff of a large Midwestern hospital for more than 20 years. Occasionally, there have been rumors of Dr. M's alcohol abuse and disruptive behavior. Until a month ago, however, the only formal report nursing administration had received was from a registered nurse, who stated that Dr. M had been verbally abusive and had embarrassed her in front of a patient and his family. Recently, nursing administration received two incident reports: one oral, the other written. Both stated that Dr. M smelled like alcohol and seemed mentally and physically impaired. The information was forwarded to the medical director, Dr. G, a hospital employee and a member of administration.

Dr. G called an emergency meeting of the medical staff executive committee, which the chief operating officer (COO) could not attend because of a professional meeting out of town. After discussing the information but without a formal investigation, the committee agreed to immediate termination of Dr. M's medical staff privileges. A registered letter was sent to Dr. M describing the action and the reasons for it. Another cardiologist was asked to treat Dr. M's hospitalized patients. Upon her return a week later, the COO was aghast to see the letter terminating Dr. M. She realized immediately that Dr. M's privileges should have been suspended, not terminated, pending an investigation.

Dr. M was enraged and retained legal counsel. The hospital withdrew the termination letter 2 weeks after it was sent and reinstated Dr. M's staff privileges pending a full investigation. Dr. M was not placated, however, and filed suit against the members of the executive committee and the hospital, alleging antitrust violations, defamation, and tortious interference with his business relationships.

Dr. G erred in terminating Dr. M's privileges; suspension pending an investigation was the appropriate disciplinary action. Dr. G acted primarily to protect patients; secondarily, he wanted to protect staff. Both actions are ethically correct. However, he mistakenly chose too punitive a disciplinary action. This error was costly for the hospital in terms of public controversy and embarrassment, legal bills, medical staff disruption, and probable lingering ill will.

The hospital erred by inadequately preparing Dr. G for his duties; furthermore, the medical staff bylaws should require an expedited review process for such actions when patient harm is not imminent. The future holds a greater risk for this hospital, however. Managers and members of the medical staff will be reluctant to act in such cases, perhaps even when the facts are more egregious. Had no action been taken and a patient been harmed because of Dr. M's impairment from alcohol, the public outcry would have been greater, however. The lesson for the hospital is that all those in managerial positions must be prepared for the demands of their jobs.

Dr. M's rights to due process were violated. His anger was justified, but it is not clear that he suffered any significant professional or economic injuries. The termination was rescinded soon after imposition. Even if the executive committee had taken the correct disciplinary action, he would have been suspended from admitting patients pending an investigation. Regardless, Dr. M was not treated fairly. He gained sympathy from physician colleagues and other staff members. This will make future disciplinary actions against him all the more difficult, should they be needed.

RELATIONS WITH NONPHYSICIAN STAFF

Like staff in nonhealth organizations, health services professionals harbor various goals, objectives, and interests. Their work in the organization is a primary focus of their lives, but the congruence between personal goals and objectives and those of the organization is likely to be less than total. Chapter 3 noted that employees must understand that they and the organization possess the same core principles of working in the patient's best interests. This attitude must be reflected in action, not just in written organizational philosophy and policies. If employees and physicians perceive that the organization places greater value on performance other than that which reflects ethical interaction with patients (e.g., increasing hospital revenues), the principles of respect for persons, beneficence, and nonmaleficence cannot be satisfied. Because the organization can act only through its staff, this lapse is serious. If staff members fear that intervening on the patient's behalf jeopardizes their relationship with their colleagues and the organization, they will be discouraged from acting as they should.

The "Uncooperative" RN

Sally Hansen, a registered nurse with 10 years' experience, works nights. At the start of her shift she noted that a urinary catheter had been ordered for a postsurgical male patient with acute urinary retention. Following established procedure, she paged the resident on duty. A first-year resident appeared and told her that he would insert the catheter. Hansen accompanied him to the patient's bedside and watched him remove the catheter from its package. He looked at the package, apparently for instructions, but found none. The resident began to insert the catheter into the patient's penis, but faltered. It was clear that he did not know what he was doing and that the patient was in great pain.

The resident turned and asked for assistance, but Hansen refused, saying that inserting a catheter was the job of a properly trained resident. "Really, you shouldn't attempt something you don't know how to do," she said. She also reminded the resident of hospital policy that prohibits a female nurse from performing certain intimate procedures on male patients. The resident yelled at Hansen and stormed off. Hansen paged the chief resident, who catheterized the patient, but offered no explanation when she described the incident with the inexperienced resident.

The next day, Hansen was awakened at home by a call from the vice president for nursing. She told Hansen that the inexperienced resident had filed a formal statement accusing her of insubordination. The resident was adamant about pressing the issue with nursing administration and the chief of his service. The vice president for nursing said she could not be sure as to the outcome.

What was Hansen's proper role in this matter? Where did her duties lie? Clearly, her duties lay with the patient and she acted properly. Even had she known how to insert the catheter, she was constrained by hospital policy from doing so. Stopping the resident protected the patient from pain and potential injury. A reprimand from nursing administration will greatly diminish Hansen's willingness to intervene to protect a patient in the future. The hospital must encourage appropriate action by all staff as it seeks to deliver high-quality care and protect the patient. Teaching is not an issue in this case; the resident was not competent to undertake the procedure—a failure of instruction, not of nursing—a failure that should be addressed with the hospital's director of medical education.

Other issues are present. One is the traditional subservient role of nurses, partly due to sexism. Poor relations between doctors and nurses do not result only from sexism, however. Anecdotal evidence suggests that the problem exists even where sexism is not a factor (e.g., male doctors–male nurses, female doctors–female nurses). A second issue is that a resident attempted a procedure beyond his training. He should have asked for help from the senior resident. Here, too, bravado, ego, and the culture of medical education may have caused an unwillingness to seek help. The third issue is that the limits of residents' clinical activities are unclear. In this regard, the procedures and safeguards in the medical education program may need review. The American Nurses Association[7] Code for Nurses requires Hansen's action: "[the nurse acts] to safeguard the client and the public when health care and safety are affected by incompetent, unethical, or illegal practice by any person." Implicit in this statement is accountability for one's actions as a nurse—a professional ethic—not merely accountability through the organizational hierarchy.

The organization must support its staff with an unequivocal commitment that encourages them to intervene when a patient is at risk. This policy should be communicated and enforced. Action in such situations may cause some individuals to accuse caregivers of spying on one another. This charge is unfounded. Spying is a negative process and has no place in health services. The focus here is on an organizationwide effort—an ethic—to protect and serve the patient. If caregivers are able to minimize their ego involvement in the care process and keep their eyes on these goals, this problem will lessen or disappear.

Ignoring problems will not solve them. This maxim is especially true if patients are at risk. As the Watergate (1970s) and Clinton-Lewinsky (1990s) political scandals showed, such problems can be ignored or covered up for a time but will come to light eventually. The public reacts to such revelations by assuming that others in the organization knew, yet did nothing. The public wonders how such situations could occur or be allowed to continue. In addition to the moral guidelines of respect for persons and the virtue to be honest in all interactions, the likelihood of discovery is a utilitarian reason for recognizing and solving such problems early.

Deadly communicable diseases and other high-risk situations raise special issues in the relationship between organization and staff. Both are ethically bound to protect patients and further their interests, but it is ethically unjustifiable for an organization, through its managers, to put clinical staff at risk by failing to properly train or equip them, for example. All potentially dangerous situations should cause managers to consider the need to protect staff from unnecessary risk; failing that, the organization cannot meet its ethical obligations to them. In turn, staff will be unable to meet their ethical obligations to patients. The paradigmatic example of human immunodeficiency virus/acquired immunodeficiency syndrome (HIV/AIDS) is discussed next and receives further attention in Chapter 8.

HUMAN IMMUNODEFICIENCY VIRUS/ACQUIRED IMMUNODEFICIENCY SYNDROME

HIV, which leads to AIDS, has proved an elusive foe. A great deal has been learned about HIV since it was identified in the early 1980s. Its spread continues but more slowly since the late 1980s. Both the pessimistic prediction of a major outbreak in the general population and the optimistic prediction that it will be eliminated have proved wrong. There have been scientific breakthroughs in understanding HIV and treating AIDS, but there is neither a vaccine to prevent infection nor a cure once infected. A second strain of HIV was isolated in the late 1980s, and a new strain entered the United States from Africa in summer 1996; it is probable there will be others. Work on a vaccine is tempered by knowledge that HIV's rapid mutation makes developing a vaccine with long-term effectiveness difficult, if not impossible. Even if a successful vaccine were developed, several years of testing and clinical trials would be required before it could become generally available. Meanwhile, the attention to prevention and education is unprecedented in modern public health. Despite these efforts, however, the incidence of HIV among homosexual males shows evidence of resurging.[8]

In late 2003, the World Health Organization estimated the worldwide prevalence (number of current cases) of HIV at 34–46 million, including 4.2–5.8 million new cases. The prevalence in North America was 790,000– 1.2 million, including 36,000–54,000 new cases. Africa remains the most severely afflicted region of the world, with two thirds of all infections and more than two thirds of all related deaths.[9] HIV and its progression to AIDS is a pandemic that threatens to destroy the economic and social fabric of whole regions of the developing world.

The prevalence of HIV in the United States in late 2003 was 750,000 to 1 million, including 11,686 new cases diagnosed in 2002.[10] People with AIDS are living longer as a result of more effective medical management using combinations of drugs and healthier lifestyles, including better nutrition and preventive measures that reduce risk of reinfection. The result may be that AIDS will become a chronic rather than an acute disease, a development with significant implications for health services organizations.

Legal Aspects of Human Immunodeficiency Virus/Acquired Immunodeficiency Syndrome

Legally, HIV/AIDS is daunting to health services organizations. By 1990, the number of AIDS-related lawsuits was already the largest attributable to any disease in United States legal history.[11] By mid-1995, half of the lawsuits filed under the Americans with Disabilities Act (ADA) of 1990 (PL 101-336) involved AIDS.[12] Federal law is buttressed by state disabilities statutes.

One major legal issue of HIV/AIDS is confidentiality. Dimensions include confidentiality of patient names and records, reporting HIV infection, and a duty to warn third parties. Legal protections against breaching medical confidentiality are well established. The AIDS epidemic caused most states to pass laws safeguarding the confidentiality and privacy of people infected or thought to be infected with HIV.[13] Like other communicable diseases, all states have made AIDS a reportable disease. Extending reporting to results of HIV antibody testing has proved more difficult, however; only about half the states require it.[14] Contact tracing, an historically important role for health departments, is belatedly being applied to HIV infection as an effective measure to diminish its spread. The American Medical Association (AMA) supports HIV testing of physicians and health care workers in appropriate situations. It opposes mandatory testing for medical staff privileges but urges physicians to voluntarily determine their HIV status and/or act as if their serostatus is positive.[15]

A second legal dimension and area of litigation results from special risks present when staff members work with AIDS patients. Under the Occupational Safety and Health Act of 1970 (OSHA), employers must provide employment and a place of employment free from recognized hazards that cause, or are likely to cause, death or serious physical harm. OSHA requires universal blood and body substance precautions.

Third are the legal concerns of the risk to staff and other patients from patients infected with HIV and the opportunistic diseases that invariably develop as HIV progresses to frank AIDS. In protecting patients and staff, health services organizations must avoid discriminating against people with HIV/AIDS, whom the law defines as having a disability. The ADA strengthened the right to full public accommodations for people with disabilities.[16] The ADA protects people with HIV or AIDS from discrimination in places of public accommodation, which include professional offices. Physicians or dentists can only refuse to treat a patient with HIV or AIDS under limited circumstances, such as where the needed care is outside the provider's expertise.[17]

Risk to staff and patients from staff infected with HIV is a fourth legal dimension. Health services organizations are subject to Section 504 of the Rehabilitation Act of 1973 (PL 93-112), which prohibits discrimination against qualified employees who have disabilities. Those protections were strengthened by the ADA, which requires that employers make reasonable accommodations for employees with disabilities. To establish a violation of either of these statutes [Section 504 of the Rehabilitation Act and Title II of the ADA], a plaintiff must prove: 1) that he has a disability; 2) that he is otherwise qualified for the employment or benefit in question; and 3) that he was excluded from the employment or benefit due to discrimination solely on the basis of the disability. Regarding the second requirement, an individual is not otherwise qualified if he poses a significant risk to the health or safety of others by virtue of the disability that cannot be eliminated by reasonable accommodation.[18]

The ADA protects HIV-positive applicants and employees. Whether such an employee is "otherwise qualified" in a health services setting is discussed next.

In 1987, the United States Supreme Court considered a case analogous to that of an HIV-positive employee. In *School Board of Nassau County, Florida v. Arline*,[19] a teacher with recurring tuberculosis was discharged because of the health risk to students. The Court determined that tuberculosis was a disability protected by Section 504 of the Rehabilitation Act of 1973 and developed a four-part test: 1) nature of the risk (how the disease is transmitted); 2) duration of the risk (how long the carrier is infectious); 3) severity of the risk (potential harm to third parties); and 4) probability that the disease will be transmitted. No HIV/AIDS case has been considered by the Supreme Court.

Cases litigating whether HIV-positive health services staff are "otherwise qualified" under the ADA turn on the potential risk of harm to patients, even when harm is remote. An HIV-positive cook in a nursing facility was found otherwise qualified. Medical evidence showed that HIV is not transmitted by preparing and serving food and beverages and that his HIV status did not restrict him from performing his job.[20] Conversely, a surgical technician with HIV who assisted in exposure-prone invasive procedures was not protected by the ADA and the Rehabilitation Act of 1973. The court determined that his HIV status disqualified him from working as a surgical technician and that he was not otherwise qualified to perform his job. Evidence showed that his duties occasionally required him to place his hands on and in surgical incisions and that this put him at risk for needle sticks and minor lacerations. Expert testimony showed the risk of transmitting HIV to a patient to be very small. Nonetheless, the trial court applied the four-part test enunciated by the Supreme Court in *Arline* and agreed with the defendant hospital that there was a real possibility of transmitting HIV and that because the consequence of infection is death, the nature, duration, and severity of the risk outweighed the fact that the chance of transmission was slight.[21]

The legal theory of a duty to warn suggests the extent to which caregivers (and, likely, organizations) may be legally obligated to protect third parties in immediate danger. *Tarasoff v. Regents of the State of California*[22] held that a psychotherapist who reasonably believes a patient poses a direct threat to a third party must warn the person in danger. The state supreme courts that have adopted *Tarasoff* limit the duty to warn to identifiable third parties at risk of real and probable harm.[23]

Protecting Staff from Human Immunodeficiency Virus

The underlying ethical premise is that health services organizations must respond to life-threatening infectious diseases by doing all they can to protect staff. This is supported by the virtue of fidelity (faithfulness, loyalty) and by the principle of respect for persons. Through its managers, the organization has a duty to provide a safe work place. Rawls's difference principle (special benefits may be given to small groups if doing so is in the interests of the least advantaged) supports this duty, as does the theory of utility (the greatest good for the greatest number). An effective work force is sustainable only with safe working conditions. The legal obligations of health services organizations discussed next reinforce this ethical duty to employees. Having identified that there is an ethical priority not to put staff at unnecessary risk, the health services organization must create and maintain an environment compatible with the obligation to provide services to the community and treat individuals with HIV or AIDS.

Although present in all body substances of those who are HIV positive, the virus apparently can be spread only by sexual intercourse or intimate contact with body substances, especially blood. Though the risk to health care workers is low, the consequences of AIDS make infection a major concern for them and the organization. The Centers for Disease Control and Prevention (CDC) and Occupational Safety and Health Administration (OSHA) guidelines for universal precautions must be used in all health services organizations.

Some physicians and staff are reluctant or unwilling to treat people with AIDS. In 1987, the AMA Council on Ethical and Judicial Affairs issued a statement that physicians behave unethically if they refuse to treat people with AIDS whose medical conditions are within their competence.[24] This continues to be its position.[25] Employees have been disciplined for refusing to treat patients with AIDS; some have been fired. Given the consequences of contracting HIV, it is likely that some staff will always be reluctant to treat people with AIDS.

In mid-1987, the American Hospital Association (AHA) issued recommendations about clinical management of AIDS patients.[26] These recommendations have not changed.[27] They are consistent with CDC guidelines and state that universal blood and body substance precautions are the best protection for caregivers. They require that all patients' blood and body substances be considered hazardous and that all patients be subject to the infection-control guidelines originally established for hepatitis and HIV. This means that isolation and biohazard precautions should be used for all patients, regardless of HIV status, and that health care workers should protect themselves against blood and body substances and patient contact. Under CDC guidelines in effect since 1987, hospitals should judge whether their patients' characteristics are such that all admissions should be tested. In late 1987, the AHA spoke out against routine testing of patients or staff and continues to hold that position.

CDC guidelines issued in 1991 require that those performing exposure-prone procedures know their HIV status; those who are HIV positive are expected to inform their patients of that fact before engaging in exposure-prone procedures. CDC has been criticized for not defining exposure-prone activities from which HIV-infected health care workers can be excluded.[28] Subsequent federal legislation required that states adopt these guidelines by regulation or legislation.

Staff compliance with the requirements for universal precautions has been and continues to be a problem and a challenge for the health services manager.[29, 30] Enhanced education can be only a small part of the answer. At this point, no caregiver can be ignorant of HIV's risk and the importance of universal precautions. Management must identify and correct structure and process inhibitors that reduce staff willingness or ability to comply with universal precautions.

In 1987, the CDC confirmed that three hospital staff had become HIV positive after occupational exposure to contaminated blood. The risk to health care workers who work with patients who are HIV positive is now well documented, and there have been 57 confirmed cases of transmission of HIV, almost all the result of percutaneous (puncture/cut injury) exposure to HIV-infected blood. In addition, 139 other cases of HIV/ AIDS have occurred among health care personnel who reported no other risk factors and reported occupational exposure but whose seroconversion after exposure was not documented.[31] Three large studies in the late 1980s estimated the risk of contracting HIV after being stuck accidentally with a contaminated needle at approximately 1 in 250.[32] Recent estimates are lower, with a finding that the average risk of HIV transmission after percutaneous exposure to HIV-infected blood is approximately 0.3% and after mucous membrane exposure is 0.09%.[33]

CDC estimated that approximately 800,000 health care workers in the United States would be injured by patient needles in 1998. Combined estimates from the CDC and EPINet—a computer-based standardized injury tracking system used by approximately 1,500 United States hospitals—suggested that more than 2,000 of those workers would test positive for new infections of hepatitis C, another 400 would get hepatitis B, and 35 would contract HIV. HIV is the most feared; but hepatitis B, for which there is a vaccine, and hepatitis C, for which there is no vaccine, are life threatening because they can lead to liver damage, cirrhosis, and cancer.[34] The CDC reports that almost 25,000 adults with AIDS have a history of employment in health care.[35] Of concern, too, are the opportunistic diseases that accompany progress to frank AIDS. These include tuberculosis and

Pneumocystis carinii pneumonia (PCP). At special risk are older adults and those with compromised immune systems.

Increasing numbers of infectious diseases in health services organizations pose special problems for managers and caregivers. As they seek to comply with legal requirements, the ethical obligations owed to staff and patients cannot be put at risk. Meeting the expectations of beneficence and nonmaleficence should always be foremost in the minds of all who deliver and manage services.

NEW RELATIONSHIPS WITH MEDICAL STAFF

Beginning in the late 1980s, significant changes occurred in relationships between physicians and health services organizations, a movement led by acute care hospitals. These arrangements are designed to add an economic dimension to relationships that emphasize clinical activities. The *MeSH (medical staff–hospital)* concept was introduced in the 1980s but gained only limited acceptance; then, the *joint venture*, which included undertakings such as medical office buildings and lease or purchase and operation of high-technology equipment, became the focus of economic relationships between organizations and practitioners. In the 1990s, both concepts were replaced by the *PHO (physician–hospital organization)* and integrated health networks, both of which focus on primary care but seek to deliver a continuum of services to a defined population. The economics of clinical practice must be tied to the organization so that each may assist the other to survive.

Such arrangements are fraught with potential ethical problems. A mildly adversarial relationship between medical staff and managers is useful because it provides checks and balances in maintaining high-quality patient care. This relationship requires that each party remember that its reason for being is to serve and protect the patient. When management and clinical practice are economically bound together, patient interests may suffer. The potential for conflicts of interest is greatly increased if the physicians involved in these arrangements are also part of the governing body. Evidence of actual conflicts of interest and fear of their potential have led to the passage of federal and state laws that regulate certain types of clinical referrals.

APPRAISAL OF MANAGERIAL PERFORMANCE

A principal role of the governing body is appraising the CEO's performance, even as the CEO appraises subordinate managers. W. Edwards

Deming rejected management by objectives (MBO) for general use in organizations. He argued that MBO pits managers against one another and leads to internal competition and suboptimization of the affected systems; ultimately, the entire organization is suboptimized. Despite Deming's concerns, MBO continues to be common in organizations.[36] In its pure form, MBO, as first conceptualized by Peter Drucker, is consistent with Deming's theory. Its use, however, has deviated from the original intent.[37]

Despite the controversy over MBO, formal appraisal of CEOs using specific criteria is appropriate. Their responsibility for the organization carries broad authority. Their interests are consistent with its optimization, and appraising them should reflect this consistency. Harvey used MBO to evaluate hospital CEOs.[38] His list of competencies necessary for managerial effectiveness included the following: planning and organizing, achieving hospital objectives, maintaining the quality of medical services, allocating resources fairly and efficiently, resolving crises, complying with regulations, and promoting the hospital. These criteria are generalizable to any health services organization in which performance is compared against predetermined measures and standards. Current theory applies similar criteria in an MBO format.[39] One study of CEOs found that 1 in 10 had *never* had a performance appraisal, despite the Joint Commission on Accreditation of Healthcare Organizations requirement and an appraisal's being an indicator of good governance.[40]

A 1990 report found that 76% of governing bodies in responding hospitals formally evaluated their CEO.[41] Ongoing informal evaluation and annual formal evaluation of CEO performance are considered essential to organizational effectiveness. Anecdotal evidence suggests, however, that relatively few CEOs are evaluated against specific criteria, especially with the specificity recommended by Harvey.

To avoid conflicts of interest when they are evaluated, CEOs must limit their role to explaining organizational performance. The CEO's performance should be reviewed without the CEO present but with feedback provided later. Like all staff, the CEO is owed fairness in the review process, especially if negative outcomes that might result in termination are possible. Problems are minimized if the governing body employs a formal process to evaluate the CEO's performance, one based on predetermined objectives that are to be attained during the period under evaluation.

CEOs evaluate the work of subordinate managers directly or in coordination with other senior managers. This includes evaluating administrative dimensions of clinical managers' work. Personal and professional relationships may interfere with objective appraisal, or, in some cases, even day-to-day management.

A Little Too Close

Sue Rosen has been a successful health services executive for more than 20 years. She is currently the CEO of an addiction treatment center that provides a full range of in- and outpatient services. Approximately 4 years ago, she experienced significant job-related stress. In addition, she had had emotional problems in her personal life, which became more complex after her divorce and difficulties with her only child.

She recognized her need for professional help and sought the services of Dr. Eisenbard, a clinical psychologist. In addition to his private practice, Eisenbard consulted for several addiction treatment centers. Rosen received 32 sessions of therapy over 2 years. Eisenbard was of great assistance and their final session occurred 2 years ago.

Recently, Rosen's clinical director, a clinical psychologist, resigned. Eisenbard responded to a blind advertisement and sent his résumé to a post office box. The director of human resources brought the résumé to Rosen, who was surprised to receive it. Rosen has high regard for Eisenbard but is concerned about the implications of his application.

There is an obvious problem here: Their previous therapeutic relationship will make it impossible for Rosen to interact effectively with Eisenbard, either as colleagues or as superior–subordinate. Rosen will never feel at ease, and, if needed, disciplinary actions against Eisenbard will be difficult, if not impossible. Eisenbard may not wish to enter into a managerial relationship with Rosen, but at this point he is unaware that she is his potential employer. Regardless of Rosen's high estimate of Eisenbard's professional abilities, this employment relationship should not be undertaken—it is problem fraught.

Governing bodies should be evaluated, and properly applied MBO is also appropriate at this level. Objectivity and comprehensiveness will be enhanced if an external expert assists in the evaluation. Important in evaluating governing body members is input from the CEO and other managers who interact with them.

PHYSICIANS AND CREDENTIALING

The process of verifying credentials begins when a physician first applies for medical staff membership and clinical privileges. All aspects of the candidate's education and training, licensure, and clinical preparation are reviewed. Regular periodic reviews ensure that physicians continue to be qualified. Renewal of privileges depends on demonstrated current competence. All clinical staff with independent access to patients receive a similar review, whether or not they are members of the medical staff. Preventing legal actions and bad publicity are important, but the primary reasons to be concerned about competence are the principles of respect for persons, beneficence, and nonmaleficence.

FRAUDULENT CREDENTIALS

Occasionally, there are reports about persons claiming to be physicians but whose credentials are partly or wholly false. The problem of overstated, misrepresented, or false credentials is extensive in the business world, and there is reason to believe health services management is infected with the same virus. Examples of misrepresented credentials include inflated job titles, responsibilities, and duties; exaggerated or falsified academic preparation and credentials; and falsified or misleading information about professional achievement and activities.[42] Such actions are dishonest and unethical.

Even a cursory check by a potential employer will usually uncover nonexistent formal credentials, such as licenses and academic degrees. More subtle and pervasive is the problem of "creative" résumé writing. One need only look at résumés produced by some employment and executive search firms to realize that it is possible to make trivial management positions appear significant. Uncovering exaggerated or overstated credentials can be difficult because specific details of employment must be verified. Even job descriptions may not adequately reflect what the incumbent actually did in a particular position. For this reason, marginal cases may slip through.

Managers who encounter an applicant who has presented dishonest credentials have one course of action—exposure and disciplinary action through the professional society. Appropriate action is less clear when it is discovered that their current employees have falsified or misrepresented their credentials. Nevertheless, action is essential. Counseling is a first step, whether or not the employee is to be retained. Beyond counseling, the action taken should be proportionate to the seriousness of the problem. Current job performance and the reasons for the falsified credentials should be considered. Serious falsifications and misrepresentations must be reported to the professional society and to the authorities if there is criminal behavior.

What action should be taken if one has personally overstated, misrepresented, or falsified qualifications? Managers with such problems should inform their superiors and offer the strongest possible rationale for the action. This is a sound course of action even when the claimed credential does not exist but was material to the hiring decision. The employer may not take drastic action, especially if the reasons for what was done are compelling. The employer is likely to consider current job performance. The manager must be prepared for termination, however. Continued concealment is unacceptable: As one rises to a more senior level, the stakes are higher and the potential for devastating damage to one's career increases. Misrepresented or falsified credentials are a burden to the individual because they will eventually be uncovered and because of the chronic, nagging fear of being caught. It is better that corrections be made when there is less to lose. This is a compelling utilitarian argument. The Kantian and virtue ethicist, however, would quickly add that it should be done because it is the right thing to do.

Discovery of significantly misrepresented or falsified credentials should cause the professional association to take disciplinary action, up to and including expulsion. Representation of a fictitious academic degree or position are significant to both employer and professional organization.

Slovenly verification by potential employers breaches their ethical obligations and adds to the ease with which false or exaggerated credentials are used. Inadequate verification is a problem even when candidates for senior management positions are considered. Managers breach their obligation if they fail to perform effective credentials checks because patients are at risk, for example, if an incompetent administrative or clinical practitioner is hired. The employer is responsible for adequately checking credentials and acting when dishonesty is uncovered.

Employers are morally obligated to accurately and comprehensively report the performance of former employees. In the case of serious problems such as drug addiction or other criminal behavior, specific information should be reported, whether or not it was requested. The legal concept of a duty to warn reinforces managers' ethical obligation to provide information about a former staff member's significant problems. Less serious problems should be communicated as part of a balanced appraisal of strengths and weaknesses.

A Massachusetts case raised questions about ethical behavior when physicians writing references neglected to include information about the character of former residents in anesthesiology.

But Is It Relevant?

The Massachusetts Medical Society investigated three physicians at a leading Boston hospital who wrote highly laudatory letters recommending a colleague only a few days after he was sentenced to jail for raping a nurse.

The convicted physician was able to use the letters to get a new job as an anesthesiologist at the Children's Hospital in Buffalo, where officials said they were unaware of his legal troubles. [He] was charged later in another Boston rape case, dating back to 1978, involving patients.

Medical officials said the case, involving physicians at the Brigham and Women's Hospital, was the most striking example they have encountered of how letters of recommendation for hospital jobs have lost their value in recent years, as physicians become cautious about writing anything critical about colleagues for fear of being sued.

Other physicians on the staff of the hospital said they believed the letters were written after consulting the attorney for the Brigham and Women's Hospital. Because the rape did not occur within the hospital, they suggested that the attorney had advised the physicians that they had no basis for being critical of (the physician's) medical performance.

In commenting on the case, B.J. Anderson, associate general counsel for the American Medical Association, said that the association advised directors of departments in hospitals to be candid when writing letters of recommendations despite the threat of lawsuits: "Too frequently hospitals that have had a problem with a physician will write a glowing letter because it is easier to export your problems across a state line than to resolve them yourself."[43]

After an investigation by the Massachusetts Medical Society, the three physicians who wrote the letters of recommendation were censured and placed on probation for a year. The controversy over the letters prompted appointment of a panel to suggest guidelines for preparing letters of recommendation. Its report advised physicians to follow a Golden Rule of letter writing: "A letter should contain the information known to the writer that he would like to have were he to receive the letter." The report also stated that "Information regarding personal character is of great importance in the case of physicians."[44]

Whether or not the physicians who wrote recommendations violated the letter of the law, they certainly failed to honor its spirit. Any health services organization hiring the physician or appointing him to its medical staff would find it relevant that he had been convicted of a crime. This is especially true of the crime of rape, which is so adverse to the intimacy of the patient–physician relationship. As with nonphysician staff and employees, the organization, through its managers, is morally obliged to report relevant information about physicians (and all staff) honestly and objectively. Reluctance to communicate information about former staff to potential new employers facilitates movement of incompetent and even dangerous clinical staff from job to job, despite spotty employment records and investigations.[45] Even state statutes that protect references if they are truthful have given limited reassurance to former employers because references tend to be subjective.[46]

CONCLUSION

This chapter identified and analyzed ethical problems managers experience in their relationships with the organization and staff. These relationships are analyzed within the context of the manager's ethical obligations to patients. Managers have access to patient and proprietary information, most of which is confidential. This accessibility suggests the potential for inappropriate disclosure, self-dealing, and misuse of insider information.

The unique relationships that senior managers, especially CEOs, enjoy with governing bodies and staff were examined within the context of various ethical duties. Managers must act to protect patients when questions of clinical competence arise. Taking this action includes having the policies, procedures, and resources needed to minimize the risk of inadequate practice and to eliminate it should it occur. Managers must establish a culture that emphasizes patient care and safety and must support all staff in their efforts to maintain this focus.

New relationships among organizations and with physicians raise ethical issues, most of which result from the potential for conflicts of interest. Emphasizing financial aspects makes it easy to forget that the patient is the primary reason for the existence of health services organizations.

The chapter concluded with an examination of falsified or overstated personal qualifications and the obligation of managers to act when these problems come to their attention. Thorough background checks and the provision of honest recommendations assist organizations in their work and maintain the integrity of the profession.

NOTES

1.   Diane M. Barowsky. (2003, September/October). Assessing cultural fit during the interview. *Healthcare Executive, 18*(5), pp. 62–63.

2. See, for example, Charles U. Letourneau. (1959). *Hospital trusteeship* (pp. 90–91). Chicago: Starling Publications; Charles U. Letourneau. (1969). *The hospital administrator* (p. 45). Chicago: Starling Publications; and Malcolm T. MacEachern. (1962). *Hospital organization and management* (pp. 87, 97). Berwyn, IL: Physicians' Record Co.

3. Jeffrey Alexander. (1990). *The changing character of hospital governance* (p. 13). Chicago: The Hospital Research and Educational Trust.

4. *Ibid.*, p. 18.

5. Paul B. Hofmann. (2003, September/October). Revealing inconvenient truths. *Healthcare Executive, 18*(5), pp. 56–57.

6. Rockwell Schulz & Alton C. Johnson. (1990). *Management of hospitals and health services* (3rd ed., pp. 87–95). St. Louis: Mosby.

7. American Nurses Association. (2001). *Code of Ethics for Nurses*. Washington, DC: Author.

8. David Brown. (2003, November 27). AIDS resurging among gay men, CDC data show. *The Washington Post*, p. A10.

9. David Brown. (2003, November 26). HIV infected 5 million worldwide this year: Study finds drop in parts of Africa. *The Washington Post*, p. A1.

10. David Brown. (2003, November 27). AIDS resurging among gay men, CDC data show. *The Washington Post*, p. A10.

11. AIDS-related lawsuits will continue to rise, report shows. (1990, April 16). *AHA News 26*, p. 3.

12. Sybil C. Pranschke & Barbara M. Wright. (1995, Third Quarter). HIV and AIDS: Employers grapple with difficult issues. *Benefits Quarterly 11*(3), p. 41.

13. Ronald Bayer & Larry Gostin. (1990). Legal and ethical issues relating to AIDS. *Bulletin of the Pan American Health Organization, 24*, p. 457.

14. Susan Okie. (1997, September 2). AIDS: Health officials launch new campaign to determine how widespread the virus is. *Washington Post Health*, p. 13.

15. American Medical Association. (2003, November 25). *Report 4 of the Council on Scientific Affairs* (p. 4). Chicago: Author.

16. Robert E. Stein. (1991, June). The Americans with Disabilities Act of 1990. *Arbitration Journal 46*, pp. 6–7.

17. Kenneth E. Labowitz. (1992, March). Refusal to treat HIV-AIDS patients: What are the legal obligations? *Trial 28*(3), p. 58.

18. Barry R. Furrow, Thomas L. Greaney, Sandra H. Johnson, Timothy S. Jost, & Robert L. Schwartz. (1997). *Health law: Cases, materials and problems* (3rd ed., pp. 487–488). St. Paul, MN: West Publishing Co.

19. School Board of Nassau County, Florida v. Arline 480 U.S. 273 (1987).

20. Raintree Health Care Center v. Human Rights Commission, 655 N.E.2d 944 (1995).

21. Mauro v. Borgess Medical Center, 886 F. Supp. 1349 (1995). The trial court decision was affirmed on appeal at 137 F. 3d 398 (6th Cir. Feb. 25, 1998). In Scoles v. Mercy Health Corporation of Southeastern Pennsylvania (887 F. Supp.765 [1994]), a federal court held that an HIV-positive surgeon was not "otherwise qualified" under Section 504 and the ADA and could be prohibited from performing exposure-prone procedures, despite the virtually nonexistent risk of infection. A federal court upheld the suspension of a

neurosurgical resident from his residency in Doe v. University of Maryland Medical System Corporation (50 F.3d 1261 [1995]) because he posed a significant risk to his patients' health and safety that could not be eliminated by reasonable accommodation.

22. Tarasoff v. Regents of the State of California, 17 Cal. 3d 425 (1976).

23. Ronald Bayer & Larry Gostin. (1990). Legal and ethical issues relating to AIDS. *Bulletin of the Pan American Health Organization, 24*, pp. 461, 462 (notes).

24. American Medical Association. (Updated June 1996 and June 1998). *E-9.131: HIV-infected patients and physicians.* Retrieved January 2, 2004, from http://www.ama-assn.org/ama/pub/category/8550.html "A physician who knows that he or she is seropositive should not engage in any activity that creates a significant risk of transmission of the disease to others. A physician who has HIV disease or who is seropositive should consult colleagues as to which activities the physician can pursue without creating a risk to patients."

25. *Ibid.*

26. American Hospital Association. (1987–1988). *AIDS/HIV Infection: Recommendations for health care practices and public policy, report and recommendations of the special committee on AIDS/HIV infection policy.* Chicago: Author.

27. Jeanette Harlow, Resource Center, American Hospital Association; personal communication, January 28, 2000.

28. Donald H. Hermann. (1994, Summer). A call for authoritative CDC guidelines for HIV-infected health care workers. *Journal of Law, Medicine, and Ethics 22*(2), p. 176.

29. Mary Koska. (1989, September 5). AIDS precautions: Compliance difficult to enforce. *Hospitals*, p. 58.

30. Cynthia Carter Haddock, Gail W. McGee, Hala Fawal, & Michael S. Saag. (1994, Fall). Knowledge and self-reported use of universal precautions in a university teaching hospital. *Hospital & Health Services Administration, 39*(3), pp. 295–307.

31. Centers for Disease Control and Prevention, Division of Healthcare Quality Promotion. (last reviewed December 11, 2003). *Surveillance of healthcare personnel with HIV/AIDS, as of December 2002.* Retrieved January 2, 2004, from http://www.cdc.gov/ncidod/hip/BLOOD/hivpersonnel.htm

32. Susan Okie. (1990, January 16). HIV-infected workers undercounted. *The Washington Post*, p. A5.

33. Centers for Disease Control. (2000, January 1). Public health service guidelines for management of health-care worker exposure to HIV and recommendations for postexposure prophylaxis. Retrieved March 15, 2004, from http://www.cdc.gov/epo/mmwr/preview/mmwrhtml/00052722.htm

34. Kathleen F. Phalen. (1998, August 11). Needle stick risk. *Washington Post Health*, p. 11.

35. Centers for Disease Control and Prevention, Division of Healthcare Quality Promotion.

36. Edward Marlow & Richard Schilhavy. (1991, January/February). Expectation issues in management by objectives programs. *IM*, pp. 29–32.

37. Philip E. Quigley. (1993, July). Can management by objectives be compatible with quality? *Industrial Engineering, 14*, p. 64.
38. James D. Harvey. (1978, Spring). Evaluating the performance of the chief executive officer. *Hospital & Health Services Administration, 23*, pp. 5–21.
39. Beaufort B. Longest, Jr., Jonathon S. Rakich, & Kurt Darr. (2000). *Managing health services organizations and systems* (4th ed., pp. 787–788). Baltimore: Health Professions Press.
40. Daniel R. Longo, Jeffrey Alexander, Paul Earle, & Marni Pahl. (1990, May). Profile of hospital governance: A report from the nation's hospitals. *Trustee, 43*(5), 7.
41. J. Larry Tyler & Errol L. Briggs. (2001, May). Practical governance: CEO performance appraisal. *Trustee, 54*(5), 18.
42. Physicians are not immune. A study by Gail Sekas and William R. Hutson of applicants to a gastroenterology fellowship found that nearly one third of the 53 applicants who said they had published articles in scientific journals misrepresented the articles ([1995]. Misrepresentation of academic accomplishments by applicants for gastroenterology fellowships. *Annals of Internal Medicine, 123*, pp. 38–41). Misrepresentations included citations of nonexistent articles in actual journals, articles in nonexistent journals, or articles noted as in press. Review of applicants to an infectious disease fellowship suggested that the problem of misrepresentation is not confined to gastroenterology. The authors of the study posit but do not answer the question of what those discovering the deception should do. They urge that guidelines be developed.
43. Fox Butterfield. (1981, September 24). Doctors' praise assailed for peer in rape case. *The New York Times*, p. A16.
44. Doctors censured in Massachusetts. (1982, February 4). *The New York Times*, p. D27.
45. Michelle Garcia. (2003, December 26). Nurse investigation expands: Five counties, 2 states to cooperate in probe of patients' deaths. *The Washington Post*, p. A4.
46. Amy Joyce. (2003, January 4). Who cares about references? Employers should—though it may be difficult to get thorough answers. *The Washington Post*, p. F5.

CHAPTER 8

ETHICAL ISSUES REGARDING PATIENTS AND COMMUNITY

This chapter identifies the special relationships between managers (and their organizations) and patients and the community. The personal duties and obligations of managers, as well as the responsibilities to their profession, were noted in Chapter 4 in the context of the moral philosophies and the ethical principles of respect for persons, beneficence, nonmaleficence, and justice, in addition to various of the virtues. That chapter highlighted the need for managers to have a well-defined personal ethic to guide their decision making on administrative and biomedical ethical problems within the context of the organizational philosophy.

This chapter reinforces the book's underlying premise that the manager is a moral agent with independent duties to the patient. Managers must juxtapose their relationship with and duty of loyalty to the organization and patient relationships. The reciprocal duties of colleagues are a part of belonging to a professional group that has expectations and demands certain behavior. In many ways, organization and manager are one. Managers must keep this in mind because their actions and decisions are judged in that context—they personify the organization. However, there are ethical limits to what the organization can expect of those working for or affiliated with it. Managers must know the limits of their personal ethic and must speak out when the organization infringes upon those limits.

MAINTAINING CONFIDENTIAL INFORMATION

Patient Records

Through their managers, health services organizations are charged with duties regarding patient information. Medical records are essential for good patient care and they must be legible, current, complete, and authenticated. The legal duty to maintain their confidentiality and security is met by providing adequate and effective personnel and systems and procedures in medical records activities and by ensuring that medical staff bylaws and rules and regulations are enforced. Much can be done to prevent or minimize unauthorized access to paper medical records. Increasing use of electronic records raises significant new confidentiality issues to be resolved.

The federal Health Insurance Portability and Accountability Act (HIPAA), passed in 1996 and effective for medical privacy as of 2003, places substantial restrictions on how health information is obtained, managed, stored, transferred, and used. Much attention is paid to the need for patients to consent for any use of their health information, including among various types of personal and institutional providers of care.

State legal requirements vary, but individuals working in health services organizations have an ethical duty to ensure the confidentiality and appropriate use of patient information. A common breach of this ethic occurs when patients are discussed with or in the presence of persons with no need to know. Hospital-based research has found significant breaches of patient confidentiality and other types of inappropriate comments such as concerns about a staffer's ability or desire to provide high-quality patient care, concerns about poor-quality care in the hospital, or derogatory remarks made about patients or their families.[1] Idle chatter, gossip, and discussing patients with those with no need to know are titillating but ethically unacceptable inside and outside the organization. Breaches of patient confidentiality can also occur through improper disposal of electronic patient records, such as computer hard drives.[2] In addition, conflicts may arise between maintaining confidential information about patients and furthering organizational interests.

Mailing Lists

University Hospital has a very active cardiac medicine section in its department of medicine. Across several decades, it has treated thousands of people with heart problems ranging from angina to congestive heart failure. Its patients have been included in several research protocols, many of them funded by the National Institutes of Health or various national heart associations.

Periodic questionnaire surveys are conducted as part of long-term patient follow-up. To complete these surveys, an extensive database and mailing lists are maintained by the cardiac medicine section. On one occasion, the development office of University Hospital used the mailing lists to solicit general contributions. On another occasion, it undertook a special fund-raising effort to assist in converting and equipping a cardiac intensive care unit. Contributions by the cardiac program's current and former patients have been excellent, primarily because the program maintains superior rapport with its patients.

The physician-director of the program and her administrative assistant have been approached by a prominent and respected national insurance company that is impressed by the results of the program. It wants to use the mailing lists to market life insurance to the program's participants. The proposal is attractive because the opportunity to obtain life insurance will benefit present and former patients, many of whom are otherwise uninsurable except at very high premiums. The proposal is also attractive because any data obtained by the insurance company will be available to the hospital at cost if the mailing lists are provided to the insurance company.

The physician-director and administrative assistant are enthusiastic about the clinical possibilities in addition to the opportunity to help patients. The director of development views the sale of mailing lists as a way to raise money for the cardiac program's activities. Both he and the physician-director spent an hour trying to convince the chief executive officer (CEO) that it is appropriate to release the mailing lists for this worthy purpose.

As stated, the proposal violates the privacy rule of the HIPAA because medical information from a covered entity—in this case, a hospital—is being used to market a product or service without the patient's written authorization.[3] Because breaking the law is unethical per se, University Hospital must obtain consent before it can use the mailing lists as proposed.

An ethical analysis produces virtually the same result as that obtained by applying HIPAA. This case suggests the legitimate but opposing and competing considerations that are a part of patient care, research, fundraising, and a limited duty of general beneficence to help patients solve problems indirectly linked to medical treatment. The case highlights the ethical problems of safeguarding the confidentiality of patient information. Using the information in the way requested violates the confidentiality of patient treatment and diagnosis. Some direct benefits may inure to patients (e.g., opportunity to obtain life insurance) and some indirect benefits may inure to the organization (e.g., improved data for epidemiological studies). Nevertheless, using the mailing lists as suggested serves no valid research purpose, nor does it directly further patients' medical treatment. Data that do not identify patients serve the same epidemiological purposes. The promise of mortality data on insurance purchasers is incidental to the research effort, and the money earned selling the mailing lists is likely to be modest. Regardless, these utilitarian arguments are irrelevant because such uses are incompatible with the principle of respect for persons, which includes confidentiality. Previous use of the lists to solicit contributions was questionable and should not be used to support making the lists available now.

A weightier ethical argument for using mailing lists could be made if all University Hospital patients were included rather than those identified by diagnoses. Mailing to all former patients identifies only that they were patients at University Hospital, but even this activity may raise concerns over confidentiality for some former patients. The problem of mailing lists can be minimized by determining on admission whether patients object to being on mailing lists used for hospital purposes, such as fund-raising.

University Hospital's use of mailing lists must be distinguished from selling or renting them. Patients must be informed if the hospital intends to use a mailing list commercially. Chapter 9 discusses several of the issues incident to obtaining consent in similar situations. Confidentiality concerns change, and patients should know that they can ask that their names be removed from a mailing list at any time. Rental or sale of mailing lists in health services settings is fraught with ethical problems and is best avoided.

MONITORING CLINICAL ACTIVITIES

Managers are agents of the organization, but as decision makers whose actions have moral implications and as members of a profession, managers are never simply instruments of the organization. Managers have duties to patients independent of those the organization has to the patient or the physician's duties to the patient. Managers' concerns and duties are not limited to problems with the business office or the quality of food but extend to clinical activities. In terms of the patient, the manager is the organization's conscience.

Nonphysician managers do not judge clinical activities as would physicians. Just as they use technical experts to develop a new computer system or prepare a loss prevention management program, managers rely on experts in nursing and medicine to assist in understanding these activities and their outcomes. Experienced managers have considerable knowledge about clinical medicine, and, in a gross fashion, this knowledge enables them to determine when problems may be present. Regardless of their clinical sophistication, their purpose is not to be junior physicians but to understand what physicians do and what they need and want. The primary reason to understand clinical activities is to help the organization serve patients safely and effectively.

The health services organization benefits most when involvement is bidirectional—managers should expect and seek physician participation in administrative decision making. Hospitals in which physicians participate in management decision making achieve superior results.

An important role of managers in clinical settings is to link the formal and informal organizations. Anecdotal evidence suggests that informal communications are helpful, perhaps critical, in identifying clinical problems, and that they are an important supplement to formal systems. Nursing is especially important as an informal link. Deficient performance by physicians is often initially identified by nurses. Information from them can alert the formal system and be a starting point for further inquiry. Disciplinary actions cannot be based on rumor, however; managers must ensure adequate follow-up and investigation in conjunction with normal monitoring of clinical outcome data. As necessary, the manager must take action to protect the patient. As a moral agent, the prudent, ethical manager cannot ignore situations that jeopardize the patient or the organization. Sometimes, however, the tables are turned.

A Different Kind of Risk

Dr. Sagatius has just returned to his office after seeing the risk manager. He was very upset and slammed the door behind him before slumping into his chair. He would not stand for it, not again, he said to himself. This was the final straw. Administration was not going to push him around!

He thought back to the two previous incidents in the pediatrics unit and considered their similarity. Now there was a third incident, this time involving a different nurse. Another one of his patients had been medicated incorrectly—actually overdosed. Luckily, Sagatius had been able to intervene once again before serious consequences occurred. The child would have to stay in the hospital several days longer because long-term consequences were possible. He had reported the first two instances to the nurse supervisor. Now he would have to take other action.

The day following the third incident, Sagatius was asked by the risk manager to stop by her office. While there, he saw the child's medical record lying on her desk. Sagatius, noticed that the risk manager had changed the medication record, which he knew had previously shown the overdose. When he asked the risk manager about it, she said that it did not matter because no apparent harm had come to the child. "Why needlessly upset the parents?" she asked. When Sagatius protested that this was dishonest, the risk manager became hostile and reminded Sagatius that a malpractice suit would hurt all those affiliated with the hospital, including the doctors, who were almost certain to be sued should the error come to light. She warned him not to discuss what happened with anyone, especially not with the parents.

Sagatius planned to tell the parents about the overdose, believing that they were owed an explanation for the extra days in the hospital. Also, they had to watch for signs of long-term effects of the overdose and seek medical treatment for the child should they occur.

Sagatius weighed his options. He knew he had to tell the parents to watch the child closely, even if he did not discuss the overdose. He retrieved the parents' telephone number from his computer.

Dr. Sagatius faces two ethical problems. The first concerns the risk manager. Ethically, Sagatius's primary duty is to protect the interests of his patient, which means that he must provide the parents with the information they need to monitor their child; doing so meets the principles of beneficence and nonmaleficence. How can he carry out this duty given the position of the risk manager? The risk manager has violated the principle of respect for persons. In addition, by covering up clinical failures, the risk manager is enabling a system that violates the principle of nonmaleficence. The dishonesty is inconsistent with a typical organizational philosophy. Furthermore, it will thwart the investigation to find the root cause of a type of problem that appears systemic.

The second ethical problem involves the nursing supervisor, who has not acted to prevent a recurrent, serious problem in the pediatrics unit. Such inaction is inconsistent with the principles of beneficence and nonmaleficence and the ethical obligations under the Code of Ethics for Nurses. Sagatius is ethically obligated to report the persistent quality problem to more senior leaders through the nursing and medical staff hierarchy or other appropriate means.

Medical record falsification is rare, even though it is human nature to want to hide failure. The manager's ethical obligations commonly become submerged in the legal dimensions of a problem, despite the fact that in this case, the risk manager's action was illegal. As a result, the patient becomes the enemy, and those in the organization move into a defensive posture. Patients and family sense this and are spurred all the more to press for an explanation, a kind word, or perhaps even an apology. Patients and their families understand that errors and mistakes can occur and it is increasingly clear that they are less likely to take legal action if they believe that they have been treated fairly and everything was done to ease the impact of the error. What they cannot understand and often will not accept are deceit and coldness. Hiding the truth and lying to patients and families angers them; angry patients and their families are much more likely to file a lawsuit. This utilitarian argument also supports the unpleasant but ethically preferred course of forthrightness and honesty with injured patients or their families, as appropriate. Doing so has been shown to be successful in some settings.[4]

Organizations that acknowledge their mistakes and strive to make things right are better served ethically—and, apparently (with limited evidence) legally—than those who fight to the end. In this regard, it is important to note that admitting an error, accepting responsibility for an error, or even admitting negligence are not the same as admitting liability. A finding of liability requires negligence (departure from the standard of care), injury (harm to the patient), and proximate cause (the harm must have been caused by the departure from the standard of care). The plaintiff has the burden of proving *all* of these elements; it is the causal relationship that remains to be proved even when negligence has been admitted.

Since the early to mid-1990s, a small number of organizations determined that their ethical duty to disclose treatment errors was greater than the potential risk of legal action against them. After acting to minimize the error's clinical consequences, they informed patients (and family, as appropriate) about what happened and why, apologized, and sought a fair solution to the medical and economic effects of the error. Money may or may not have changed hands.

Being honest with patients gained momentum in 2001, when the Joint Commission on Accreditation of Healthcare Organizations (Joint Commission) amended its patient safety and medical and health care error reduction standards. The changes require that patients and families, as appropriate, be informed of unanticipated outcomes, including medical error. Medical error was defined as "an unintended act, either of omission or commission, or an act that does not achieve its intended outcome." The Joint Commission addresses medical error by requiring that "Patients and, when appropriate, their families are informed about the outcomes of care, treatment, and services, including unanticipated outcomes." This information is provided by the responsible licensed independent practitioner or designee.[5] Honestly admitting mistakes carries potential harms, as well as benefits to patient and practitioner.[6]

All members of the organization have a shared responsibility to scrutinize the services delivered and take action as necessary. If this is seen as "ratting" or being a "stool pigeon," the organization's culture is in need of change. Identifying problems should be an important part of the culture and everyone should be committed to correcting them once identified.

This type of culture will make whistleblowing unnecessary. Such a negative interpretation is possible only if one ignores the reason for being of the organization and those who work there. Both exist to further the interests of patients. When problems occur in the delivery of services, the organization and its managers must act to minimize loss and injury and do whatever is possible to make the patient whole. The manager must be involved, as necessary, to eliminate or reduce the recurrence of problems.

WHISTLEBLOWING

When an employee reveals information about illegal, inefficient, or wasteful action that endangers the health, safety, or freedom of the public it is called *whistleblowing*.[7] This definition is broad enough to include revelations of mismanagement, including nonfeasance, misfeasance, and malfeasance. Many contemporary discussions of whistleblowing narrowly focus on fraud and abuse or other illegal activities under state and federal law. Here, however, the broad definition is used.

Whistleblowing affects the private and public sectors and includes disclosing information both internal and external to the organization. Generally, internal whistleblowing is much more likely to be seen as positive because the organization has the opportunity to correct the problem. External whistleblowing usually occurs after internal reporting has proved fruitless; it may have significant negative effects on the organization. Negative reaction from managers is likely to be a function of the perceived or real level of embarrassment and threat to them and the organization. Whistleblowing results from activities of individuals and those of the organization.

An example many health services managers will recognize is an organization that harbors a clinical or management staff member whose incompetence or incapacitation is known, except, of course, to those outside of the organization. Despite this knowledge, nothing is done. The organization's culture discourages acting against those "in the club," or the lack of support in remedying the problem and the fear of retribution make the price too high. Thus, the problem continues until a catastrophe occurs or the situation becomes intolerable to a critical mass of managers and staff, forcing action. Much of the stimulus is fear of public exposure and the embarrassment or disciplinary action that is likely to result. Such motivation is not the stuff of moral agents, who act because it is right to do so.

Three types of activities result in whistleblowing: clear illegality, potential illegality or danger, and the organization's social policy.[8]

Clear illegality occurs when the law is knowingly violated. Examples include falsifying information reported to the government, bribing inspectors, making illegal campaign contributions, falsifying audits, deliberately violating labor laws, discriminating in employment because of race or gender, and improperly disposing of hazardous wastes.[9]

The second type of activity affected by whistleblowing involves *potential illegality or danger*. A growing body of regulations and case law protects employee health, patient safety, public health, and the environment. In addition, managers and employees are moral agents who are obligated to take action when there is reason to believe that patients are at risk, regardless of other requirements. In most situations in which whistleblowing occurs or should occur, the whistleblower acts in the belief that a given practice, process, or result is either not in compliance with accepted standards or places the patient unnecessarily at risk. "In any well-run enterprise, management should be seriously concerned about such violations and should welcome warnings by its own employees."[10]

The third type of activity affected by whistleblowing involves the *organization's social policy*. An employee may become concerned about the morality of a management policy and its effect on patients or society. For example, an employee may believe that the net revenue of a not-for-profit health services organization is excessive or spent inappropriately and that too little is used for indigent care. Speaking out or refusing to participate is likely to be protected by conscience clauses in state or federal statutes or by the U.S. Constitution, if state action is involved. Assuming the policy is legal, employee protest raises two issues: the employee's right to free speech and the employee's responsibility as a moral agent. Employees are entitled to the same constitutionally protected right of free speech as are other individuals. Furthermore, as moral agents, they have an ethical duty to speak out when policies and actions could or do adversely affect patients or society. The controversy usually arises when an employee exercises the right of free speech or the duty of moral agency by speaking publicly against an organization's lawful policy, thereby harming its reputation and market advantage.[11]

Health services organizations create a paradox when they encourage managers and staff to act responsibly in all situations without causing unnecessary disruption. When the organization or individuals in it act illegally, inefficiently, or wastefully, staff are expected to be loyal and not speak out. This paradox is less easily resolved as organizations become more competitive because employees are asked to deal aggressively with external competitors but to be complacent internally.

An important dimension of whistleblowing is found in federal law. In 1986, Congress amended the False Claims Act, which was originally passed during the Civil War to reduce fraud in federal contracting. The amendments added important protections and rewards for individuals who blow the whistle. These whistleblowers are known as *relators*. The lawsuits they can bring are known as *qui tam* actions (*qui tam*, from the Latin *who as well for the king as for himself sues in the matter*). The law protects relators against wrongful dismissal, and they are allowed reinstatement with seniority, double back pay, and compensation for discriminatory treatment.[12] When relators file suit, the case is sealed for 60 days while the U.S. Department of Justice (DOJ) decides whether it will intervene. If the DOJ does not intervene, the whistleblower may proceed independently. Assuming a successful outcome (and a significant role on the part of the relator), the whistleblower may receive 15%–30% of any double or triple damages and fines that are imposed.[13] The vast amounts of money spent by the federal government in programs such as Medicare and Medicaid result in significant potential for fraud, and many *qui tam* suits have been brought in the health services sector. The value of *qui tam* suits is shown by the fact that since 1988, almost $2 billion has been recovered under the statute.[14] Federal false claims law is supplemented by state laws.

Examples of Whistleblowing

When considering these cases, it is important to bear in mind that employees and managers are moral agents with an ethical duty to speak out when policies and actions could or do affect patients or society adversely. This is true regardless of other requirements, such as the law.

How Sweet It Is!

Dr. A. Grace Pierce joined the research staff of Ortho Pharmaceutical Corporation in 1971. In 1975 she was part of a team developing a prescription drug known generically as loperamide. The drug was used to treat acute and chronic diarrhea in infants, children, and older adults. Saccharin was used to make it palatable by masking its bitter taste.

The research team agreed that the formula was unsuitable because it substantially exceeded U.S. Food and Drug Administration (FDA) saccharin limits. Management was informed of this fact but decided nevertheless to file a new drug application with the FDA. Other members of the research team continued development, but Dr. Pierce refused. Although she was offered work in other projects at no decrease in pay, she resigned her position, apparently believing her refusal had irrevocably damaged her career at Ortho.

Later, she sought relief in the courts, alleging wrongful discharge. The New Jersey Supreme Court ruled that Ortho had not acted illegally and that there were no grounds for a cause of action.[15]

The court placed substantial weight on the fact that there was no imminent harm to the public. The court ruled that the ethic of the Hippocratic oath did not contain a clear mandate of public policy that would have prevented Dr. Pierce from continuing her research. Similar cases have occurred in organizations that deliver health services.

It's Really Only an X-ray

Frances O'Sullivan was an X-ray technician employed by several radiologists and a hospital. She brought suit for breach of an employment contract after she was fired. She alleged she was fired for refusal to perform catheterizations, a procedure she had not been trained to perform. O'Sullivan could not legally perform catheterizations in New Jersey, where only licensed nurses and physicians may do so. The issue involved was unique because the plaintiff had been asked to perform an illegal act. The superior court denied the defendant physicians' and hospital's motion to dismiss.[16]

Denying the motion to dismiss meant that O'Sullivan was entitled to a trial on the merits of the case. No report exists that this occurred, and it may be assumed that the case was settled before trial. In light of the illegality of what O'Sullivan was asked to do, she acted properly.

Don't Speak Now and Forever Hold Your Peace

Linda Rafferty was a psychiatric nurse at a state institution in which the conditions were appalling. The abuses Rafferty claimed to have observed included the staff failing to protect patients from sexual abuse by other patients and from sexual exploitation by outside employees, providing improper non-psychiatric medical care, allowing patients to keep medications in their rooms, locking up fire extinguishers, leaving blank prescription forms that were signed in advance by physicians in unlocked drawers for nurses to fill out on weekends, and hospital medical staff being chronically absent from work. Rafferty repeatedly complained to her superiors but resigned when her protests brought no change.

She was hired at another institution, Community Mental Health Center, as supervisor of nurses. Before she began work, she gave an interview to a Philadelphia newspaper in which she was sharply critical of treatment at the state institution. The morning after the story appeared, she was fired from her new position because "staff members were upset about the article." No other reasons were given until trial, when the Community Mental Health Center alleged inadequate job performance in addition to the previous reason.

Rafferty brought suit alleging she had been deprived of her constitutional rights. The court ruled that she be reinstated and be awarded over $3,000 in back pay.[17]

These whistleblowing cases resulted in court decisions. The types and number of whistleblowing cases are legion, and many are reported in the professional literature and the media. Senior administrators at the University of California–Irvine Medical Center were fired for allegedly retaliating against employees who had reported physician misconduct at the center's fertility clinic. Whistleblowers said that physicians were implanting eggs and embryos into patients without donor consent. An internal investigation supported the whistleblowers' allegations and showed that after they reported the wrongdoing, they were treated badly by medical center management and clinic physicians and subsequently fired.[18] Another whistleblower case alleged that 132 research center hospitals conspired to deliberately miscode procedures and manipulate patient records so as to obtain $1 billion in federal reimbursement for the use of investigational devices, which are not covered under Medicare and Medicaid guidelines. The hospitals argued that diagnosis-related groups pay by diagnosis rather than by products used, and thus payment was due regardless of treatment. The facts suggest that this is a *qui tam* case brought under the False Claims Act.[19]

A clear example of a *qui tam* suit occurred at a community hospital in Pineville, Kentucky, at which a new physician found that several physician colleagues were not performing some patient histories, physical examinations, and other services listed in patient records. Hospital medical records clerks wrote histories and physicals based on information in the medical records or, sometimes, by interviewing patients. The document created by the clerk was used to bill Medicare. At discharge, clerks used the medical record to prepare a discharge summary, which was stamped with the physician's signature and used by the physician's office to bill Medicare for a discharge examination and treatment plan. After repeated efforts to change the practice, the new physician brought a *qui tam* suit. The hospital settled the case for $2.3 million; each physician paid $100,000. Had they been imposed, maximum damages and penalties could have totaled $31 million. Allegedly, hospital administration hindered efforts to end the fraudulent practices. Not unexpectedly, the whistleblower was seen as the problem by many at the hospital and in the community.[20]

Other *qui tam* cases include a settlement in which TAP Pharmaceuticals agreed to pay nearly $600 million over allegations of kickbacks to physicians and false Medicare claims regarding treatment of their patients. Another case found Beverly Medical Care paying $175 million to settle allegations that employees of its nursing homes were exaggerating claims of time spent attending Medicare patients.[21]

These cases highlight the three significant issues relating to whistleblowing as an ethical problem in health services organizations. The first is staff responsibility and accountability, something that applies to all employees, whether or not they are managers. The second is fair practices. To encourage responsibility and accountability, due process procedures are necessary to protect employees who consider themselves moral agents and are courageous enough to speak out. Due process regarding employee disciplinary actions (both in terms of procedure and substance) is necessary, whether the organization is one to which federal or state constitutional protections apply. Being bound by such requirements will also encourage others to act when they should. Methods must be developed to balance the individual's duty to the employer against the duty to the public. This can be difficult because "many of the rights and privileges . . . so important to a free society that they are constitutionally protected . . . are vulnerable to abuse through an employer's power."[22] The third issue is how to encourage employees to speak out in appropriate ways in order to meet their independent duty to the patient, without causing unnecessary damage to the indispensable cooperative and trust relationships that exist within the organization as well as between them and their communities.

Negative Aspects of Whistleblowing

Several negative aspects temper what is positive about whistleblowing: Determining the accuracy of whistleblowing charges is not always easy. Whistleblowers may be incorrect in what they allege to be the facts of management's misconduct. The danger exists that incompetent or inadequate employees may become whistleblowers to avoid facing justifiable disciplinary actions. Employees can blow the whistle in unacceptably disruptive ways, regardless of the merits of their protest. Some whistleblowers are not protesting unlawful or unsafe practices but social policies by management that the employee considers unwise or unethical. The legal definitions of a safe product, danger to health, or improper treatment of employees are often not clear. The efficiency and flexibility of human resources management could be threatened by the creation of legal rights to dissent and legalized review systems. Risks to the desirable autonomy of the private sector are possible because a review of allegations by whistleblowers will expand government's role too deeply into internal business policies.[23]

Courses of Action

Managers with the authority to remedy a problem are morally bound to do so. If persons in authority will not act, there are alternatives consistent with the duty of loyalty managers and staff have to the organization, even if these alternatives ultimately involve public disclosure. It is ethically appropriate to act early, even at the risk of embarrassing an organization, than to await further corruption, with its attendant greater risk of harm to others as well as the organization. The alternatives involve whistleblowing of various types. Regrettably, whistleblowing has a bad connotation for many. It suggests disloyalty to the group, if not to the organization—the person who blows the whistle is considered a "stool pigeon" or an informer, a betrayer. Despite the pervasiveness of this attitude, its reasoning is perverse. How, for example, could one be considered a traitor by informing senior management of illegal or incompetent actions that risk the health of patients or staff? The negative perception of whistleblowing persists, nonetheless. Establishing a culture that makes whistleblowing unnecessary is a major challenge that management must take up. Making the environment risk free in terms of retribution against those who are willing to speak up (i.e., internal whistleblowers) is an essential first step.

One type of whistleblowing involves stimulating action by approaching those in authority directly. Working with persons of like mind—finding allies and strength in numbers—can reinforce and stimulate the need to act. In an environment of fear, anonymous communication with those who are able to remedy the problem may be necessary to produce the desired result.

It is crucial that there be a change in the atmosphere typically found in an organization—the "I win, you lose" (*zero-sum*) approach to whistleblowing. Responsible reporting will benefit employees, employers, and, most important, the patient. As Bowman, Elliston, and Lockhart[24] pointed out, "Directing corrective efforts to [whistleblowers] instead of the policy or practice they protest will not alter the conditions that make whistleblowing necessary." This attitude was pervasive at Pineville when the whistleblower was perceived by many people to be the problem.

Place of Whistleblowing

Leading commercial companies have created ombudsman programs in which one person receives, investigates, and responds to employee complaints. Such programs are important for employees who believe illegal or improper conduct is occurring. The problem is that the ombudsman may lack the authority to solve problems in line departments. The ombudsman may not be empowered to deal with senior managers who actively promote illegal or improper conduct as an organizational imperative.[25]

Even where employees are protected by law, as in federal employment, they fear reprisals. A 1992 survey by the U.S. Merit Systems Protection Board found that 50% of employees who said they knew firsthand of illegal acts or waste in federal government failed to report it. Only 13% of whistleblowers were given credit by management for doing the right thing; 71% said their supervisors or upper management became unhappy with them. Of whistleblowers, 37% said they had experienced or had been threatened with retaliation. The retaliation included poor performance appraisals, being shunned by co-workers and managers, and verbal harassment or intimidation.[26] These findings are confirmed by a 1998 survey showing that 25% of employees believe that their agency will not protect them from retaliation for whistleblowing.[27] Research on whistleblowing in the private sector has similar findings. Half of management accountants who observed wrongdoing did not report it.[28]

The concept of moral agency and the willingness to speak and act as necessary remain central, recurring themes for managers and caregivers alike. Professional dissent is critical to the field of health services administration and the delivery of health services. No morality exists without action; ethics will survive only if people speak out when it matters. Professionals are distinguished by the ability to recognize ethical problems and to act as moral custodians of the organization in which they work.

Doorway Consultations

A consulting ethicist for a large nursing facility was asked by a nurse to discuss a problem concerning a physician, several of whose patients are residents in the facility. The nurse said she had an ethical quandary and was not sure what to do. She continued by describing how the physician routinely looked into his patients' rooms from the doorway and then made chart entries indicating he had had a professional visit with them. The nurse said that she had heard of physicians who would "survey" the dining room at mealtime and then make chart entries indicating a professional visit. The nurse said that behavior was only slightly worse than what she had seen. In fact, she said, one of her patients asked if her doctor was coming in because she had questions for him. "What should I do?" asked the nurse.

Quality of care questions aside, the physician is acting unethically. If he is billing for his visits—almost a certainty—he is committing fraud, which makes him subject to criminal prosecution. Billing a government program for care not provided subjects him to penalties for fraud as well. Nursing's Code of Ethics and this nurse's apparent personal ethic requires that she report her concerns within the nursing administration hierarchy, that she become an internal whistleblower. Failing action, the nurse should consider external whistleblowing or a *qui tam* action.

Organizational Culture

The word *whistleblowing* is itself unfortunate terminology. In historical perspective, it suggests a police officer who used a whistle to stop criminal activity and summon assistance. It would be far better to make the concept one of highlighting the compliant culture that emphasizes quality—one in which calling attention to a problem is considered positive, not negative. An open culture that stresses honesty, integrity, quality of care, fairness, and concern for employees and patients—an ethical environment with a shared values orientation—will produce proper treatment of staff and patients, a safe work and clinical environment, and honest billing practices, the result of which is compliance with the law. This makes a compliance officer and compliance program largely redundant. Even if both are deemed necessary, their roles will be to communicate information, educate staff, and assist in establishing policies and procedures that enable compliance. Assigning "ethics" to an individual or a program is foolhardy and will never create a culture of shared values. It bears repeating that meeting the law's demands (compliance) is only the base expectation for an organization. An ethical organization, through its managers, holds itself to a higher standard of performance. Larson noted this in the following excerpt:

> Take the example of a homeless person who repeatedly comes into the ER for care. Compliance dictates only that the patient be stabilized, then released or transferred. Ethics ask us: What can we do for this patient? . . . Do we pass the buck or is it our turn? Should we do

more? Compliance is the minimum, but ethics mean addressing all that is necessary.[29]

Managers must work to establish and nurture a largely risk-free culture in which problems of nonfeasance, malfeasance, or misfeasance are easily communicated and action taken. Such a culture is the ounce of prevention that is worth a pound of cure. The acculturation begins in the recruitment and selection processes and continues with new employee orientation. Later, it must be reinforced by the example of formal and informal leaders. The importance of example setting from the governing body down through all of the management ranks cannot be overstated.

This culture of responsibility, openness, and commitment on the part of management is essential to developing a meaningful internal policy on whistleblowing. Also essential is drafting the principles and policy statements that apply management's intention throughout the organization and communicating the policy to employees. The importance of middle and line managers must be stressed. Not only must they be knowledgeable about the policy but also evaluation must ensure their adherence to it.

Identifying, communicating, and solving problems are made easier if fear and fault finding are removed from the equation, an approach consistent with the philosophy of W. Edwards Deming. Even Deming recognized that a small percentage of problems is caused by the employee but that the greatest gain in quality will occur by improving the process. In the case of impairment because of substance abuse or other willful acts with negative effect, however, focusing on the individual is a necessary first step.

ASSESSING AND IMPROVING QUALITY OF CARE

Through their organizations, health services managers are charged with the weighty responsibility of assessing and improving the quality of patient care. Managers cannot directly assess clinical quality but are ethically bound to support and encourage the efforts of experts who can. Sometimes, managers must stimulate quality assessment and corrective action. More important, managers are key in leading the organization to adopt the philosophy and concepts of quality improvement and to apply its methods.

Consistent with the manager's duties of beneficence and nonmaleficence—as well as virtues such as courage, compassion, discernment, and conscientiousness—is to discourage or actively oppose establishing or continuing clinical services that expose patients to unnecessary clinical risk. One source of risk occurs when health services organizations perform low volumes of a surgical procedure or treat few patients with a specific medical condition. Early studies suggested that successful cardiac surgery was correlated positively with the number of procedures and that hospitals performing few procedures had poorer outcomes than hospitals performing many. Explanatory factors may have included patient acuity and a willingness to accept higher risk patients, but their contributions were not examined. Absent explanation of the differences, the studies recommended closure of low-volume/high-risk programs.[30]

Data published in the mid-1990s supported these recommendations and included physician and geographic area volumes, as well as improved outcomes and lower costs.[31] Research published in 2000, 2002, and 2003 has further supported the proposition that there is a positive relationship, albeit variable, between higher volume providers and better outcomes, including better results for high-risk patients. These studies analyzed a broad range of surgical procedures; one also showed similar benefits for high-volume site treatment of HIV.[32]

Thus, evidence of the link between volume and quality of clinical outcome continues to mount. There is a clear ethical imperative for managers whose organizations either have a low-volume service or are considering undertaking a service that is likely to remain low volume.

Higher-Risk Procedures

Teaching Hospital was established in 1907 with a grant from a wealthy local industrialist. The star of its long history of educating nurses and physicians is a surgical residency program, a key element of which is cardiac surgery. Two years ago, the cardiac surgery program was set back substantially by the death of the chief of cardiac surgery and the departure of a member of the team. Referrals declined markedly, and the volume of open heart procedures dropped to five per month. This occurred despite significant efforts to build referral volume.

The quality assessment department performs special studies for various clinical services. Recently, it reviewed mortality data from cardiac surgery and found that mortality rates were more than double the rates found in the literature. The director of quality assessment expressed concern as she discussed the report with the CEO. She noted that the literature reported an inverse relationship between mortality rates and the number of procedures performed. It seemed that technical competence could be gained only by performing a high volume of procedures.

Soon after, the CEO saw the medical director at lunch. During their conversation, the CEO asked whether he had any reason to believe that the cardiac surgery program was of lower quality than it had been in the past. The medical director replied, "As far as I know, things are fine." When she inquired as to the reason for the concern, the CEO replied that the frequency of performing cardiac procedures had declined and the literature suggested that this had implications for the quality of care. In fact, the hospital's review had confirmed this information. The medical director said she would look into it. The discussion moved to other matters.

The ethical issue for Teaching Hospital and its patients is apparent. An ethical problem exists because patients undergoing cardiac surgery there are at higher risk than they would be in a high-volume hospital, and this violates the principle of nonmaleficence. The CEO may not ignore what is happening; to do so is inconsistent with the manager's role as a moral agent as well as that of a professional with an independent duty to protect patients. What is the next step? Discontinuing the program immediately may be politically and economically impossible, but steps must be taken now to gain the support of the medical staff and to apprise the governing body of the problem. Whether or not the medical staff lends its support, the CEO must urge the governing body to suspend the program.

What happens if working within the organization proves fruitless because no one will listen? What if the problem is acknowledged but those in authority will not act? This situation is a significant test of the manager's ethic because it poses a true ethical dilemma: The manager is confronted with conflicting moral duties. On the one hand, information about the cardiac surgery program is confidential and the manager has a duty of loyalty to the organization. On the other hand, organization inaction places patients at special risk. Weighing these conflicting duties should lead the manager to conclude that the higher duty is that of protecting patients. The manager must press and pursue, even to the point of releasing information outside the organization if corrective action is not taken. Going public with such damaging information (whistleblowing) is a last resort and an act of great moral courage. External whistleblowing will make the manager a pariah in the organization, someone likely to be terminated for what will be seen as an act of betrayal.

The CEO might consider two other options that are more pragmatic but ethically less desirable. One option is to ignore the short-term implications of the decline in quality of care and find ways to build on program strengths to increase volume and quality. Another option is to determine the types of procedures with better results and focus on performing them. Both approaches place patients at unnecessary risk. This option seems unconscionable in terms of the virtues of caring, trustworthiness, and integrity, and the principles of beneficence and nonmaleficence. Absent an emergency or triage situation, one cannot justify the harm to some (patients) because of benefit to others (surgeons and residents; hospital income and status). Using patients as a means to an end is morally wrong.

Other clinical quality issues go beyond reviewing and ensuring a clinician's competence. These include ensuring the adequacy of support staff and equipment, evaluating the patient's clinical appropriateness for a procedure, and acting when a clinician's abilities decline. Often, the problem is apparent only retrospectively. Some processes allow concurrent quality control, however, and it should be used.

Operating Beyond His Skill?

Jim Hudson picked up the form that had been delivered by the operating room (OR) scheduling clerk and began to review the procedures scheduled for 2 days hence. Hudson's job is to ensure that surgical packs, equipment, time, and personnel are adequate to meet the demands of any scheduled surgery. The list included a procedure that Hudson had never seen scheduled before. Looking at the column that showed whether special equipment was needed, Hudson saw a note that the attending surgeon would provide the items. This notation puzzled him because it was the responsibility of the OR supervisor or the purchasing department to provide everything needed for a surgical procedure. Hudson called the chief of surgery, to whom OR staff reported clinically. He was unavailable, but his secretary promised he would return the call.

When the chief of surgery called, he was noncommittal. "If the procedure is scheduled," he said, "it's probably okay for it to be done." The clear implication was that the surgeon would not perform a procedure with inadequate preparation.

Hudson was not sure what to do. Not being a physician, any further action by him would certainly be seen as meddling. Nevertheless, further checking is crucial.

This case focuses on a problem of clinical quality. Hudson must do more than ponder the problem. Hudson should query the attending surgeon, and if that does not produce satisfactory information, the problem should be taken higher up the administrative hierarchy. Additional information may clear up the questions; it may also cause the procedure to be canceled.

To obtain routine information on quality of services, health services organizations establish systems to review the content of clinical and administrative activities. Table 2 shows examples of quality measures. The two have many parallels. It should be stressed, however, that these are primarily

Table 2.   Some measures of hospital quality

Feature	Measures of patient care quality	Measures of administrative quality
Structure	Accreditation	Accreditation
	Medical staff qualifications	Administrative staff qualifications
	Professional staff qualifications	Employee development programs
	Professional staff training	Staff per occupied bed
	Special care unit availability/ utilization	Services provided
Process	Medical staff peer review	Use of management studies
	Average length of stay	Occupancy rate
	Autopsy rate	Management planning activities
	Community involvement	Community involvement
Outcome	Patient outcome	Cost per unit of output
	Surgical procedures assessment	Staff hours per patient-day
	Adjusted death rate	Financial stability
	Hospital-acquired infections: reported/treated	Compliance
	Malpractice suits	
Attitude	Expert evaluation of patient care	Expert evaluation of administrative performance
	Patient satisfaction (dissatisfaction)	Employee satisfaction (dissatisfaction)

From Grimes, R., & Moseley, S. (1976, Fall). An approach to an index of hospital performance. *Health Services Research, 2,* 289; adapted by permission.

objective functions and measures. The judgments and conclusions of individuals reviewing the data are also required. It is these conclusions that trigger action.

MAINTAINING RELATIONS WITH THE COMMUNITY

The health services organization is usually considered quasi-public, regardless of ownership. It has a service orientation and an ethical obligation to meet community health needs. This relationship necessitates building and retaining community confidence, and it means taking steps to act in the interests of people in the community who are as yet only potential patients. If potential patients risk acquiring an infection or are in danger because the facility is operating with physical plant or life safety code deficiencies, the organization has special obligations to them.

Protecting Patients and Community from Staff with Human Immunodeficiency Virus

Chapter 7 provided the background to the human immunodeficiency virus/ acquired immunodeficiency syndrome (HIV/AIDS) issue and set out the legal dimensions, as well as the obligations health services organizations owe to staff and physicians. Clinical developments in the 1990s allow health services organizations to treat patients with AIDS more effectively. Generally, staff are better prepared and have developed specialized clinical skills. These advances, in addition to new drugs, will increase longevity for persons with AIDS. The result will be more episodes of hospitalization as well as treatment at other types of organizations, especially nursing facilities.

The AIDS pandemic raises significant ethical issues for the organization and its managers. Protecting staff who are providing care to patients with HIV was discussed in Chapter 7. Protecting patients and staff from infected staff and maintaining the confidentiality of staff and patients with HIV/AIDS are addressed here. A critical context for analysis is that for reasons unknown, the probability that caregivers will become infected when exposed to blood and body substances from patients who are HIV positive is several magnitudes greater than that patients will become infected from caregivers who are HIV positive. With two *possible* exceptions, there are no known cases in which a caregiver with HIV has infected a patient. There have been prominently reported instances of surgeons and other physicians with frank AIDS performing exposure-prone and invasive procedures, but screening their patients found no transmission of HIV. This suggests unique aspects of HIV and the likelihood of cofactors in transmissibility as well as infectivity and progression to frank AIDS, cofactors not present in the general population. The Centers for Disease Control and Prevention (CDC) defines an invasive procedure as "surgical entry into tissues, cavities, or organs, or repair of major traumatic injuries" and identifies treatment locations and types of procedures.[33] An explanation of *exposure prone* follows:

> Characteristics of exposure-prone procedures include digital palpation of a needle tip in a body cavity or the simultaneous presence of the health care worker's fingers and a needle or other sharp instrument or object in a poorly visualized or highly confined anatomic site.[34]

These definitions make it clear that although many clinical staff will perform or participate in invasive procedures, few will undertake exposure-prone procedures. Health services organizations must take care in assigning duties to staff consistent with these definitions.

Significant, too, is that HIV may induce neuropsychiatric problems, such as impaired coordination and cognitive difficulties, that may occur before physical symptoms are apparent. Subtle diminutions in competence greatly complicate use of clinical staff who have HIV. The ethical (and legal) duty of employers to monitor staff and safeguard patients is well established.

The ethical (and legal) problems for health services organizations are complicated further by the fact that some caregivers who are HIV positive but do not have frank AIDS wish to continue treating patients. The American Medical Association (AMA) and American Dental Association (ADA) have retreated from their positions in the early 1990s, which stated that ethics *required* (emphasis added) practitioners with HIV to either inform their patients of their HIV status or refrain from performing exposure-prone invasive procedures.[35] Currently, the AMA advises physicians and other health care workers with HIV to disclose their serostatus to a state public health official or to a local review committee to establish practice limitations. The review committee will determine which activities can be continued without risk of infecting patients. The current policy recommends that physicians *should* (emphasis added) refrain from conducting exposure-prone invasive procedures or "perform such procedures with permission of the local review committee and the informed consent of the patient. HIV-infected physicians . . . must err on the side of protecting patients."[36] The ADA's approach is similar:

> A dentist who becomes ill from any disease or impaired in any way shall, with consultation and advice from a qualified physician or other authority, limit the activities of practice to those areas that do not endanger the patients or members of the dental staff.[37]

Most states require patient notification for exposure-prone invasive procedures when the physician is HIV positive; many also require notification for invasive procedures that are not exposure prone.[38]

In meeting their ethical duties, clinical staff should want to know whether they pose a risk to patients and other staff. Because of the opportunistic diseases they contract as HIV progresses to frank AIDS, infected staff may pose a risk to patients, many of whom are immunocompromised or physically weakened. Staff members with AIDS may also pose risks to other employees and to visitors. These risks should cause managers to err in favor of caution in assigning staff. As staff who are HIV positive become increasingly immunocompromised, infectious diseases common in health services organizations will pose risks to them. If the organization is to discharge its ethical obligations to staff, it must be able to consider such information in job assignment. Given how much is *not* known about trans-missibility of the virus, staff who are HIV positive should be encouraged to accept nonpatient care assignments. Physicians who wish to continue performing exposure-prone invasive procedures pose a special problem, but as noted in Chapter 7, the law is generally well settled. Given the unknown but possible risk to patients, it is prudent to prohibit physicians and other staff who are HIV positive from performing exposure-prone invasive procedures, as reasonably defined. Protecting confidentiality to the greatest extent possible is crucial to the success of any such effort.

Despite some legal uncertainty, health services organizations should know the HIV status of all staff who engage in exposure-prone invasive procedures. It is ethically appropriate (and legally prudent) to prohibit those who are HIV positive from performing exposure-prone invasive procedures, a policy consistent with CDC guidelines. Such a rule meets the ethical principle of nonmaleficence, which is that the caregiver's first duty is "do no harm." That there have been only two cases of HIV transmission from care giver to patient—one is "confirmed" but challenged and the other is "not entirely conclusive"—suggests that the risk of being infected by a health care worker with HIV is infinitesimally small.

The CDC has determined that dentist David Acer infected six patients with HIV. It is still unknown how he transmitted the virus to them. Acer was confirmed as the source after investigators found that the patients' HIV contained genetic material matching his and learning that he did not follow infection-control procedures.[39] The CDC maintains that its investigation was competent and thorough in all respects. There is, how-ever, evidence suggesting that the infected patients had unreported and undetected risk factors for HIV and that the molecular analyses used to determine that Acer and his patients had the same strains of HIV had potentially serious flaws.[40] Since the Acer case in 1990, the CDC has evaluated 22,000 patients of 63 physicians, surgeons, and dentists with HIV and found no similar cases of transmission in the United States.[41]

In early 1999, a French study provided strong evidence that an infected orthopedic surgeon transmitted HIV to a patient during surgery. Of the almost 1,000 patients on whom the orthopedist had performed surgery who were tested, only one had contracted HIV. "The evidence . . . is not entirely conclusive, but provider-to-patient transmission during orthope-dic surgery is the most plausible explanation for the . . . infection."[42]

The CDC has estimated that the risk that an infected surgeon will transmit HIV during an exposure-prone invasive procedure is between 1 in 40,000 and 1 in 400,000 and that the risk of transmission from an infected dentist is between 1 in 200,000 and 1 in 2,000,000.[43] By way of context, hepatitis B virus (HBV) is a greater threat to patients than HIV. In 1996, a thoracic surgeon was found to have transmitted HBV to 19 patients during surgery despite evidence that he used adequate infection control procedures.[44] This incident, plus that of a Spanish cardiac surgeon who infected five of his patients with hepatitis C (HCV), supports mandatory testing for HBV, HCV, and HIV among caregivers who perform exposure-prone invasive procedures.[45]

Something Must Be Done, But What?

Stunned, Carolyn Aubrey, the CEO of Metropolitan Hospital, sank into her chair and stared out the window for a very long time. She realized that something was afoul when Dr. Midmore's wife had angrily insisted on seeing the CEO. Even in her worst nightmares Aubrey had never imagined that Mrs. Midmore would tell Aubrey that she was suing her husband, an orthopedic surgeon, for divorce because he had given her AIDS. As Mrs. Midmore left Aubrey's office, she had turned back and said, "I was sure you'd want to know. Surely you'll have to do something."

Aubrey thought Mrs. Midmore's statements might be nothing more than the ravings of an angry, vindictive wife, but that was not likely. As she considered what she had just learned, she recalled an incident several years ago involving Dr. Midmore and a male orderly. In retrospect, it suggested that Dr. Midmore might be bisexual. Aubrey also thought about the department of surgery meeting last year when there had been a long discussion about the desirability of knowing the HIV status of all surgical patients. The special risks to surgeons of torn gloves and cuts during orthopedic surgery had been described in detail.

Now it seemed that Dr. Midmore's patients might be at risk. Aubrey called operating room scheduling and learned that Dr. Midmore was maintaining a full surgical load. Aubrey asked her secretary to call the hospital attorney and the medical director and set up an emergency meeting for 7:00 the following morning. Mrs. Midmore had been right, thought Aubrey. We'll have to do something, but what?

This case suggests several ethical (and legal) issues. Protecting patients is key, and Midmore's surgical privileges must be suspended immediately. Once Midmore no longer poses a risk to patients, further action can follow in an orderly and deliberate manner. Meeting the principle of justice requires that the investigation be fair to Midmore in terms of process and substance. If Midmore is HIV positive, the hospital may choose from two courses of action: 1) allow Midmore to continue performing surgery if he follows CDC guidelines that physicians who are HIV positive notify their patients before performing exposure-prone invasive procedures or 2) terminate Midmore's surgical privileges. The first choice maximizes patient autonomy, but the hospital must ensure that Midmore actually informs patients that he is HIV positive and that patients understand the implications of this information. As a practical matter, few patients are likely to allow him to perform their surgery after learning his HIV status. The second choice meets the principle of nonmaleficence by preventing potential harm to patients but is paternalistic by not allowing Midmore's patients to make their own choice. Prudence, however, demands terminating his surgical privileges. All actions must be consistent with protecting patients and meeting the requirements of the medical staff bylaws and state and federal law.

Confidentiality regarding Dr. Midmore's HIV status must be safeguarded. Such efforts can never compromise patient safety, however. The issue of confidentiality takes on further complexity if Midmore leaves the staff and applies for surgical privileges elsewhere. The hospital is ethically bound to communicate what it has learned in the course of its investigation.

Maintaining Confidentiality   Health services organizations must be alert to the special problems of confidentiality when treating patients with HIV/AIDS. Within the constraints of state law, however, the first obligation must be to safeguard staff and other patients. Identifying patients who are HIV positive may be an important additional stimulus that will encourage staff to comply with universal precautions.

Early in the HIV/AIDS epidemic, it was asserted that identifying patients as HIV positive would lead to a two-class medical system. This prediction has proved baseless. The potential for this problem has existed since HIV was first identified and patient charts and rooms were marked with biohazard notices and other less transparent codes. Thus far, there is no evidence that the HIV positive or those with AIDS receive care different from that accorded other patients.

Protecting staff confidentiality to the greatest extent possible is crucial to the success of any such effort and, consistent with the ethical principle of respect for persons, health services organizations must be alert to the special problems of confidentiality when treating patients with AIDS. Within legal constraints, however, the organization's first obligation is to safeguard staff and other patients.

HIV/AIDS is only one of numerous infectious disease that raise ethical (and legal) problems for health services organizations and their managers. The experience of University Hospital suggests another.

Protecting the Community

University Hospital plays a unique role in the community. It is a tertiary referral hospital for the region and a major source of health care to the community.

In 1977, it experienced an outbreak of legionnella (Legionnaires' disease). A number of patients contracted the disease; several died.

Legionnella is a bacterial infection of the respiratory tract and lungs that may result in death if not diagnosed and treated early. It is especially dangerous for older adults and people with medical problems that weaken their general resistance. A factor requiring even greater caution on the part of hospital management is that at the time of the outbreaks, the process for identifying the organism in the laboratory took several days. Thus, patients were at greater risk until a confirmatory diagnosis was obtained.

Epidemiological studies showed a relationship between the fine aerosol mist that the hospital's air conditioning cooling tower gave off and the spread of the disease through the aerosol. Employees exposed directly to the aerosol contracted severe cases of legionnella. Chlorinating the water in the cooling towers eliminates the organism. Although the cooling tower was suspected in the 1977 outbreak at University Hospital, the relationship was never confirmed. The hospital's infection control committee did not develop any standing orders or policies after the first outbreak.

In May 1982, there was evidence of another outbreak of legionnella. The cooling tower water was immediately chlorinated and the number of new cases dropped dramatically. However, an undetected failure in the chlorination system brought a second outbreak in early June.

When the first cases were detected in May 1982, the hospital administrator was notified. He met with various staff members, including physicians. It was decided that information about the outbreak should be kept from the community, lest a panic and sudden drop in patient census occur, as well as loss of public confidence. A confidential letter was sent to staff physicians advising them of the problem and asking that they keep in mind the potential for infection when making admissions decisions. Admissions were not limited to emergencies, however, and there was neither a prospective review of elective admissions to determine whether patients at risk for pulmonary infections such as legionnella should be sent elsewhere nor a review of indications for and necessity of admission. The medical staff developed a protocol stating that unexplained, acute-onset pneumonias were to be treated immediately with a potent antibiotic known to be effective against legionnella. However, no provision was made for effective review to determine that the protocol was actually followed.

The administrator at University Hospital faced several problems, all with ethical dimensions:

1. The medical staff wanted to continue elective admissions.

2. The community could lose confidence in the hospital if it learned that there was an epidemic of a potentially deadly disease.

3. The administrator and management staff could lose face, even their jobs, should the infection become common knowledge.

4. There was potential legal liability.

Solving this ethical problem is difficult but not impossible. Similar situations arise in nursing facilities that are threatened with closure because their physical plants violate fire safety requirements and in hospitals in which outbreaks of meningitis or salmonella occur in the nursery. How does the organization protect current as well as potential patients in such situations? More important, what is the manager's role?

One feature that distinguishes this legionnella outbreak from other, similar cases is the difference in duty owed to potential rather than actual patients. The law recognizes a difference. Generally, unless there is a special relationship with potential patients, one has no duty to act on their behalf. In this case, however, there would be a duty to warn elective admissions who are at risk from legionnella.

The legal distinction is useful in ethical analysis. The duty toward actual patients is immediate and more compelling than the duty owed potential patients. Potential patients should be put at risk of legionnella only if their medical condition puts them at greater risk outside the hospital. Inpatients who might benefit from a continued stay but who are at greater risk by remaining in the hospital should be discharged. It is incumbent on the managerial and clinical staff to make caregivers understand the obligation to protect the patient.

The argument that the administrator has a duty to protect the reputation of the organization in the community has merit because individuals needing hospitalization should have no fear about receiving it and because of the significant psychological component in health care. Furthermore, individuals may be at greater risk by not obtaining treatment for their medical problems than they are from legionnella. Yet, they may defer care because they are frightened or lack confidence in the facility.

On admission, potential risk becomes actual risk. Emergency admissions pose no ethical problem if an alternative source of care is unavailable and the risk of no care is greater than that of harm from contracting legionnella.

Elective admissions are quite different, however. At the very least, the organization, led and prompted by its managers, should have developed and applied policies and procedures separating high- from low-risk elective admissions and made special provisions either to send the former group elsewhere or to take special precautions regarding them. Ethically, it could not rely only on the discretion of the admitting physician. As with any quality assessment activity, management has a responsibility to review decision making about care and do so in a fashion consistent with the level of risk. Here, concurrent review is required.

Obvious potential conflicts of interest exist. It is natural for managers to protect their positions and reputations. They do so out of loyalty to the organization but also out of selfish motives. A typical response is to cover up. Concealment seems an easy way to reduce the risk of personal and professional damage. Experience suggests, however, that from both an ethical and a pragmatic standpoint honesty is the best policy. Rumors will be carried into the community by staff and patients, and the potential tarnish to the organization's reputation may last much longer than if the community is informed that there is a problem and that steps are being taken to protect patients from infection. This tactic may raise questions about the cause of and responsibility for the problem, but the community will not distrust the organization. Furthermore, in terms of guiding ethical principles, the organization must treat individuals in the community with respect and dignity by being truthful, and managers must live by the virtues of trustworthiness and conscientiousness.

CONCLUSION

Just as they rely on computer programmers or wage and salary experts for reports, advice, and counsel, health services managers rely on technical expertise and assistance to monitor, review, and maintain the quality of clinical activities. Managers provide clinical staff with the systems, procedures, and resources needed to be effective in delivering and monitoring clinical services. Beneficence and nonmaleficence—as well as the virtues of compassion, caring, and courage—demand that managers are sufficiently aware of what is expected and how that expectation is measured to determine that the goal of delivering quality health services is being met. Managers are remiss in meeting their ethical (and legal) duties if they occupy themselves exclusively with nonclinical activities and claim that clinical matters lie outside their ken and range of responsibilities. The manager is accountable to the governing body for all activities, and this requires active involvement and effective partnerships between managers and clinicians.

This chapter identified and examined several generic ethical problems arising from the duties owed by managers to patients and community. The duties are not always clear and may be further obscured by accompanying problems, such as bureaucratic inertia and medical staff relations. They become clear if managers focus on the primary reasons for the organization's existence—serving and protecting the patient and community.

NOTES

1. Peter A. Ubel, Margaret M. Zell, David J. Miller, Gary S. Fischer, Darien Peters-Stefani, & Robert M. Arnold. (1995, August). Elevator talk: Observational study of inappropriate comments in a public space. *American Journal of Medicine, 99,* pp. 190–194; Simone N. Vigod, Chaim M. Bell, & John M.A. Bohnen. (2003, November 1). Privacy of patients' information in hospital lifts: Observational study. *British Medical Journal, 327,* pp. 1024–1025.

2. Amy Daoust. (2002, May 23). Privacy breach: VA patients' records fund on surplus computers. *Industry Beat Archive.* Retrieved December 3, 2003, from http://www.superiorconsultant.com/Pressroom/superiorHealth/Industry Beat/2002/052302_Privacy.asp

3. HortySpringer. (2003, July 10). *Question of the week.* Retrieved July 2003 from http://www.hortyspringer.com

4. Steve S. Kraman & Ginny Hamm. (1999, December 21). Risk management: Extreme honesty may be the best policy. *Annals of Internal Medicine, 131*(12), pp. 963–967.

5. Joint Commission on Accreditation of Healthcare Organizations. (2004). Ethics, Rights, and Responsibilities. In *Hospital Accreditation Standards* (p. 110). Oakbrook Terrace, IL: Author.

6. Albert W. Wu, Thomas A. Cavanaugh, Stephen J. McPhee, Bernard Lo, & Guy P. Micco. (1997, December). To tell the truth: Ethical and practical issues in disclosing medical mistakes to patients. *Journal of General Internal Medicine, 12,* pp. 770–775.

7. James S. Bowman, Frederick A. Elliston, & Paula Lockhart (Eds.). (1984). *Professional dissent: An annotated bibliography and research guide: Vol. 2* (p. 3). New York: Garland Publishing.

8. Alan F. Westin. (1981). *Whistle blowing! Loyalty and dissent in the corporation* (p. 140). New York: McGraw-Hill.

9. *Ibid.,* p. 139.

10. *Ibid.,* p. 140.

11. *Ibid.*

12. Whistle-blowing. (2001). *The Columbia Encyclopedia* (6th ed.) [as cited on Bartleby.com]. Retrieved November 7, 2003, from http://www.bartleby.com/65/wh/whistlebl.html

13. Qui Tam FYI. (2003.) *What is the reward for blowing the whistle on fraudulent action?* Retrieved November 7, 2003, from http://www.quitamfyi.com/whistleblower_rewards.html

14. Shelley R. Slade. (2000, August 23). *Health care fraud: How far does the False Claims Act reach?* Retrieved November 7, 2003, from http://www.quackwatch.org/02ConsumerProtection/fca.html

15. Pierce v. Ortho Pharmaceuticals, 84 NJ. 58, 417 A.2d 505 (1980).
16. O'Sullivan v. Mallon et al., 160 NJ. Super. 416, 390 A.2d 149 (1978).
17. Commonwealth of Pennsylvania ex rel. Rafferty et al. v. Philadelphia Psychiatric Center, 356 R Supp. 500 (E.D. Pa. 1973).
18. Louise Kertesz. (1995, July 3). Execs fired in whistleblower case. *Modern Healthcare*, p. 11.
19. Lisa Scott. (1995, August 21). Whistleblower suit alleges patient records doctored. *Modern Healthcare*, p. 34. Another example of a *qui tam* suit occurred in *United States ex rel. Brandimarte v. Wurtzel*, Civ. Action No. 94-2398 (E.D. Pa. Nov. 3, 1995), in which defendants settled allegations of making false and fraudulent claims for psychotherapy services under the Medicare and Medicaid programs by paying $500,000 to the United States government and $50,000 toward whistleblower's legal fees and costs.
20. Berkeley Rice. (1995, August 7). When a doctor accuses colleagues of health fraud. *Medical Economics*, pp. 172–174, 177–179, 183–184, 189–190.
21. Qui Tam FYI.
22. Lawrence Blades. (1967, December). Employment at will vs. individual freedom: On limiting the abusive exercise of employer power. *Columbia Law Review*, 67, p. 1407.
23. Westin, pp. 133–136.
24. Bowman et al., p. 4.
25. Westin, p. 144.
26. Stephen Barr. (1993, October 19). Whistleblowers sound alarm on their superiors' reprisals. *The Washington Post*, p. A21.
27. U.S. Merit Systems Protection Board. (1998). *Adherence to the merit principles in the workplace: Federal employees' views* (p. 12). Washington, D.C.: Author.
28. John P. Keenan & C.A. Krueger. (1992). Whistleblowing and the professional. *Management Accounting*, pp. 21–24.
29. Laurie Larson. (1999, September). The right thing to do: An ethical framework helps trustees lead the way. *Trustee*, 59(2), p. 10.
30. Edward L. Hannan, Joseph E. O'Donnell, Harold Kilburn, Jr., Harvey R. Bernard, & Altan Yazici. (1989, July). Investigation of the relationship between volume and mortality for surgical procedures performed in New York State hospitals. *Journal of the American Medical Association*, 262(4), pp. 503–510; Harold S. Luft, John P. Bunker, & Alain C. Enthoven. (1979, December). Should operations be regionalized? *The New England Journal of Medicine*, 301(25), pp. 1364–1369; Spencer Rich. (1984, April 26). Hospitals doing more operations lose fewer patients. *The Washington Post*, p. A2.
31. Regionalizing cardiac surgery facilities contributes to improved outcomes and lower costs. (1996, January/February). *Research Activities 190*, pp. 1–2; Volume of procedures for physicians, hospitals, and geographic areas linked to outcomes for angioplasty and bypass patients. (1995, July/August). *Research Activities, 186*, pp. 1–3.
32. John D. Birkmeyer, Andrea E. Siewers, Emily V.A. Finlayson, Therese A. Stukel, F. Lee Lucas, Ida Batista, H. Gilbert Welch, & David E. Wennberg. (2002, April 11). Hospital volume and surgical mortality in the United States. *The New England Journal of Medicine 346*(15), pp. 1128–1137; R. Adams

Dudley, Kirsten L. Johanson, Richard Brand, Deborah J. Rennie, & Arnold Milstein. (2000, March 1). Selective referral to high-volume hospitals: Estimating potentially avoidable deaths. *Journal of the American Medical Association 283*(9), pp. 1159–1166; Philip P. Goodney, F.L. Lucas, & John D. Birkmeyer. (2003). Should volume standards for cardiovascular surgery focus only on high-risk patients? *Circulation, 107*, pp. 384–387.

33. Recommendations for preventing transmission of human immunodeficiency virus and hepatitis B virus to patients during exposure-prone invasive procedures. (1991, July 12). *MMWR Recommendations and Reports.* Retrieved January 23, 2004, from http://www.cdc.gov/mmwr/preview/mmwrhtml/00014845.htm. An invasive procedure is defined as "surgical entry into tissues, cavities, or organs, or repair of traumatic injuries" associated with any of the following: 1) an operating or delivery room, emergency department, or outpatient setting, including both physicians' and dentists' offices; 2) cardiac catheterization and angiographic procedures; 3) vaginal or cesarean delivery or other invasive obstetric procedure during which bleeding may occur; or 4) the manipulation, cutting, or removal of any oral or perioral tissues, including tooth structure, during which bleeding occurs or the potential for bleeding exists.

34. *Ibid.*

35. Ronald Bayer. (1991, May). The HIV-infected clinician: To exclude or not exclude? *Trustee 44*(5), p. 16.

36. American Medical Association. (2001, December). *Report 4 of the Council on Scientific Affairs (A-03), Consolidation of the AMA House Policies on HIV/AIDS* (p. 8). Chicago: Author.

37. American Dental Association. (2003). *Resource manual for support of dentists with HBV, HIV, TB and other infectious disease.* Retrieved March 25, 2004, from http://www.ada.org/prof/resources/topics/hiv/legal.asp

38. How to balance interests of physician, patients, and your organization when physician is HIV-positive. (2003, August). *Credentialing & Peer Review Legal Insider*, p. 1.

39. Joyce Price. (1996, February 9). 2 of 6 who got HIV from dentist are alive. *The Washington Times*, p. A7.

40. Stephen Barr. (1996, January 15). The 1990 Florida dental investigation: Is the case really closed? *Annals of Internal Medicine, 124*(2), pp. 250–254.

41. Centers for Disease Control and Prevention. (1999, July). *HIV and its transmission.* http://www.cdc.gov/hiv/pubs/facts/transmission.htm

42. Susan Okie. (1999, January 12). French surgeon gave a patient AIDS virus. *The Washington Post/Health*, p. 9.

43. Bayer, p. 17.

44. Rafael Harpaz, Lorenz von Seidlein, Francisco M. Averhoff, Michael P. Tormey, Saswati D. Sinha, Konstantina Kotsopoulou, Stephen B. Lambert, Betty H. Robertson, James D. Cherry, & Craig N. Shapiro. (1996, February 29). Transmission of hepatitis B virus to multiple patients from a surgeon without evidence of inadequate infection control. *The New England Journal of Medicine 334*(9), pp. 549–554.

45. Juan I. Esteban, Jordi Gomez, Maria Martell, Beatriz Cabot, Josep Quer, Joan Camps, Antonio Gonzalez, Teresa Otero, Andres Moya, Rafael Esteban, & Jaime Guardia. (1996, February 29). Transmission of hepatitis C virus by a cardiac surgeon. *The New England Journal of Medicine 334*(9), pp. 555–559.

SECTION IV

BIOMEDICAL ETHICAL ISSUES

Section IV analyzes consent and issues at the end of life, the biomedical ethical issues most commonly confronted by health services managers and their organizations. Myriad other biomedical ethical issues affect some managers: genetic engineering, screening, and counseling; reproductive technologies; psychosurgery and behavior control; the right to health care; personhood, fetal rights, and abortion; implants and transplants; and mental illness and involuntary commitment.

The thorny issue of consent is addressed in Chapter 9. Consent affects managers in all types of health services organizations. The law defines acceptable relationships between provider and patient; for managers this is but a starting point, one that builds on their moral agency and the organization's expected philosophy.

Chapter 10 addresses ethical issues arising at the end of life, often called the *ethics of dying and death*. Changes occurring since the 1970s, many caused by new technology, raise new questions. The chapter includes ways of defining death, the application of life-sustaining treatment (using the example of infants with impairments), the withdrawal of treatment, futility policies and guidelines, and the ethics of terminal illnesses. Health services organizations are affected by some or all of the ethical issues that arise at the end of life. As with consent, there are major implications for managers.

Chapter 11 explores the relationships among physician-assisted suicide (PAS), autonomy, and the organization. PAS is an ethical issue with deep historic roots in medical practice, even though it is prohibited by the Hippocratic tradition. Links to European views and actions regarding PAS are explored.

CHAPTER 9

CONSENT

C onsent is an ethical imperative of great importance to managers and clinicians. In the early 1980s research by the President's Commission for the Study of Ethical Problems in Medicine and Biomedical and Behavioral Research made it clear that patients want more involvement in medical decision making, a finding that suggests both a problem and a goal for health services providers.

The concept of consent in medical care evolved to protect patients from nonconsensual touching. Although the ethical and legal dimensions overlap, the legal requirements of consent are minimal. The ethics of consent are grounded in the principle of respect for persons, specifically the element of autonomy, which reflects a view of the equality and dignity of human beings. In addition, the ethics of consent reflect the special relationship of trust and confidence between physician and patient and between organization and patient. This fiduciary relationship is supported by the principles of beneficence and nonmaleficence. The manager's virtues of trustworthiness, honesty, integrity, and candor also support the ethics of consent.

According to the law, failure to obtain consent can support a legal action for battery, an intentional tort. Beyond this, an action for negligence can be brought if the physician breaches the duty to communicate information necessary for the patient to give informed consent.

Paternalism stems from beneficence and is the ethical value that competes with patient autonomy in implementing consent. Paternalism arises naturally from the relationship between physician and patient because psychologically, technically, and emotionally, the physician is in a position of superior knowledge and is expected to choose the best course of action for the patient. This reflects the ethics of care discussed in Chapter 1. The paternalism inherent in the physician–patient relationship was first described in the Hippocratic oath. Beneficence, nonmaleficence, and paternalism continue to be important, implicit elements of the practice of medicine. The revisions of the Principles of Medical Ethics adopted by the American Medical Association (AMA) in 1980 moved organized medicine from paternalism toward autonomy and patient rights, themes that continued in the 2001 revision. The AMA's Council on Ethical and Judicial Affairs amplified these themes by its statement Fundamental Elements of the Patient–Physician Relationship. This document and the 2001 Principles of Medical Ethics are reproduced in Appendix B.

Specialized codes, such as the Declaration of Helsinki, which guide biomedical research, also recognize the importance of consent. The emphasis on patients' rights or sovereignty in documents such as these are ideals toward which managers and organizations should strive.

LEGAL ASPECTS

Legally, consent must be voluntary, competent, and informed. The law presumes that persons unable to give consent in an emergency want to receive treatment. The presumption of wanting treatment can be rebutted if it is declined by a competent patient or if the person requiring treatment has an advance directive, such as a nonhospital do-not-resuscitate order. In addition, if that person's attorney-in-fact (e.g., someone who holds a durable power of attorney) is present, consent must be obtained. When minors or persons considered mentally incompetent are patients and those who speak for them refuse to give consent when withholding treatment is not in the patients' best interests, the organization is usually successful in persuading a court to order treatment.

Even in nonemergencies, general consent for treatment is implied by the patient's presence and apparent desire to be treated. Noninvasive elective treatment of a routine nature requires only general consent. Special consent is necessary, however, for invasive, surgical, or special procedures, or when the patient is part of an experiment. Consent for the invasive procedures common in intensive care units is problematic, for example, especially because they are often performed as emergencies and patients may not be able, or their surrogates may not be available, to give informed consent.[1] Oral consent is legally binding, but staff changes, faulty memories, and prudence dictate consent in writing. The George Washington University Medical Center's general and special consent forms are shown in Figures 8 and 9, respectively.

To be *voluntary*, consent must be given free of duress. Whether duress is present depends on the facts, but threats or force constitute duress. Persons with diminished autonomy are unable to make voluntary choices;

PATIENT AUTHORIZATION FORM

80010

PATIENT IDENTIFICATION

GENERAL POLICY: All patients shall be treated, admitted and assigned accommodation without distinction to race, religion, color, national origin, sexual orientation, age or handicapping condition.

CONSENT TO TREATMENT: I have come to The George Washington University Hospital for medical treatment. I ask the health care professionals at the Hospital to provide care and treatment for me that they feel is necessary. The undersigned consents to the procedures, which may be performed during this hospitalization, or on an outpatient basis including emergency treatment or services. I consent to undergo routine tests and treatment as part of this care. These may include but are not limited to laboratory, radiology, medical or surgical tests, treatments, anesthesia or procedures as directed under the general and special instruction of the physician or surgeon. I understand that I am free to ask a member of my health care team questions about any care, treatment or medicine I am to receive. Because The George Washington University Hospital is a teaching hospital, I understand that my health care team will be made up of hospital personnel (to include nurses, technicians, and ancillary staff) under the direction of my attending physician and his/her assistants and designees (to include interns, residents, fellows and medical students). I am aware that the practice of medicine is not an exact science and admit that no one has given me any promises or guarantees about the result of any care or treatment I am to receive or examinations I am to undergo.

PHYSICIANS NOT AS EMPLOYEES: I understand that each physician is an independant contractor who is self employed and is not the agent, servant or employee of the hospital. I understand that I may receive separate billing from each of these providers for services rendered.

_____initials

RELEASE OF INFORMATION: The George Washington University Hospital is authorized to release any information necessary, including copies of my hospital and medical records, to process payment claims for health care services which have been provided, and to duly authorized local and federal regulatory agencies and accrediting bodies as required or permitted by law. George Washington University Hospital is further authorized to release demographic information to organizations performing patient satisfaction surveys. Such records may include information of a psychological or psychiatric nature, pertaining to my mental condition or treatment for conditions relating to the use of alcohol or drugs. In addition, I authorize my insurance carrier, employer or person otherwise responsible for payment to provide The George Washington University Hospital information necessary to determine benefits or process a claim. This release will be valid for the period of time to process the claim or until consent is revoked by myself. I release and forever discharge The George Washington University Hospital, its employees and agents, and my attending physician from any liability resulting from the release of my medical records or information from them for payment purposes. I understand that my name will be displayed in the signage system outside my hospital room.

PERSONAL VALUABLES: THE GEORGE WASHINGTON UNIVERSITY HOSPITAL WILL NOT BE RESPONSIBLE FOR LOSS OR DAMAGE TO CLOTHES, PERSONAL PROPERTY OR VALUABLES.

NON-SMOKING POLICY: In accordance with regulatory agency standards, the Hospital is a non-smoking facility.

FINANCIAL AGREEMENT/ASSIGNMENT OF BENEFITS: I assign any and all insurance benefits payable to me to The George Washington University Hospital. I understand that I am responsible for payment for services rendered at the Hospital including excluded services from my insurance either because the plan deems such services not medically necessary, or for any other reason including pre-certification requirements, second opinions or preexisting conditions. Should the account be referred to any attorney or collection agency for collection, I understand that I will be responsible for attorney or collection expenses. I give permission to my insurance provider(s), including Medicare and Medicaid, to directly pay The George Washington University Hospital for my care instead of paying me. I understand that I am responsible for any health insurance deductibles and co-insurance and non-covered services.

I, the undersigned, state that the information that I have provided The George Washington University Hospital is correct to the best of my knowledge. I acknowledge by my signature that I have read and received a copy of this statement. I understand that by signing it, I am agreeing to it.

X _____
       Signature of patient or responsible party

Unable to sign
( ) Serious Condition
( ) _____

_____   _____   _____   _____
Date   Witness   Hospital Representative   Date

ADVANCE DIRECTIVE (Only If Inpatient, Day Surgery, or Emergency Room Visits)
Do you have an Advance Directive
   (Living Will/Health Care Power of Attorney)?   __ Yes __ No
If yes, did you bring it with you?   __ Yes __ No
If you did not bring it with you, is there
someone we can contact to obtain a copy?   __ Yes __ No
Name _____ Tel. _____
Your Advanced Directive wishes must be on your chart.

By my signature below, I consent to laboratory studies (HIV, HBV, HCV) in the event a health care worker is exposed to my blood or body fluids. I also agree to the disposal or use of any tissue or part removed from my body and/or to the taking of photographs during my treatment for research, teaching, or scientific purposes as long as my identity is not disclosed.

80-010 (1/03)

MEDICAL RECORDS

Signature _____ Date _____

Figure 8.   A general consent form. (From The George Washington University Medical Center. Copyright © 2003. Reprinted by permission.)

PATIENT'S REQUEST FOR PROCEDURE OPERATION AND TREATMENT

76519

(PATIENT IDENTIFICATION)

1. I, _____ PATIENT _____ (, or _____ as ☐ Parent   ☐ Representative
   _____ ☐ Guardian   (Check One)
   acting on his/her behalf,) request the procedure/operation/treatment set out below.

2. I have requested Dr(s). _____ perform
   and supervise my procedure/operation/treatment which has been explained to me to be:

   _____

   My doctor's explanation informed me about my medical condition as well as the common foreseeable benefits and risks of the procedure/operation/treatment as well as of its reasonable alternatives, if any.

3. I know, too, that during my procedure/operation/treatment it may become apparent to my doctor that in his/her professional judgement further procedures, operations, or treatments may be necessary. I therefore authorize modification or extension of this consent to include those additional procedures which in my doctor's professional judgement are medically necessary under these special circumstances and for my benefit with the exception of (check one): ☐ type of procedure _____ ☐ no exceptions

4. I understand that if a member of the Department of Anesthesiology is to participate in my care, for general, regional, or monitored anesthesia care, a separate consent will be obtained for these services.

5. If my doctor has indicated to me that I will require a local anesthetic as part of my procedure/operation/treatment, I authorize its administration. I acknowledge that my doctor has explained the benefits and risks of my receiving a local anesthetic as well as a reasonable alternative, if any. Potential risks may include but are not limited to pain at the injection site, or very rarely allergic reaction to the anesthetic. Further, I understand that during my procedure/operation/treatment, unforeseen circumstances may require alternative methods of anesthesia, such as general, and I therefore authorize modification of anesthesia administration which my doctor's professional judgment indicates to be necessary under the circumstances.

6. If it is anticipated that I may require transfusion of blood or blood products during my procedure, I will be required to sign a separate INFORMED CONSENT TO BLOOD TRANSFUSION AND/OR BLOOD COMPONENT ADMINISTRATION form. If in the event of an unanticipated emergency during my operative care and based on the medical judgement of my physician, I require the transfusion of blood or blood products, I understand they will be administered and agree to such action being taken.

7. Knowing that the George Washington University Hospital is a teaching institution, I understand that along with my doctor and his/her assistants and designees, other Hospital personnel such as residents, trainees, nurses, and technicians will be involved in my procedure/operation/ treatment and care. I understand and agree to the presence of appropriate observers for the advancement of medical education and care.

8. I consent to appropriate routine tests and treatment as part of my medical care associated with this procedure/operation/treatment.

9. I agree to the appropriate disposal of any tissue or part removed from my body, to the taking of photographs during the procedure/operation/ treatment for research, teaching, or scientific purposes as long as my identity is not disclosed, and to participate in the _____ research protocol/program.

PATIENT AFFIRMATION

By signing this request form, I am indicating that I understand the contents of this document and agree to its provisions. I know that if I have concerns or would like more detailed information, I can ask more questions and get more information from my attending physician. I am also acknowledging that I know that the practice of anesthesiology, medicine and surgery is not an exact science and that no one has given me any promises or guarantees about the designated procedure/operation/treatment or its results. I fully understand what I am now signing of my own free will.

WITNESS TO AFFIRMATION AND SIGNATURE _____ DATE _____ TIME _____ PATIENT SIGNATURE (or Parent, Guardian or Representative) _____ DATE/TIME _____

SIGNATURE OF PHYSICIAN OBTAINING INFORMED CONSENT _____ DATE _____ TIME _____

PHYSICIAN ATTESTATION

I, Dr. _____ , attest that this patient or the representative named above has been informed about the common foreseeable risks and benefits of undergoing the procedure/operation/treatment as well as its reasonable alternative(s),if any. Further questions with regard to this procedure have been answered to his/her apparent satisfaction.

PHYSICIAN SIGNATURE _____ DATE/TIME _____

76-519 (11/97)

Figure 9.   A special consent form. (From The George Washington University Medical Center. Copyright © 1997. Reprinted by permission.)

military personnel or prisoners are examples. Historically, the military and prisoners were important for research involving human subjects. Negative publicity and public indignation virtually eliminated experimentation in such settings.

Competent consent means that the person understands the nature and consequences of the course of treatment. The law presumes minor children to be incompetent. In addition, persons whose mental illness or cognitive disability have resulted in a legal determination of incompetence may not decide about medical treatment or experimentation, and others must make such decisions. Judging mental competence is complex when patients are terminally ill, depressed, or suicidal; expert opinion is required.

Consent must be *informed*. The law requires full disclosure of the nature of the patient's condition and treatment proposed, available alternatives, and consequences and difficulties that may likely result from treatment or nontreatment. The courts are about evenly split between those holding that patients should receive as much information as the reasonable physician would provide under the same or similar circumstances and those using a standard based on what the reasonable patient would want to know. A legal criterion used by a few courts—and one oriented to patient sovereignty—is what that particular patient would have wanted to know.

Historically, cases involving Jehovah's Witnesses, a religion that prohibits even homologous (self-donation) transfusions of whole blood or components, have been problematic for hospitals. Potential legal liability for transfusing or not transfusing the patient has resulted in numerous court cases. In early cases, courts often overrode the patient's wishes and ordered transfusions when patients, especially mothers, were charged with significant family responsibilities. These cases showed that judges considered more than liberty rights (autonomy) when important societal interests were present. Developments in bloodless medicine and surgery in the 1960s and 1970s were spurred in the mid-1980s by problems with the blood supply, such as transmission of the human immunodeficiency virus. The result of these developments has been a complete rethinking of the use of blood and blood products—transfusions are avoided, if possible. The right of competent persons to refuse treatment is well established in the law:

> Thus, on the basis of either the common law liberty right to be free from unwanted treatment or by statute, competent adults, incompetent adults who have clearly expressed their wishes, and even older minors with adult-like decision-making capacity can legally refuse unwanted

blood transfusions. As for minor children generally, although parents may not deprive their children of necessary care, if the parents have a choice between two or more effective treatment options, the state has no *parens patriae* interest in mandating treatment entailing the use of blood simply because it is the popular or standard approach. If the child's health problem can be effectively managed without the use of homologous blood, the parents should be free to choose that treatment option without governmental interference.[2]

An ethic that emphasizes autonomy and respect for persons can significantly affect the patient–caregiver relationship. Fully expressed, patients alone choose the level of involvement they want. In the early 1980s, the President's Commission stated that patient sovereignty with complete participation in the process is a desirable, if not a readily achievable, goal.[3] The principle of respect for persons cannot be realized, nor participation achieved, absent truthfulness and the organization's consistent efforts. Autonomy means patients may not agree with caregivers' recommendations and assessments. Sometimes, clinicians and organizations find this concept threatening.

Some patients choose not to participate in decision making. Explicitly or implicitly, they want to remain ignorant of their medical problems and excluded from decision processes. They prefer paternalism and choose to delegate decision making to caregivers to do what they think is best. This relationship between patient and caregivers is neither the one envisioned as ideal by the President's Commission nor that demanded by contemporary patient rights advocates. Patient autonomy, however, is also violated if the patient is forced to participate. Caregivers and managers should consider a decision not to participate to be acceptable and work to make it a reality. Delegating to others the authority to make decisions may be the ultimate expression of autonomy.

The law and medical ethics include the concept of *therapeutic privilege*, which permits physicians to withhold information from patients when the physician believes it serves patients' best interests. States recognize therapeutic privilege in several ways; a general rule is difficult to formulate. Some reference the danger that full disclosure may cause to the patient's physical or mental health; others focus on patient best interests. Such paternalism is supported by the principles of beneficence and nonmaleficence and the virtue of caring. The therapeutic privilege exception is pragmatic and avails physicians of a range of actions. It is desirable that physicians possess the latitude to make such judgments, especially if the alternative is probable harm to the patient. In these cases, beneficence takes precedence.

ETHICAL ASPECTS

The premise for a discussion of the ethics of consent is that the ethical standard is significantly higher than the legal standard. This expectation arises from exercising the principles of respect for persons (autonomy) and nonmaleficence—which are based on Kantian deontology (see Chapter 1), natural law, and rule utilitarianism—and is supported by virtue ethics as expressed by virtuous managers.

The nuances inherent in duress and inducement are important in determining whether consent is *voluntary*. In these cases, ethical considerations and duties extend well beyond the standard in the law. Can patients suffering from a fatal disease make medical decisions voluntarily? Are patients' decisions free of duress if they fear losing their physicians' friendship and loyalty because they prefer an option the physician opposes? Clinical staff talk about "bad" patients, usually defined as uncooperative patients. Such patients are not intentionally harmed or mistreated, but they may not receive the same attention as "good" or pliable patients. Patients sense this attitude and it affects their volition. Patients are also heavily influenced by family and friends and may make decisions because of them. Similarly, family members may ask clinicians to behave in ways that may be unwanted by a patient who is considered incompetent or that, under the principle of beneficence, do not serve the patient's interests.

Such considerations suggest that consent may never be entirely voluntary. It has been argued that patients' personal freedom to accept or reject medical treatment has been so reduced that it is only a right to veto unwanted procedures.[4] This argument is bolstered by the increasingly complex relationships in medical care and its delivery, all of which preclude simple answers and easy determinations as to the voluntariness of consent. Managerial and clinical staff must understand the difficulties of consent and make all efforts to further patient autonomy.

In determining the voluntariness of consent, some groups present special problems. As noted, in the past, healthy persons with diminished autonomy, notably military personnel and prisoners, participated in experimentation that was nontherapeutic—meaning it had no benefit for them. The consent of persons in such groups has since been seen as nonvoluntary and using them as healthy subjects has virtually ceased. Voluntariness may also be reduced because inducements are so significant that prudence is cast aside. Money or other incentives may be offered to those who participate in high-risk experimentation; for example, some persons may be persuaded by payments that for them are significant. Students who participate in experiments are unique in this regard and may fit into several categories. Often, they are economically disadvantaged. In addition, some faculty encourage students to participate in experiments by exempting them from other, seemingly more onerous requirements such as term papers or examinations. Occasionally, there is implicit, or even explicit, coercion by faculty who control the students' academic (and sometimes economic) destiny and who unethically use this position to "encourage" consent.

Ethical considerations regarding whether one is *competent* to consent are usually easier than those regarding voluntariness. Competence is assumed in adults. Medical personnel can usually determine when a patient's mental capacity is questionable and seek expert opinion. Absent such evidence, there should be an explicit assumption in the organization's policies that patients are autonomous in making decisions. It is incumbent on managers to assist in this process through staff education and the support provided by appropriate systems and procedures.

The third element of consent is that it be *informed*. Some commentators inaccurately refer to the concept of "informed consent" as though it were the only criterion for consent. Because of the complexity of informed consent, whether the patient was *adequately informed* receives the most attention. Some states have statutes designed to ensure that patients obtain adequate information to make informed medical decisions. A Virginia law, for example, was prompted by reports that physicians performed radical mastectomies when removal of malignancy would have sufficed and that women were not given enough information to make an intelligent choice.[5]

Wait a Little Longer, We'll Do it Then

The emergency department at County Hospital has a typical caseload: some true emergencies and urgent medical conditions but many sniffles and other nonemergencies. The hospital contracts with an emergency medicine group, but administrative activities, including systems, procedures, and personnel, are managed by the hospital. The process for obtaining consent is typical: Unconscious patients are treated as their conditions necessitate. Competent patients who are able to communicate sign a consent form authorizing treatment. Parents and other family members are involved as needed and as available.

Early one afternoon, a conscious, middle-age man who had been in a car accident was brought in. He was diagnosed with internal injuries that required immediate exploratory surgery. He was asked to sign the consent form but refused on the grounds that as a Christian Scientist, receiving medical treatment violated his religious beliefs. He asked for a Christian Science practitioner.

The physician-director of the emergency department was paged, and, after reviewing the chart, she felt certain she could obtain his consent for surgery. She discussed the situation with the patient, who clearly understood that without surgery death was likely. He continued to refuse and repeatedly asked for a Christian Science practitioner. The physician-director left the treatment area very agitated; her mouth and chin shook in anger. She said, "This man is throwing his life away, all in the name of some religion that denies scientific medicine to its followers. I can't believe he's doing it!" She turned to the nurse and whispered, "Let me know when he's unconscious and we'll save his life, despite his silly ideas."

Such deception rides roughshod over the patient's clearly expressed wishes. The patient is competent, he has been informed, and his refusal is voluntary. In addition to violating the principle of respect for persons (autonomy), the physician is ignoring the AMA's Principles of Medical Ethics and the AMA's Council on Ethical and Judicial Affairs's Fundamental Elements of the Patient–Physician Relationship, which are reproduced in Appendix B. Such methods are unconscionable.

The organizational philosophy should consider the issues presented here prospectively. The results could reflect the approach used for Baby Boy Doe, whose case is discussed in Chapter 1. That chapter suggested that the organization might have intervened by petitioning a court to order life-saving surgery. Such intervention gives less weight to the principle of respect for persons (autonomy) and more to beneficence (and its corollary, utility) and paternalism. Increasing focus on liberty rights such as autonomy by the courts make it unlikely that the Christian Scientist will be forced to undergo surgery, which is true even if he has a family that is dependent on him. The principle of nonmaleficence supports action by the hospital. However, forcing treatment is paternalistic and significantly limits individual autonomy. The competing ethical principles of such cases pose ethical dilemmas for organizations and managers.

ROLE OF THE ORGANIZATION

What is the organization's role in consent? Patients should give informed, voluntary, and competent consent before treatment—a simple ethical concept. As is often true, difficulties arise in operationalizing the concept; it is instances such as these that the criteria for consent may be more often violated than met. Since the 1970s, organizations have focused greater attention on consent, an emphasis that reflects more a fear of legal problems than a desire to do what is ethically correct. Before the 1970s, organizations were less concerned about consent because they adopted and amplified the historic paternalistic view of the patient, a view consistent with the Hippocratic concept of the physician–patient relationship.

Policies and procedures consistent with the organizational philosophy must at minimum be established for obtaining consent, and their application must be systematically monitored. If, as it should, the philosophy emphasizes patients' rights, actions and efforts to perfect those rights will be encouraged and actions and efforts to contravene them will be restricted. Specific means exist for allowing patients to assert their rights, but these means are costly and can result in adversarial relationships. One method is to provide an advocate for each patient. Another is to establish an ombudsman office to review problems.

Often, the circumstances of consent are complicated because of the many parties involved, as shown in the following case.

When Is Consent Consent?

Henry Franklin was an emergency admission to University Hospital. He was diagnosed with mild cardiac failure by an attending physician. Because he was 78 years old and had complicating medical problems, a dispute arose as to the proper course of treatment. The consulting cardiologist recommended that Franklin be treated medically and given the best quality of life possible. The cardiologist estimated that Franklin had 6 months to live.

The cardiac surgeons who also consulted on the case saw things differently. They recommended replacing the aortic and mitral valves and estimated that this procedure would provide at least 2 years of useful life. When the options were described to Franklin, he was told the probability of surviving the surgery was 50%. He decided he would work with the cardiologist.

After hearing his decision, the surgeons intervened directly with Franklin's family, with whom they had had previous conversations. The family agreed with the surgeons and put great pressure on Franklin. He finally agreed to the procedure. Franklin's body could not withstand the rigors of surgery; he died in the operating room.

Even if informed and competent, Franklin's final decision was made under duress. The coercive circumstances greatly reduced his autonomy. In such situations family and physicians press for what they assert are the patient's best interests. However, sometimes both groups are driven by motives that conflict with the patient's self-expressed decision. Family may have various psychological and financial motives; physicians may act out of technological daring or hubris.

The challenge managers face is ensuring patient autonomy. Patients may choose a course of action that is not their first choice or even in their best interests as they view them because they defer to the wishes of others. They may fear abandonment or caregivers' anger if they choose a course of action other than what caregivers suggest or what they think caregivers want. An added complexity is that patients are often uncertain about what to do; they vacillate between wanting and not wanting aggressive treatment. Preserving patient autonomy in these circumstances is difficult, perhaps impossible, but must be attempted, nonetheless.

The surgeons were important in the Franklin case. They may have allowed bravado to cloud their judgment, especially given the probability of success. Franklin's family was also important. Health services organizations interfere in situations that reflect family dynamics at their peril, even though their duty clearly lies with the patient.

What is the role of the organization in determining that patients have consented in a way that meets ethical criteria? Obvious coercion is likely to be noticed by staff. A patient advocate program may minimize duress. Complicating efforts to ensure that consent meets the criteria is that the private attending physician has an independent ethical duty to inform patients about the procedure's nature, consequences, risks, and alternatives. The attending physician also primarily determines that the patient is competent to give consent and does so voluntarily. Some health services organizations see their ethical duty as independently determining or verifying that the criteria of consent have been met. Others ask only that patients sign an authorization that verifies that they have been informed about the procedure by the physician and that permits the hospital to participate in rendering the care to which patients have consented.

Unless it is certain that patients have been informed about the treatment in a way that meets organizational criteria, the ethically preferred course is that staff be involved, at least to the extent of verifying that the patient is informed and competent. The manager must fulfill the organization's positive ethical duty to monitor consent, which includes processes and procedures to assist and guide staff as necessary. Physician and nonphysician staff will also benefit from education about the ethical (and legal) dimensions of consent.

The case of Henry Franklin is distinguishable from that of the Christian Scientist. Franklin had more time to consider his decision, and his decision was likely influenced by his age. The other patient was middle age, with the potential for decades of life remaining. Beyond these apparent differences, both cases raise questions about patient autonomy and its relationship to the principles of beneficence and nonmaleficence. The weight given these principles in the organizational philosophy determines the outcome.

Managers of nursing facilities face ethical issues regarding consent similar to those of their counterparts in acute care hospitals. Decision making in nursing facilities is more likely to be complicated by factors such as competence or abandonment of patients. Thus, the process requires special attention.

I Intend to Be Independent

Oliver Harris is 82 years old and has been a resident at Five Oaks Nursing Home for 7 years. When he first sought admission, Harris had been evaluated and found to be only marginally in need of the care provided at Five Oaks. Because he was a private-pay patient, management decided to admit him. For 5 years his health was such that he needed minimal nursing care. In the sixth year, he began to show evidence of dementia. Medical evaluation found that he had experienced several small strokes. Harris likes to visit with other residents as he walks around the facility. His declining physical condition has resulted in several falls, which caused cuts and bruises but no broken bones as yet.

Harris's case was discussed at a staff conference. It was the consensus to physically restrain him so that he could not ambulate independently. Under federal guidelines, this was possible only with an order from Harris's physician. Staff doubted the physician would agree, but they believed that if Harris continued to walk unassisted, it was only a matter of time before he fell and sustained a fracture. Staff also believed that even if his physician ordered restraints, Harris would fight them: When the issue was discussed with Harris, he was adamant that he not be restrained. His daughter, however, agreed that physical restraint was wise.

Staff and management face a dilemma: How can they meet their duty of nonmaleficence to Harris while maximizing his autonomy under the principle of respect for persons? Harris is competent to decide about restraints. It is clear to staff (and Harris comprehends) that his well-being is at risk. A major fracture will likely result in rapid deterioration of his general health. Staff do not seem very creative in finding a way to allow him to ambulate safely. Such options should be explored first. Alternatively, various possibilities should be tested for short periods. If Harris cannot be persuaded to accept restraints, he should be allowed to ambulate freely in the facility.

MEDICAL EDUCATION

The case of Richard Weidner in Chapter 7 involved problems of consent in the context of medical education. Weidner was admitted to the hospital for a cardiac catheterization following recurrent chest pain. His cardiologist allowed him to think that she would perform the procedure, but a cardiology resident actually did the catheterization. The misrepresentation violated Weidner's right to autonomy and informed decision making and angered him greatly. There is significant tension between medical education's legitimate needs and the rights of patients to be treated with dignity and respect. The two are not incompatible, however.

Medical education is a primary source of problems in consent, especially as to patient knowledge about who will provide treatment. The conclusions of a New York State Assembly task force were based on interviews with chiefs of surgery, attending surgeons, residents, and anesthesiologists at 34 hospitals in the state. It reported the following:

- Private surgical patients in teaching hospitals are usually not operated on by the attending surgeon they retained, but by residents. Between 50% and 85% of the surgery in teaching hospitals is done by residents.

- Although most residents operated only under the close supervision of attending surgeons, some residents performed surgery without supervision, and some attending surgeons left the room while the operation was still in progress or before the incision was closed.

- Most patients are unaware of the degree to which residents participate in their surgery, and consent forms that name the attending surgeon and "such assistants as he shall select" do not give patients meaningful notice that a resident may do the actual cutting or suturing.[6]

The authors of the report stressed that there was no evidence that allowing residents to be active participants in surgery caused harm to patients. However, other researchers were less certain. They suggested that harm to patients from care rendered by physicians in training may be much more common than is generally known.[7] Whether harm occurs is a utilitarian measure. Kantians do not consider outcomes but only determine whether actions meet the criterion of respect for persons. Misleading patients or lying to them violates this principle.

The report addressed the disclosure necessary for informed consent and sufficient supervision to ensure patient safety. It also recommended that physicians be required to obtain the patient's consent for each person who participates in the surgery and that vague phrases such as "such assistants as the surgeon may select" be deleted from consent forms. The recommendations encouraged adequate supervision by limiting the number of patients a surgeon could treat and the number of operating rooms surgeons could reserve at one time.[8]

The AMA and the American College of Surgeons (ACS) have addressed the question of medical education and consent. They agree that if a resident—rather than the surgeon retained by the patient—actually performs the surgery, the patient must be made aware of that fact and consent to the substitution. *Report of the Council on Ethical and Judicial Affairs of the AMA* states the following:

> A surgeon who allows a substitute to operate on his or her patient without the patient's knowledge and consent is deceitful. The patient is entitled to choose his or her own physician and should be permitted to acquiesce in or refuse to accept the substitution.
>
> Under the normal and customary arrangement with patients, and with reference to the usual form of consent to operation, the operating surgeon is obligated to perform the operation but may be assisted by residents or other surgeons. With the consent of the patient, it is not unethical for the operating surgeon to delegate the performance of certain aspects of the operation to the assistant provided this is done under the surgeon's participatory supervision, i.e., the surgeon must scrub. If a resident or other physician is to perform the operation under nonparticipatory supervision, it is necessary to make a full disclosure of this fact to the patient, and this should be evidenced by an appropriate statement contained in the consent. Under these circumstances, it is the resident or other physician who becomes the operating surgeon.[9]

The ACS devotes the first of its Statements on Principles to (I.) Principles of Patient Care:

> A. The responsibility of a surgeon includes preoperative diagnosis and care, the selection and performance of the operation, and postoperative surgical care.

A surgeon may delegate part of the care of patients to associates or residents under his or her personal direction, because modern surgery is often a team effort. However, the surgeon's personal responsibility must not be delegated or evaded. It is proper for the responsible surgeon to delegate the performance of part of a given operation to assistants, provided the surgeon is an active participant throughout the essential part of the operation. If a resident is to operate upon and take care of the patient, under the general supervision of an attending surgeon who will not participate actively in the operation, the patient should be so informed and consent thereto.

It is unethical to mislead a patient as to the identity of the doctor who performs the operation.[10]

These statements are unequivocal. The patient must be informed about a resident's participation. Regrettably, the evidence suggests that these principles are often violated. Learning by doing is most apparent in surgical training. There is no ethical difference, however, between a surgical resident wielding a scalpel and a medical resident ordering a treatment or medication if patients have not given consent for them to participate in their care.

Patient consent in medical education settings generally receives inadequate attention. Examples range from conducting pelvic examinations on anesthetized women (37% of medical schools taught pelvic exams in this manner) without their consent to performing procedures (for educational purposes) on dead bodies without family members' consent. Almost half of accredited emergency medicine programs permitted physicians in training to perform procedures on dead bodies; three quarters admitted that they almost never obtained consent from family members.[11] Such breaches are all the more unacceptable because there is no therapeutic benefit derived by the "patient."

Failure to obtain patient (or family) consent for purposes of medical education occurs despite the review of accreditation bodies such as the Joint Commission on Accreditation of Healthcare Organizations and the Liaison Committee on Medical Education. The failures of the accreditors puts even greater importance on the need for increased attention by the organization itself through its managers.

Medical education and patient consent are compatible, but medical educators apparently fear that obtaining explicit consent will diminish educational opportunities and thus the quality of the educational program. Patients and families are likely to cooperate if asked to help with teaching needs.[12] In addition, patients will likely cooperate if they know that physicians in training will play a role in their care.[13] If patients do not consent to residents' participation in their care, they should have the right to seek care elsewhere. Ignoring this right shows that an ethical commitment to patient rights and autonomy is lacking, that the organization and staff violate their obligations, and that managers violate the expressions of virtues such as honesty and trustworthiness.

CONCLUSION

This chapter addressed ethical issues raised by consent. Health services organizations and their managers should consider legal requirements a minimum. It is on the basis of ethical principles that the organization should build a strong relationship with the patient. This independent relationship is the basis for the autonomy and respect owed to the patient.

Operationalizing patients' desire to be further involved in the consent process will require managerial attention to consent processes—not an easy task. Doing so means overcoming a long history of medical paternalism and educating patients as well as encouraging and assisting them to become involved.

A significant ethical problem is providing information about treatment to patients in health services organizations in which teaching occurs. Managers face many barriers in convincing attending staff that fully informing patients will not lead to diminished "clinical material" for teaching. No evidence suggests that many patients will refuse to participate after they have been informed, and there is every reason to believe that patients will overwhelmingly agree to the involvement of medical and surgical residents in their treatment. Regardless, the need for patients to consent cannot be ignored.

NOTES

1. Nicole Davis, Anne Pohlman, Brian Gehlbach, John P. Kress, Jane McAtee, Jean Herlitz, & Jesse Hall. (2003, April 16). Improving the process of informed consent in the critically ill. *Journal of the American Medical Association, 289*(15), pp. 1963–1968.
2. Donald T. Ridley. (1995, February). Working with Jehovah's Witnesses on treatment issues. *Hospital Law Newsletter, 12*(4), p. 6.
3. President's Commission for the Study of Ethical Problems in Medicine and Biomedical and Behavioral Research. (1982). *Making health care decisions: A report on the ethical and legal implications of informed consent in the patient–practitioner relationship. Volume 1: Report.* Washington, DC: U.S. Government Printing Office.

4. Jay Katz. (1977, Winter). Informed consent—A fairy tale. *University of Pitts-burgh Law Review, 39*, pp. 137–174.

5. Breast cancer law opposed in Richmond. (1983, August 12). *The Washington Post*, p. A4.

6. Margaret Keller Holmes. (1980, May). Ghost surgery. *Bulletin of the New York Academy of Medicine, 56*(4), p. 414.

7. Toby Cohen. (1983, September 20). The high cost of bad medicine. *The Washington Post*, p. A15.

8. Holmes, p. 415.

9. American Medical Association Council on Ethical and Judicial Affairs. (1994). *Code of medical ethics: Current opinions with annotations* (pp. 121–122). Chicago: Author.

10. American College of Surgeons. (1997, October). *Statements on principles*. Chicago: Author.

11. Robin Fretwell Wilson. (2003, August 17). Law would prohibit unauthorized exams on hospital patients. *The Buffalo News*. Retrieved August 20, 2003, from http://www.buffalonews.com/editorial/20030817/1051339.asp

12. *Ibid.*

13. Martin L. Kempner. (1979). Some moral issues concerning current ways of dealing with surgical patients. *Bulletin of the New York Academy of Medicine, 55*(1), pp. 62–68.

CHAPTER 10

DYING AND DEATH

Dying and death are fundamental to human existence. As in abortion, the ethical questions involved prompt emotional responses from the public and many health professionals. Ethical issues in dying and death arise in ways such as treating neonates with severe disabilities who are unlikely to survive and caring for children or adults who are terminally ill and unable to express personal autonomy.

Technology is at the heart of the matter. Since the 1970s, technology such as renal dialysis, mechanical ventilation, cardiac medications, and intensive care units have made it possible to postpone the end of life. Similar developments allow neonates who would have died in the 1980s to survive. Sometimes an ethical dilemma occurs when a person asks the organization to assist in achieving pain-free death. A great deal has been written about the questions such technology raises, but there are few widely accepted courses of action.

Adding complexity to these ethical issues is that many are poorly developed in the law. Deliberately shortening a patient's life raises obvious ethical and legal questions. Judges and juries are reluctant to convict, even when violent means have been used to end the painful life of someone terminally ill.

Chapter 9 noted that in the early 1980s, the President's Commission for the study of Ethical Problems in Medicine and Biomedical and Behavioral Research recommended a physician–patient relationship that maximizes patient sovereignty, with the patient fully participating in the decision process. Often, by the time crucial medical decisions must be made, the patient can no longer participate effectively and may not be competent. If available, advance medical directives are helpful, but they are often disregarded by families and caregivers. A medical ethic dedicated to preserving life and staving off death controls, and it is typical that the technological imperative results in expending all efforts, many times with marginal results. The economic, emotional, and psychological costs are obvious.

Managers may feel uneasy discussing dying and death. They are likely to consider decision making at the end of life to be clinical, a situation in which they play no role. Certainly, physicians are the lead actors in these dramas, but the effect of such issues on the organization requires that managers be knowledgeable about them and participate in developing and implementing policies and procedures. Managers also must be involved in the work of relevant committees.

In the mid-1980s, a distinction was drawn between treatments that were life prolonging and those that were life sustaining. Since then, however, the two concepts have merged and are simply called *life-sustaining treatments*. Life-sustaining treatment is "any treatment that serves to prolong life without reversing the underlying medical condition. Life-sustaining treatment may include, but is not limited to, mechanical ventilation, renal dialysis, chemotherapy, antibiotics, and artificial nutrition and hydration."[1]

DEATH DEFINED

Historically, death was defined as the stoppage of blood circulation and the cessation of circulation-dependent animal and vital functions, such as respiration and pulsation. New technology proved this definition inadequate. Table 3 summarizes definitions of death. Definitions based in law and theology provide limited guidance for contemporary clinicians.

In 1968, a Harvard Medical School committee defined *irreversible coma*, a development that solved some problems but created others. The Harvard criteria were accompanied by a report stating that the patient's condition can be determined only by a physician and that when the condition is found to be hopeless certain steps are recommended:

> Death is declared and *then* the respirator is turned off. The decision to do this and the responsibility for it are to be taken by the physician-in-charge, in consultation with one or more physicians who have been directly involved in the case. It is unsound and undesirable to force the family to make the decision.[2]

This quotation is noteworthy because of changes in society's attitudes and perceptions that have occurred since 1968, including emphasis on patient autonomy and natural death acts, family involvement in decision making,

Table 3. Definitions of death

Concept of death (Philosophical or theological judgment of the essentially significant change at death)	Locus of death (Place to look to determine whether a person has died)	Criteria of death (Measurements physicians or other officials use to determine whether a person is dead—to be determined by scientific empirical study)
1. Irreversible loss of flow of vital fluids (i.e., the blood and breath)	Heart and lungs	Visual observation of respiration, perhaps with the use of a mirror Feeling of the pulse, possibly supported by electrocardiogram
2. Irreversible loss of the soul from the body	Pineal body (?) (according to Descartes) Respiratory tract (?)	Observation of breath (?)
3. Irreversible loss of the capacity for bodily integration	Brain	Unreceptivity and unresponsivity No movements or breathing No reflexes (except spinal reflexes) Flat electroencephalogram (to be used as confirmatory evidence) All tests to be repeated 24 hours later (excluded conditions: hypothermia and central nervous system depression by drug)
4. Irreversible loss of consciousness or the capacity for social interaction	Probably the neocortex	Electroencephalogram

Adapted from Veatch, R.M.S. (1976). *Death, dying, and the biological revolution: Our lost quest for responsibility* (p. 53). New Haven: Yale University Press. Used with permission. This table has been modified using material from the 1989 second edition.

Note: Death is defined as a complete change in the status of a living entity characterized by the irreversible loss of those characteristics that are essentially significant to it. The possible concepts, loci, and criteria of death are much more complex than the ones provided here. These concepts are simplified models used to define death. It is obvious that those who believe that death means the irreversible loss of the capacity for bodily integration (3), or the irreversible loss of consciousness (4), have no reservations about pronouncing death when the heart and lungs have ceased to function. This is because they are willing to use loss of heart and lung activity as shortcut criteria for death, believing that once the heart and lungs have stopped, the brain or neocortex will necessarily stop, as well.

Note: In the table, (?) signifies uncertainty.

and establishment of institutional ethics committees (IECs). These changes have reduced the physician's primacy in decision making.

Near the time that the Harvard criteria were issued, a Virginia state court issued one of the first rulings accepting brain death.[3] The case raised issues of consent, appropriate criteria and process for determining death, conflicts of interest, beneficence, nonmaleficence, and organizational philosophy and managerial ethics. The physicians involved tried to use a brain death standard but failed to meet the Harvard criteria because there was no electroencephalogram to verify brain activity and the respirator was turned off *before* the patient was pronounced dead. Despite the lapses, the court accepted a determination that the patient was dead using a brain death criterion, thus making legal history.

The Uniform Determination of Death Act (UDDA) was developed by the National Conference on Uniform State Laws in 1980 in cooperation with the American Medical Association (AMA) and American Bar Association (ABA), who officially approved the UDDA in 1980 and 1981, respectively.[4] It provides alternative definitions of death. One uses the traditional definition—that is, irreversible cessation of pulsation (circulatory and respiratory functions); the other uses whole brain death. By 2003, some version of the UDDA had been enacted in 40 states.[5] The uniform act states the following:

> An individual who has sustained either (1) irreversible cessation of circulatory and respiratory functions, or (2) irreversible cessation of all functions of the entire brain, including the brain stem, is dead. A determination of death must be made in accordance with accepted medical standards.[6]

The uniform determination of death act is endorsed by the National Kidney Foundation, the North American Transplant Coordinators Association, and the American Nephrology Nurses' Association.[7]

Brain death, as shown in (2) in the preceding UDDA definition, or some variation, as stated following, is now a commonly used alternative criterion for death:

> The three cardinal findings in brain death are coma or unresponsiveness, absence of brainstem reflexes, and apnea. The clinical examination of the brainstem includes testing of brainstem reflexes, determination of the patient's ability to breath spontaneously, and evaluation of motor responses to pain.[8]

Definitions vary slightly, but the concept of whole brain death—defined as irreversible cessation of all functions of the brain, including the cortex and the brain stem—has been endorsed by the AMA, the ABA, and the American Academy of Neurology. Use of the whole brain death concept is law in 46 states.[9, 10]

As scientific developments permit increasingly sophisticated assessments of a patient's condition, especially prognosis, brain death criteria may be superseded by those that incorporate psychosocial factors. Prominent among the criteria proposed is the capacity or potential capacity for social interaction. This definition raises ethical issues and jeopardizes persons with no capacity for typical social interaction (e.g., persons with significant cognitive disabilities). A definition that includes a lack of the potential for typical social interaction was applied when infants with mental retardation, such as Baby Boy Doe, were allowed to die. Federal regulations since the 1980s specifically prohibit applying quality-of-life criteria to infants with disabilities who have life-threatening medical conditions, but there is evidence that quality-of-life criteria are commonly, if implicitly, used in decision making for other types of patients.

ADVANCE MEDICAL DIRECTIVES

When the federal Patient Self-Determination Act (PSDA) of 1989 took effect December 1, 1991, efforts to achieve patient participation in and control of their health care decisions gained a significant impetus. PSDA requires that hospitals, nursing facilities, hospice, home health agencies, and managed care organizations that participate in Medicare and Medicaid give all patients written information about their rights under state law to accept or refuse medical or surgical treatment and to formulate advance medical directives (AMDs). Adult patients must also be given the provider's written policies about implementing these rights. Medical records must document whether a patient has executed an AMD. Providers must also educate their staffs and communities about AMDs. Despite PSDA and the fact that all 50 states have laws authorizing some type of AMD (e.g., living wills, health care agents, medical powers of attorney),[11] problems continue in operationalizing patient involvement in decision making about AMDs, and relatively few patients execute them. It is estimated that only 20% of Americans have AMDs.[12] As few as 5% of individuals older than age 65 *may* have them.[13] The Joint Commission on Accreditation of Healthcare

Organizations requires accredited hospitals to address the wishes of patients relating to end-of-life decisions. Adults must be given written information about their right to accept or refuse medical or surgical treatment, including forgoing or withdrawing life-sustaining treatment or withholding resuscitative services.[14] The decisions that patients should consider in their AMDs include specific types of life-sustaining treatment that they want used or withheld. Examples include cardiopulmonary resuscitation (CPR), elective intubation, mechanical ventilation, surgery, dialysis, blood transfusions, artificial nutrition and hydration, diagnostic tests, antibiotics, and other medications and treatments, as well as future admission to the intensive care unit. Patients tend to choose more restrictions on treatment as diseases progress.[15]

Living Wills

The living will was developed so that persons unable to participate in decision making could guide caregivers. The words *living* and *will* seem contradictory. Traditionally, a will is the legal mechanism by which a deceased person's wishes as to disposition of property are carried out. Living wills allow persons unable to communicate with caregivers to express their wishes about the extent of treatment they wish to have applied. Living wills allow persons to limit what is done for and to them and to control the technological imperative, regardless of its potential benefit. Absent state legislation or case law, living wills have no legal status; patients must rely on the willingness of caregivers to follow the directives in them. Generic living wills are useful only in states without specific requirements.

State Statutes

Interest in living wills and public reaction to cases in which seemingly excessive treatment was provided led to rapid enactment of state laws recognizing the patient's right to control treatment processes. These laws are variously known as living wills laws, advance medical directives, natural death acts, or death with dignity laws. In early 1983, there were 14 states with such laws; by 1985, there were 35 states and the District of Columbia; by 2002, the total was 47.[16] The Virginia Advance Medical Directive form is shown in Figure 10.

Generally, these statutes recognize a patient's right to direct physicians to withhold or withdraw life-sustaining treatment. When statutory requirements are met, the directives are legally binding on caregivers. The laws tend to be drafted narrowly and apply when a physician has determined

VIRGINIA ADVANCE MEDICAL DIRECTIVE

This form, with slight variations, is the form approved by the Virginia General Assembly in the Health Care Decisions Act. The form contains a "Living Will" portion, a portion in which you may appoint an agent to make health care decisions for you, and a portion in which you may appoint an agent to make an anatomical gift. You may complete any one or all of these portions of the form. Virginia law does not require the use of this particular form in order to make a valid advance directive. If you have legal questions about this form, or would like to develop a different form to meet your particular needs, you should talk with an attorney. You must sign your advance medical directive in the presence of two witnesses who are not blood relatives or your spouse. It is your responsibility under Virginia law to provide a copy of your advance directive to your attending physician. You should also provide copies of the directive to close relatives and/or friends.

ADVANCE MEDICAL DIRECTIVE made this _____ day of _____ , _____
                                                                              Month   Year

I,_____ , willfully and voluntarily make known my desire and do hereby declare:

(Cross through this box if you do not want to make a living will in this form.)
"Living Will" Portion of Advance Medical Directive

If at any time my attending physician should determine that I have a terminal condition where the application of life-prolonging procedures would serve only to artificially prolong the dying process, I direct that such procedures be withheld or withdrawn, and that I be permitted to die naturally with only the administration of medication or the performance of any medical procedure deemed necessary to provide me with comfort care or to alleviate pain. (OPTION: I specifically direct that the following procedures or treatments be provided to me:_____

_____.)

In the absence of my ability to give directions regarding the use of such life-prolonging procedures, it is my intention that this declaration shall be honored by my family and physician as the final expression of my legal right to refuse medical or surgical treatment and accept the consequences of such refusal.

(Cross through this box if you do not want to appoint an agent to make health care decisions for you.)
Appointment of Agent to Make Health Care Decisions

I hereby appoint the following as my primary agent to make health care decisions on my behalf as authorized in this document:

Name of Primary Agent	Telephone Number
Address	City, State, Zip Code

If the above named primary agent is not reasonably available or is unable or unwilling to act as my agent, then I appoint the following as a successor agent to serve in that capacity:

Name of Successor Agent	Telephone Number
Address	City, State, Zip Code

Rev. 3/2004   **Page 1 of 3**

(continued)

Figure 10.   An example of an advance medical directive. (*Source:* Virginia Department for the Aging, 2004.)

that the patient who signed the declaration is terminally ill and has no prospect of recovery. Some statutes require that the directives must be reaffirmed when patients know they are terminally ill. Some include penalties against caregivers and the organization if directives are ignored. In

Figure 10   *(continued)*

"Appointment of Agent to Make Health Care Decisions" continued:

I hereby grant to my agent, named on the previous page, full power and authority to make health care decisions on my behalf as described below whenever I have been determined to be incapable of making an informed decision about providing, withholding or withdrawing medical treatment. The phrase "incapable of making an informed decision" means unable to understand the nature, extent and probable consequences of a proposed medical decision or unable to make a rational evaluation of the risks and benefits of a proposed medical decision as compared with the risks and benefits of alternatives to that decision, or unable to communicate such understanding in any way. My agent's authority hereunder is effective as long as I am incapable of making an informed decision.

The determination that I am incapable of making an informed decision shall be made by my attending physician and a second physician or licensed clinical psychologist after a personal examination of me and shall be certified in writing. Such certification shall be required before treatment is withheld or withdrawn, and before, or as soon as reasonably practicable after, treatment is provided, and every 180 days thereafter while the treatment continues.

In exercising the power to make health care decisions on my behalf, my agent shall follow my desires and preferences as stated in this document or as otherwise known to my agent. My agent shall be guided by my medical diagnosis and prognosis and any information provided by my physicians as to the intrusiveness, pain, risks and side effects associated with treatment or nontreatment. My agent shall not authorize a course of treatment which he/she knows, or upon reasonable inquiry ought to know, is contrary to my religious beliefs or my basic values, whether expressed orally or in writing. If my agent cannot determine what treatment choice I would have made on my own behalf, then my agent shall make a choice for me based upon what he/she believes to be in my best interests.

Further, my agent shall not be liable for the costs of treatment pursuant to his/her authorization, based solely on that authorization.

OPTION: Powers of my agent. (Cross through any language you do not want and add any language you do want.)

The powers of my agent shall include the following:

A.   To consent to or refuse or withdraw consent to any type of medical care, treatment, surgical procedure, diagnostic procedure, medication and the use of mechanical or other procedures that affect any bodily function, including but not limited to artificial respiration, artificially administered nutrition and hydration, and cardiopulmonary resuscitation. This authorization specifically includes the power to consent to the administration of dosages of pain-relieving medication in excess of recommended dosages in an amount sufficient to relieve pain, even if such medication carries the risk of addiction or inadvertently hastens my death;

B.   To request, receive and review any information, verbal or written, regarding my physical or mental health, including but not limited to medical and hospital records, and to consent to the disclosure of this information;

C.   To employ and discharge my health care providers;

Rev. 3/2004   Page 2 of 3

addition to statutes, appeals court and state supreme court decisions affect how the laws are interpreted and how life-sustaining treatment is withheld or withdrawn.

These laws solve some of the issues of control (autonomy), patient role, and, to an extent, organizational and provider efforts to comply with

"Powers of My Agent" continued:

D. To authorize my admission to or discharge (including transfer to another facility) from any hospital, hospice, nursing home, adult home or other medical care facility for services other than those for treatment of mental illness requiring admission procedures provided in Article 1 (§37.1-63 et seq.) of Chapter 2 of Title 37.1;

E. To make decisions about who may visit me, subject to physician orders and policies of any institution to which I am admitted; and

F. To take any lawful actions that may be necessary to carry out these decisions, including the granting of releases of liability to medical providers.

Other powers of my agent: _____

_____

_____

_____

(Cross through this box if you do not want to appoint an agent to make an anatomical gift or organ, tissue or eye donation for you.)
Appointment of Agent to Make Anatomical Gift

Upon my death, I direct that an anatomical gift of all my body or certain organ, tissue or eye donation may be made pursuant to applicable Virginia law governing anatomical gifts (§32.1-289 et seq.) and in accordance with my directions, if any. I hereby appoint _____ as my agent, of
                                                        Name of Agent

_____
Address   City, State, Zip Code   Telephone Number
to make any such anatomical gift or organ, tissue or eye donation following my death. I further direct that:
(Declarant's decisions, if any, concerning anatomical gift or organ, tissue or eye donation, written below.)

_____

_____

This advance directive shall not terminate in the event of my disability. By signing below, I indicate that I am emotionally and mentally competent to make this advance directive and that I understand the purpose and effect of this document.

_____   _____
Signature of Declarant   Date

The declarant signed the foregoing advance directive in my presence. I am not the spouse or a blood relative of the declarant.

_____ _____   _____ _____
Witness #1   Date   Witness #2   Date

Rev. 3/2004   **Page 3 of 3**

---

the patient's wishes. Even when there is an AMD, caregivers may not comply. Fragmentation of care among several health services providers and organizations further complicates patients' use of AMDs and poses a special challenge to managers in the organization to which the patient has been transferred. For example, an AMD in a nursing facility medical record may not accompany the patient to the hospital, especially in an emergency. A study of older patients hospitalized for acute illnesses found that in 75% of cases the medical record did not indicate that physicians had consulted the patient's living will or designated proxy before making treatment decisions, including whether to resuscitate. The problem was attributed to several factors: nursing facilities failed to transfer the information, patients were not asked or did not volunteer the information, and the hospital staff failed to ask or to ensure that such documents were part of the record. Once documented in the hospital medical record, AMDs influenced treatment decisions in 86% of cases involving patients who were judged incompetent.[17]

There are other problems with AMDs, including determining mental status and whether the patient comprehends the effect of what is being done and establishing the presence of a terminal illness. Of course, ethical issues arise for organizations when the patient has not met statutory requirements or there is no statute and no AMD.

The challenge for the organization is to provide processes that promote the completion of AMDs. Completion rates for AMDs can be markedly improved by altering the time when information is distributed to patients entering hospitals for planned admissions. Patients were far more likely to complete an AMD at a hospital that distributed information several days before admission rather than only on the day of admission. Patients were much more likely to read the information provided when it was available before hospitalization. The most common reason given for not completing an AMD was that it was not seen or was not read, a problem more common in hospitals that did not provide information in advance.[18] Other data suggested that providing reminders, education, and feedback to attending physicians and a new documentation form used by physicians for AMDs can greatly increase the percentage of patients with AMDs. The study also found that 87% of physician-attested directives agreed with the treatment preferences of patients interviewed. Other results showed that physicians' attitudes and interest in AMDs improved.[19] Other research suggested that changes in the care of dying patients may not have kept pace with national recommendations, in part because many physicians and nurses disagreed with and may have been unaware of some key guidelines, such as the permissibility of withdrawing treatment.[20]

Surrogate Decision Making

Surrogate decision making occurs when decisions about health care are made by someone other than the patient. A form of surrogate decision making called *substituted judgment* occurs when someone makes decisions for a patient who is unable to do so and the surrogate's decisions are based on what the surrogate believes the patient would want were the patient able to make a decision. Surrogates are needed to make decisions when patients are too young or otherwise legally incompetent or have a physical or mental infirmity and no AMD. Historically, surrogates have been appointed by courts upon a petition that a person was incompetent to make health care decisions. To avoid the cost and delay of court proceedings, states enacted laws that established a priority list of relatives who could make decisions for someone with no AMD. In 2001, only 28 states had statutes specifically authorizing surrogate decision making.[21]

Powers of attorney are another type of surrogate decision making. Powers of attorney are prepared before the fact and are a delegation of decision-making authority by a competent person, who is called the *principal*. Powers of attorney may be *general* (broad powers to act for the principal) or *limited* (authority to act for the principal for a specific purpose). Powers of attorney are *durable* when the grant of authority extends beyond the principal's incapacitation. Capacity (competence) is an important issue in health care decision making. Health care agents are persons who have been granted durable powers of attorney to make health care decisions for the principal. The states may use different names for these limited, durable powers of attorney. At the end of 2001, all 50 states had statutes recognizing appointment of health care agents.[22] Figure 10, the Virginia Advance Medical Directive form, includes appointment of a health care agent. In all such undertakings, care must be taken to meet state requirements.

Do-Not-Resuscitate Orders

The do-not-resuscitate (DNR) order is a type of AMD that is used at the point of service delivery. Many patients have neither living wills nor AMDs complying with state requirements. This point emphasizes the organization's need for policies and processes about resuscitating patients who are terminally ill and patients for whom life continuation decisions must be made (e.g., a patient in persistent vegetative state [PVS]).* Health services organizations usually have DNR policies affirming the legal right of a patient (or a surrogate, as appropriate) to direct caregivers. The DNR policy should identify the chemical and mechanical technologies included

---

*Commonly, the word *permanent* is used instead of *persistent* after a vegetative state has continued longer than a year.

and the specific instances in which they will be applied. Patients with DNR orders may require surgery and anesthesia management for palliative care, for relief of pain or distress, or to improve the patient's quality of life. DNR orders present unique ethical problems that should be addressed prospectively by the organization.[23]

In the 1990s, state laws began to recognize nonhospital DNR orders that allowed persons to refuse resuscitation when medical emergencies occurred. By 2003, more than half the states had such laws.[24] Often, these are known as emergency medical services do-not-resuscitate (EMS DNR) orders. EMS DNR orders make the patient's wishes legally binding in the home or a similar setting and override state laws that require EMS technicians to undertake CPR.

A study of three Houston teaching hospitals without DNR policies reported inconsistent application of DNR orders.[25] The study found that some patients with DNR orders underwent chemotherapy and surgery and were admitted to the intensive care unit while others received inadequate hydration and nutrition. Staff are often confused about what type of care patients with DNR orders should receive, perhaps because they disagree with decisions. The study found that in 10% of cases, no decision had been reached about keeping the patient alive. This finding indicates that efforts to decide about resuscitation before a crisis commonly fail. In most no-decision cases, the subject of DNR had not been broached with the patient or family. Other studies of DNR orders report similar findings.[26] A key aspect of DNR is whether patient wishes about CPR are clear to physicians. One study found that in nearly one of three cases, the patient's preference not to be given CPR was at odds with the doctor's perception of what the patient wanted.[27]

Summary

It has been suggested that the widespread use of AMDs, such as natural death act declarations, may encourage systematic rationing of health care to older adults. If a right to die becomes a duty to die, the living will and its progeny, the natural death act declaration, will become a Frankenstein monster. Indeed, the suggestion by former Governor Richard Lamm of Colorado, as well as by officials at the U.S. Department of Health, Education, and Welfare (now called the Department of Health and Human Services [DHHS]), that older people should be required to have living wills raised a storm of protest. Regardless of true motives, such suggestions are often seen as motivated by economics.

It has been suggested that treatment may end because physicians assume it is not in a patient's interest or because physicians believe the patient would not want it.[28] Others, however, assert that physicians are caught up in the same ethos of death as failure as patients and family and are focusing on what has been called the riddle—physicians' determination to diagnose and cure the disease. When there is no longer a riddle—when death is inevitable—physicians' interest may decline or be lost entirely, and having lost the major battle, they may try to maintain some authority by controlling the dying process of their patients.[29] If correct, these views neither consider patients as independent decisions makers nor as involved participants and, thus, physicians may be acting other than in the patients' best interests, as determined by the patient. Both suggest significant ethical problems in meeting the wishes of terminally ill patients.

It seems logical that surrogate decision makers will accurately reflect patient's wishes about life-sustaining treatments. That appears not to be true, however. Even those who know patients well are not highly accurate in predicting their life-sustaining treatment preferences. Chronically ill patients are more satisfied with their primary care physicians and the care they deliver when AMDs are discussed.[30] Neither AMDs nor discussion of directives significantly improved the accuracy of surrogate substituted judgment, however.[31] Family members were more accurate in making substituted judgments than are physicians but still fell short of complying with patients' wishes. The presence of AMDs assisted hospital-based physicians but not primary care physicians in their decisions as surrogate decision makers.[32] Furthermore, end-of-life care needs improvement in meeting patients' wishes to die at home (rather than in an institution) and in the quality of palliative care.[33] These and numerous other studies show that a great deal of work remains for health services organizations if they are to provide health services that are consistent with AMDs and patients' wishes for end-of-life care.

The organization must be alert to the ethical issues of AMDs, which are present regardless of a natural death act statute or a living will. Health services organizations and their managers must consider these issues prospectively and develop policies that respect patients' wishes, consistent with the organizational philosophy.

Improving care of the dying in health services organizations should include the following: reaffirming patients' rights to palliative care, providing adequate pain and symptom management, improving policies and procedures to ensure that AMDs are available as needed, ensuring a well-functioning IEC, improving access by all concerned to the IEC, enhancing community outreach education, ensuring timely referrals to hospice and family support services, and encouraging medical education in dying and ethics.[34]

EUTHANASIA

The term *euthanasia* comes from the Greek *eu* and *thanatos*, or good death. In the context of the Hippocratic tradition, which prohibits physicians from administering a deadly drug, euthanasia describes care that makes an inevitable death pain-free.

In contemporary parlance, however, euthanasia describes situations in which active steps cause death. Such word use blurs important distinctions. Providing comfort care and pain control without purposefully hastening death allows persons to die with dignity and free of pain. This discussion uses the contemporary definition of euthanasia as active steps to cause death—that is, mercy killing. Actively intervening to end life is illegal in all states.[35]

Morphia Somnolence

Henrietta Morrow was diagnosed with inoperable cancer 18 months ago. Chemotherapy was ineffective. The lymph system had spread the disease throughout her body, and Morrow was in severe pain. Initially, she received care through a home hospice care program. As the disease worsened she became an inpatient at the hospice. She was expected to live less than 3 months.

Morrow received nutrition, hydration, and comfort care. The morphine used for pain control was increased as the disease progressed and her pain worsened. A staff member asked the medical director about the depressant effect that morphine would have on Morrow's respiration. She worried about depressing respiration so much that death would result. Her concern was expressed in both legal and ethical contexts. The medical director assured her that there were no legal problems and described the ethical considerations, including ordinary versus extraordinary care, active and passive euthanasia, voluntary versus involuntary euthanasia, and the rule of double effect.

Ordinary versus Extraordinary Care

Hastening or bringing about death by increasing the morphine beyond that needed to control pain would be euthanasia, an unethical and illegal act. For Morrow, comfort care and pain relief would have the hope of benefit to provide a comfortable and pain-free dying process and thus would be considered ordinary care. Because the hope of benefit is virtually nil, further chemotherapy would be considered extraordinary. Normal hydration and nutrition are always considered ordinary care. Artificial hydration and nutrition (AHN) is ordinary care, too, if there is hope of benefit from administering it. AHN becomes extraordinary when a patient's condition is such that there is no hope of benefit from AHN. Some assert that AHN is never extraordinary, however. The principle of nonmaleficence provides a distinction:

> Ordinary means are all medicines, treatments, and operations which offer reasonable hope of benefit and which can be obtained and used without excessive expense, pain, or other inconvenience. Extraordinary means are all medicines, treatments, and operations which cannot be obtained or used without excessive expense, pain, or inconvenience, or which, if used, would not offer a reasonable hope of benefit.[36]

Simply put, continuing a course of treatment (including AHN) that offers no hope of benefit only prolongs the dying process and inflicts unnecessary suffering and discomfort on the patient.

Ordinary and *extraordinary* are not defined as usual and unusual, respectively. This interpretation could be confusing because there is variation even among similar hospitals as to which treatments are usual or unusual. The usual emergency treatment in a shock trauma unit is different from that provided in a community hospital emergency room. Instead, the criterion is hope of benefit as compared with excessiveness of expense, pain, or other inconvenience. Absent hope of benefit, any medicine, treatment, or operation is extraordinary. If there is hope of benefit, use of the same medicines, treatments, and operations is not excessive.

Some ethics literature uses benefits to, and burdens on, the patient—the proportionality of treatment. Some writers suggest that *proportionate* and *disproportionate* are more clear and descriptive than *ordinary* and *extraordinary*. The criteria used to measure proportionate and disproportionate care are like those used for ordinary and extraordinary but are stated somewhat differently. The type of treatment, its complexity or risk, cost, and appropriateness are studied and compared with results to be expected, taking into account the state of sick persons and their physical and moral resources.[37] Using this calculus, it is ethical to provide the treatment if the potential benefit justifies the burden. Like ordinary and extraordinary, proportionate and disproportionate are primarily qualitative measures of the ethical appropriateness of treatment. Crudely summarized, ordinary/

extraordinary and proportionate/disproportionate mean "Does the benefit justify the burden?"

Types of Euthanasia

Euthanasia has four permutations: voluntary active, voluntary passive, involuntary active, and involuntary passive. *Voluntary* means that the person has freely consented. *Involuntary* means that the person either has not freely consented or cannot freely consent but is presumed to want to die. *Active* means that positive steps are taken to bring about death, an action that should be called killing. *Passive* means that nothing is done to hasten death; the natural course of the disease causes death. All types of euthanasia include providing comfort care and pain control.

Active or Passive Euthanasia

Active or Passive Euthanasia   The case of Henrietta Morrow raises questions about the concept of euthanasia: Does increased morphine for pain control constitute euthanasia that is active or passive or voluntary or involuntary? Active euthanasia occurs when someone's death is purposely hastened. Intentionally giving Morrow more morphine than needed to control pain is active euthanasia, an act that is both unethical and illegal. Passive euthanasia occurs when the patient is allowed to die and no extraordinary means are used to sustain life or when extraordinary means for sustaining life are withdrawn and the patient dies as the result of the natural course of the disease. Withholding or withdrawing life-sustaining treatment does not preclude providing comfort care and pain control. Artificial nutrition and hydration can be extraordinary (disproportionate) care, however, if they offer no hope of benefit.

Voluntary or Involuntary Euthanasia   Voluntary and involuntary euthanasia refer to patient decisions about treatment. It is unknown whether Morrow is aware that increasing the amount of morphine may shorten her life and, if knowing, that she agrees. It is reasonable to assume that she prefers to live pain-free despite morphine's other effects. The organization emphasizing patient autonomy will involve, to the fullest extent, the competent patient in decisions regarding all treatment, including pain control.

Rule of Double Effect   Morrow's situation suggests application of the moral rule of double effect (RDE). Like ordinary and extraordinary care, double effect is a subset of nonmaleficence.

> Classic formulations of the RDE identify four conditions or elements that must be satisfied for an act with double effect to be justified. Each

is a necessary condition, and together they form sufficient conditions of morally permissible action.

1. *The nature of the act*—The act must be good, or at least morally neutral (independent of its consequences).

2. *The agent's intention*—The agent intends only the good effect. The bad effect can be foreseen, tolerated, and permitted, but it must not be intended.

3. *The distinction between means and effects*—The bad effect must not be a means to the good effect. If the good effect were the direct causal result of the bad effect, the agent would intend the bad effect in pursuit of the good effect.

4. *Proportionality between the good effect and the bad effect*—The good effect must outweigh the bad effect. That is, the bad effect is permissible only if a proportionate reason is present that compensates for permitting the foreseen bad effect.[38]

The rule of double effect allows ethical use of morphine, even in increasing quantities, to ease Morrow's pain.

PATIENT DECISION-MAKING PROCESS

Competent Patients

Persons who are competent have an ethical and a legal right to decide what treatments they will accept. This precept applies equally to withholding and withdrawing treatment. Consent is discussed in Chapter 9. Anecdotal evidence suggests that staff find it easier to withhold than withdraw treatment. Reluctance to discontinue treatment may be driven by fear of legal liability as well as by uncertainty as to the ethically correct choice.

The Henninger Case   Decided by the New York Supreme Court, the appellate division in New York State, this case involved 85-year-old G. Ross Henninger, who was confused, depressed, and irritable and was hospitalized for treatment of fever and infection. His medical problems were compounded by a stroke, arthritis, heart disease, and hardening of the arteries. The court stated it would not "go against (Henninger's) wishes and order this 85-year-old person to be operated on, or be force fed, or to be restrained for the rest of his natural life."[39] The decision followed a hearing in which attorneys for Henninger and the nursing facility where he lived petitioned the court to determine the legality of the facility allowing him to starve to death, which was his wish. Henninger died the day following the decision.

The case of Henrietta Morrow suggests the similarity of decisions about dying and death in various types of health services organizations. Nursing facilities, hospice, and home health agencies must prospectively address the ethical issues end-of-life decisions raise. This focus entails a review from organizational philosophy down to operational policies. The philosophy and policies regarding matters such as life-continuation decisions and AHN must be communicated to patients and potential patients and their families.

Somebody Changed the Rules!

In 1996, Ruth Mittlemann was admitted to the Hebrew Home, a nursing facility. Mittlemann suffered from amyotrophic lateral sclerosis, or Lou Gehrig's disease. Her condition deteriorated gradually. By late 1999, it was clear that she would soon be unable to swallow and thus could not take food and water by mouth. Before entering the facility, Mittlemann had executed a living will expressly stating that she did not want to receive artificial hydration or nutrition; she wished to be kept comfortable and treated for pain when she could no longer swallow. At the time Mittlemann entered the Hebrew Home, her living will posed no problem because the facility had no organizational policy on this issue.

In early 1998, the Hebrew Home's board of trustees began work on a policy regarding artificial nutrition and hydration. It was the most rancorous issue the board ever considered. Several members resigned because of the intense debate, which sometimes degenerated into personal attacks. The result was a policy adopted in late 1998, which stated that the sanctity of life had to be respected and that only if death were imminent could patients or their surrogates direct that such basic human care as food and water be stopped.

Mittlemann learned of this new policy only when she was informed that it would be necessary to place a nasogastric tube so that she could be hydrated and fed. She protested vehemently and reaffirmed her living will. She did not want to move to another nursing facility in the area, she liked where she was. She only objected to being forced to receive treatment that she did not want.

On its face, this change is fundamentally unfair to Mittlemann. She is caught in a situation not of her making and beyond her control. The organization also faces a dilemma: acceding to Mittlemann's wishes causes the organization to violate its new values statement about the sanctity of life.

The principle of respect for persons—specifically, fidelity (promise keeping)—governs the Mittlemann case. The organization is obliged to apprise patients of policies that affect them. Because the Hebrew Home had no written policy on AHN when Mittlemann was admitted, the trust she placed in the organization when she chose it is being violated. Moving her elsewhere does not eliminate the home's duty. As distasteful as it may be to the organization and its board, Mittlemann's wishes must be an exception to the policy.

Formerly Competent Patients

In theory, patients retain the right to determine what care they receive and when it will be discontinued. However, treatment decisions, even for competent inpatients, often become psychologically and physically overwhelming. The processes and the persons who apply them dominate; the patient loses control. Patients (or their advocates) may be forced to bring legal action to reassert their autonomy.

Instructions from a Formerly Competent Patient

Constance Emerson had lived a full life. She had been active in the community. She worked as a volunteer at Homer House, a noted settlement house, where she developed educational programs for children of working mothers. Emerson is 92 and lives in a nursing facility. In 1995 she fell and sustained a cerebral hemorrhage. Her mental faculties remain impaired even after extensive therapy.

After her injury, Emerson's husband cared for her until his own health deteriorated and it became impossible for him to continue. Emerson has long had diabetes. She requires a special diet and insulin. She eats only soft foods or liquids and is bedridden, blind, and deaf. Emerson experiences occasional respiratory infections that respond well to treatment. Her heart is strong. Except for mild arthritis, she has no pain. She sometimes recognizes her husband when he visits, but her speech is often unintelligible.

Three years before her injury, Emerson gave a talk on the miseries of prolonging life for older adults who are dying. Having experienced the agony of deterioration in her relatives, she made an eloquent plea for a "dignified and simple way to choose death." She showed the manuscript to her husband and mentioned publishing it but had not done so. Her husband now fears speaking to her about what she had written or how she feels about her life because she might infer that he wants her to die. The Emersons' son visits her weekly and feels they should not disturb the care she is receiving.[40]

This case illustrates the ethical problems of caring for older people who are infirm and no longer mentally competent. The care provided to Emerson maintains her life; her brain injury is irreversible. The evidence as to Emerson's views about people in a situation like hers is several years old.

Her mental state precludes knowing her current wishes. Even if Emerson could direct her care or had an AMD, she could not force the organization to help her end her life.

Applying the criteria of ordinary and extraordinary care to Constance Emerson, who needs a special diet, insulin, and occasional antibiotics, leads to the conclusion that nothing being done is extraordinary. All care offers reasonable hope of benefit without excessive expense, pain, or inconvenience. Reasonable hope of benefit is not based on an expectation that she will regain her former cognitive and physical condition but that she will have the life of a 92-year-old woman who has sustained a brain injury. She is not terminally ill; discontinuing treatment is unethical.

It is instructive to apply the final definition of death in Table 3 (see p. 231) to Emerson. Is she "alive" if a social interaction criterion is applied? The case notes that she sometimes recognizes her husband when he visits. Whether she has the capacity for social interaction could be determined. If she is not capable of social interaction, this definition of death would allow the organization to withhold antibiotics or insulin, thus rapidly hastening her death. Given the facts in this case, however, the only ethical action is to continue hydration, nutrition, and medication.

Noncompetent Adult Patients

The Quinlan Case   Karen Ann Quinlan was 21 years old in mid-1975 when she became comatose after overdosing on alcohol and tranquilizers. On appeal, the New Jersey Supreme Court permitted Karen's father to be appointed her guardian.[41] The court authorized Quinlan to discontinue all extraordinary measures to sustain life if the family and physicians agreed that there was no reasonable possibility that Karen would emerge from her vegetative state and if there was consultation with the hospital ethics committee. This ruling was among the earliest enunciations of an ethics committee's role, and it stimulated New Jersey hospitals to establish them. It is clear that the court intended it to be a prognosis committee, a role very different from that of present-day ethics committees.

After her father ordered the respirator disconnected, Karen was successfully weaned and able to breathe unaided. She was discharged to a nursing facility, where she remained until her death in mid-1985. When she died, she weighed 66 pounds, and her body was locked in a fetal position.

In addition to the New Jersey courts, courts in Massachusetts and New York have been especially active in cases similar to Quinlan. The cases have been brought by families seeking to regain control from the organization or by managers wanting protection from legal claims. Not all similar cases follow Quinlan, however. Some patients continue to receive treatment absent hope of benefit. In others, painful treatment of little benefit was withheld. With court guidance, health services organizations are attempting to solve the problem of when to withdraw life-sustaining treatment. The courts are a necessary final arbiter in settling legal questions that arise, especially when there is dissonance in the ethics of those involved, including the organization. Court decisions aid persons and organizations in developing and refining their ethic. They should be a last resort, however.

The Cruzan Case   A landmark legal case on withdrawing life-sustaining treatment was handed down by the U.S. Supreme Court in 1990. Nancy Cruzan was a young adult who sustained severe injuries in a 1983 automobile accident. She was subsequently diagnosed as being in PVS. A permanent gastrostomy tube provided hydration and nutrition. When it became apparent that Cruzan had virtually no chance of regaining her cognitive faculties, her parents asked the Missouri state hospital caring for her to end AHN. The staff refused to do so without court approval. A state trial court found that someone in Cruzan's condition had a fundamental right under state and federal constitutions to refuse treatment or direct the withdrawal of "death-prolonging procedures."

The Missouri Supreme Court reversed the trial court's decision and ruled that the state constitution included no right to privacy that would support an unrestricted right to refuse treatment. The court found that Missouri's living will statute embodied a policy strongly favoring preservation of life and that Cruzan's statements to her housemate that she would not want to continue her life unless she could live "halfway normally" were unreliable in determining her intent.[42] The court concluded that her parents could not withdraw medical treatment because no one can make that choice on behalf of an incompetent person absent the formalities required by the state's living will statute or clear and convincing evidence of the patient's wishes.

In mid-1990, the U.S. Supreme Court affirmed the Missouri decision.[43] It held that the U.S. Constitution does not forbid Missouri to require that an incompetent person's wishes about withdrawing life-sustaining treatment be proved by clear and convincing evidence. The Court distinguished the rights of competent persons, who it assumed have a constitutionally protected right to refuse life-sustaining hydration and nutrition, from those of incompetent persons. It noted that the state had established procedural safeguards to ensure that a surrogate's action conforms as closely as possible to wishes expressed while the person was competent. The Court granted broad latitude to the states to protect and preserve human life and recognized their right to require a standard of clear and convincing evidence as to a person's intentions regarding life-continuation decisions. It noted that the state is entitled to guard against potential abuses by surrogates who may not act to protect the patient's interests. In addition, states may decline to judge the quality of a person's life and simply assert an unqualified interest in preserving human life to be weighed against the constitutionally protected interests of the individual. The Cruzan case makes it clear that the Court is unwilling to extend to incompetent persons (through surrogates) the same constitutional right of self-determination available to competent persons.

In November 1990, Cruzan's parents were granted a second hearing in state court, which Missouri did not oppose. New evidence convinced the judge that Nancy Cruzan would not have wanted to live in PVS. In late 1990, he ordered the feeding tube removed. Anti-euthanasia groups unsuccessfully sought to intervene, but the state did not appeal the decision. Cruzan died of dehydration two weeks later, 8 years after her accident.[44]

The Cruzan decision granted the states broad latitude to legislate in such situations. Health services organizations are guided by state law. In addition, they shoulder a special burden: advising patients about their legal rights regarding AMDs. The organization must go beyond informing and assisting patients to actually ensuring that the guidance is part of the medical record and is applied in the process of care. Health services organizations meet that challenge as part of their commitment to the principles of respect for persons, beneficence, and nonmaleficence.

Cases such as *Henninger* and *Cruzan* have not settled the issue of withdrawing life-sustaining treatment for those in PVS. The case of Terri Schiavo in Florida[45] and other cases are fueling the debate about whether health services organizations and their clinical staff are ethically and legally obliged to provide AHN to patients in PVS. When patients must be sedated or restrained to endure tube feedings or intravenous lines, the burdens are significant and it must be asked whether care in this context is required.[46] Another way to state the issue is whether life-sustaining hydration and nutrition for this type of patient is extraordinary (disproportionate) care, although under usual circumstances nutrition and hydration are ordinary (proportionate) care.

Some may question whether feeding and hydrating patients who are terminally ill or in PVS is or should ever be considered extraordinary (disproportionate) care. The AMA addressed this issue in the mid-1980s when it stated that it was not unethical for physicians to discontinue "life-prolonging" medical treatment from patients with terminal illness or irreversible coma when the physician determined that the burdens of treatment outweighed its benefits. Treatment was defined to include medication and artificially or technologically supplied respiration, nutrition, or hydration.[47] There were protests from those who feared that the new policy might cause physicians to discontinue nutrition and hydration when *they* considered it in the patient's best interests, even though patients believed their interests were furthered by continuing these treatments but could not communicate this decision. The AMA maintains this position but with greater emphasis on patient autonomy and surrogate decision making, where necessary, rather than on a physician determination of benefits and burdens.[48]

The goals of AHN are often unclear. When initiated, the hope is that AHN will sustain the patient until improvement or recovery occur. Subsequently, however, the situation is often allowed to drift so that AHN continues without an identified end point. Here, the greater reluctance of clinicians (and family) to withdraw treatment than withhold it has been identified. Furthermore, in dying patients, AHN may not prolong life but may worsen suffering. Of the many potential complications of AHN, the largest risk is fluid overload. It is recommended that a defined therapeutic goal for AHN is firmly stated and agreed upon before intervention; family members should be part of the decision process and the evaluation of results of AHN.[49]

A common question for patients denied hydration and nutrition has been whether it is inhumane because of the pain they are believed to experience. The issue may not be entirely settled, but the weight of evidence is that prolonged dehydration and starvation produce no pain and that ice chips or swabs will relieve the limited discomfort from a dry mouth. Problems with excessive secretions, edema, or incontinence can be alleviated.[50] As Sullivan[51] stated,

> In the setting of dehydration and starvation, death can occur from a multitude of causes. Arrhythmia, infection, and circulatory system collapse due to volume depletion are common terminal events. The clinical course of each should be rapid and, ideally, not associated with perceived discomfort by the patient.

Sullivan's conclusion is supported by nurses' assessments that patients who refused food and water had "good deaths," generally within 2 weeks, with little pain or suffering, thus refuting the popular assumption that such a death is painful and gruesome.[52] Some organizations insist on continuing hydration even though nutrition is stopped, an action that seems pointless and only prolongs the dying process.

Objections to this ethic are heard less often than in the mid-1990s, although most people are likely to find themselves discomforted by failing to provide food and water, the staples of human life. Regardless of debate at the theoretical level, an ethic must be applied at the bedside. What is the ethically correct action for a particular patient? This may begin the debate anew.

Infants

The Baby Doe cases added an important dimension to what began with the Quinlan case in the mid-1970s. The name Baby Doe derives from court proceedings in several states in the early 1980s. All cases involved parents who decided to forgo life-sustaining treatment of their newborn infants with treatable genetic anomalies. Publicity surrounding the subsequent deaths of two such infants prompted the DHHS to issue regulations in April 1982 prohibiting hospitals that receive federal funds from withholding life-sustaining treatment from infants with disabilities. Authority for this action was claimed under Section 504 of the Rehabilitation Act of 1973 (PL 93-112), which prohibits discrimination on the basis of disability. The regulations were challenged by health services organizations on procedural grounds, and an injunction suspending implementation was issued. Another attempt to promulgate a modified version of the regulations followed in 1983. Like the first regulations, they mandated telephone hotlines to report alleged cases of withholding life-sustaining treatment from newborns with serious illnesses. Signs containing information about the need to treat such newborns had to be posted. For providers, the hotlines were the most hated and controversial requirement. Opponents claimed the regulations turned providers into spies. An important modification in the 1983 revision was that impossible or futile acts or therapies that merely prolong the dying of an infant born terminally ill are not required. Opponents of the regulations successfully obtained judicial relief preventing implementation.

In June 1985, the U.S. Supreme Court agreed to hear a U.S. Justice Department appeal of a lower court decision that invalidated the Baby Doe regulations. This was surprising because the actions of Congress and the DHHS had eliminated the need for the first regulations. In June 1986, the high court agreed with the lower court in an opinion that struck down the Baby Doe rules. It agreed that Section 504 of the Rehabilitation Act of 1973 did not empower the DHHS to force hospitals to treat infants with severe disabilities over parental objections. The Court's decision displeased some disability advocacy groups, who claimed that there are major enforcement problems with the Child Abuse Prevention and Treatment Act Amendments of 1984 (PL 98-457), both procedurally and because of a basic antidisability bias held by some physicians and child protective services agencies. They contended that these biases will result in do-not-treat decisions in large numbers of cases.

Child Abuse Amendments

The original controversy surrounding the Baby Doe cases prompted Congress to address the question of newborns with serious disabilities in the Child Abuse Amendments of 1984. Subsequent regulations established treatment and reporting guidelines for care of newborns with significant disabilities. Withholding medically indicated treatment from infants with disabilities is illegal except when:

> In the treating physician's (or physicians') reasonable medical judgment any of the following circumstances apply:
> (i) the infant is chronically and irreversibly comatose; or
> (ii) the provision of such treatment would merely prolong dying, not be effective in ameliorating or correcting all of the infant's life-threatening conditions, or otherwise be futile in terms of the survival of the infant; or
> (iii) the provision of such treatment would be virtually futile in terms of the survival of the infant and the treatment itself under such circumstances would be inhumane.[53]

The definition of *medically indicated treatment* includes appropriate care, such as nutrition, hydration, and medication.[54] The regulations do not allow decisions based on subjective opinions about the future quality of life of a person with mental retardation or another disability.[55]

Under the law, affected health services organizations must designate persons who will report suspected problems to state child protective services agencies. The agencies coordinate and consult with those persons and, after notification of suspected medical neglect, may initiate legal action.

CONCLUSION

Ethical issues arising from end-of-life decisions are among the most common that health services organizations and their clinical and managerial staffs encounter. Technology is central to the ethical and legal problems surrounding dying. New technology may solve some problems, but if history is a guide, technology is as likely to create ethical dilemmas as it is to solve them. For treatments such as tube feedings, which extend life using low technology, the issue is more basic. Food and water are fundamental to human existence. It is likely, however, that both will be seen as extraordinary treatment when continuing to provide them artificially offers no hope of benefit.

NOTES

1. American Medical Association. (1994, June). *E-2.20: Withholding or withdrawing life-sustaining medical treatment.* Retrieved March 15, 2004, from http://www.ama-assn.org/ama/pub/category/8457.html

2. A definition of irreversible coma: Report of the Harvard Medical School Ad Hoc Committee to Examine the Definition of Brain Death. (1968, August). *Journal of the American Medical Association, 205*(6), pp. 337–338.

3. Robert M. Veatch. (1972, November). Brain death: Welcome definition or dangerous judgment? *The Hastings Center Report, 2*(6), p. 10.

4. National Conference of Commissioners on Uniform State Laws. (1980). *Uniform Determination of Death Act.* Retrieved Chicago: Author. December 2, 2003, from http://www.law.upenn.edu/bll/ulc/fnact99/1980s/udda80.htm

5. *Ibid.*

6. National Conference of Commissioners on Uniform State Laws, 1980.

7. National Conference of Commissioners on Uniform State Laws, 2003.

8. Eelco F.M. Wijdicks. (1995, May). Determining brain death in adults. *Neurology, 45*, p. 1005.

9. Ascension Health, Inc. (2003, October 17). *Brain death.* Retrieved from http://www.ascensionhealth.org/ethics/public/issues/brain.asp

10. The American Academy of Neurology (AAN) adopted the Uniform Law Commissioners' definition of whole brain death in 1978. "For legal and medical purposes an individual with irreversible cessation of all function of the brain, including the brain stem, is dead. Determination of death under this act shall be made in accordance with reasonable medical standards." American Academy of Neurology, personal communication, May 17, 1996.

11. Partnership for Caring. (2001, February). *Facts about surrogate decision making law.* Retrieved October 28, 2003, from http://www.partnershipforcaring.org/Resources/pdf/surrogate.pdf

12. *Ibid.*

13. Center for Bioethics at the University of Minnesota–Twin Cities. (2003, October 21). *Advance directives* (p. 3). Retrieved March 15, 2004, from http://www.bioethics.umn.edu/resources/topics/advance_directives.shtml

14. Joint Commission on Accreditation of Healthcare Organizations. (2004). Ethics, rights, and responsibilities. In *Hospital accreditation standards* (p. 109). Oakbrook Terrace, IL: Author.

15. Richard J. Ackermann. (2000, October 1). Withholding and withdrawing life-sustaining treatment. *American Family Physician, 62*, p. 1556.

16. Choice in Dying, Inc. (1996, March). *State statutes governing living wills and appointment of health care agents.* New York: Author; Partnership for caring. (2001, December 31). *Summary of state statutes. State statutes governing living wills and appointment of health care agents.* Retrieved March 15, 2004, from http://www.partnershipforcaring.org/Resources/developments_set.ht ml

17. R. Sean Morrison, Ellen Olson, Kristan R. Mertz, & Diane E. Meier. (1995, August 9). The inaccessibility of advance directives on transfer from ambulatory to acute care settings. *Journal of the American Medical Association, 274*(6), pp. 478–482.

18. Anna Maria Cugliari, Tracy Miller, & Jeffery Sobal. (1995, September 25). Factors promoting completion of advance directives in the hospital. *Archives of Internal Medicine, 155*, pp. 1893–1898.

19. Brendan M. Reilly, Michael Wagner, C. Richard Magnussen, James Ross, Louis Papa, & Jeffrey Ash. (1995, November 27). Promoting inpatient directives about life-sustaining treatments in a community hospital. *Archives of Internal Medicine, 155*, pp. 2317–2323.

20. Mildred Z. Solomon, Lydia O'Donnell, Bruce Jennings, Vivian Guilfoy, Susan M. Wolf, Kathleen Nolan, Rebecca Jackson, Dieter Koch-Weser, & Strachan Donnelley. (1993, January). Decisions near the end of life: Professional views on life-sustaining treatments. *American Journal of Public Health, 83*(l), pp. 14–21.

21. Partnership for Caring, 2001 (February).

22. Partnership for Caring, 2001 (December).

23. Bonnie S. Jacobson. (1994, September). Ethical dilemmas of do-not-resuscitate orders in surgery. *AORN Journal, 60*(3), pp. 449–452; Proposed AORN position statement on perioperative care of patients with do-not-resuscitate (DNR) orders. (1994, October). *AORN Journal, 60*(4), 648, 650; Statement of the American College of Surgeons on advance directives by patients: "Do not resuscitate" in the operating room. (1994, September). *ACS Bulletin*, p. 29; Judith O. Margolis, Brian J. McGrath, Peter S. Kussin, & Debra A. Schwinn. (1995). Do not resuscitate (DNR) orders during surgery: Ethical foundations for institutional policies in the United States. *Anesthesia and Analgesia, 80*, pp. 806–809.

24. Partnership for Caring. (2003, November 25). *States are creating a new form called a "nonhospital DNR order." Here's why.* Washington, DC: Author.

25. Andrew L. Evans & Baruch A. Brody. (1985, April). The do-not-resuscitate order in teaching hospitals. *Journal of the American Medical Association, 253*(15), pp. 2236–2239.

26. Susanna E. Bedell & Thomas L. Delbanco. (1984, April). Choices about cardiopulmonary resuscitation in the hospital: When do physicians talk with patients? *The New England Journal of Medicine, 320*(17), pp. 1089–1093.

27. Joan M. Teno, Rosemarie B. Hakim, William A. Knaus, Neil S. Wenger, Russell S. Phillips, Albert W. Wu, Peter Layde, Alfred E. Connors, Neal V. Dawson, & Joanne Lynn, for the SUPPORT Investigators. (1995, April). Preferences for cardiopulmonary resuscitation: Physician–patient agreement and hospital resource use. *Journal of General Internal Medicine, 10*, pp. 179–186.

28. Susan Morse. (1985, July 15). Final requests: Preparing for death. (Quoting ethicist Robert Veatch.) *The Washington Post*, p. B5.

29. Sherwin B. Nuland. (1995). *How we die: Reflections on life's final chapter* (pp. 248, 258–259). New York: Vintage Books.

30. William M. Tierney, Paul R. Dexter, Gregory P. Gramelspacher, Anthony J. Perkins, Xiao-Hua Zhou, & Frederic D. Wolinsky. (2001, January). The effect of discussions about advance directives on patients' satisfaction with primary care. *Journal of General Internal Medicine, 16*(1), pp. 32–40.

31. Peter H. Ditto, Joseph H. Danks, William D. Smucker, Jamila Bookwala, Kristen M. Coppola, Rebecca Dresser, Angela Fagerlin, R. Mitchell Gready, Renate M. Houts, Lisa K. Lockhart, & Stephen Zyzanski. (2001, February 12). Advance directives as acts of communication: A randomized controlled trial. *Archives of Internal Medicine, 161*(3), pp. 421–430.

32. Kristin M. Coppola, Peter H. Ditto, Joseph H. Danks, & William D. Smucker. (2001, February 12). Accuracy of primary care and hospital-based physicians' predictions of elderly outpatients' treatment preferences with and without advance directives. *Archives of Internal Medicine, 161*, pp. 431–440.

33. Andis Robeznicks. (2002, December 9). End-of-life care receives failing grades. *AMANews*. Retrieved November 14, 2003, from http://www.ama-assn.org/amednews/2002/12/09/prsd1209.htm

34. Lois LaCivita Nixon & Lori Roscoe. (1999, June). How can you improve end-of-life decision making? *Trustee, 52*(6).

35. Carrie Gordon Earll. (2001, February 27). Status of physician-assisted suicide law. *CitizenLink: Focus on Social Issues*. Retrieved November 4, 2003, from http://www.family.org/cforum/fosi/bioethics/euthanasia/a0028006.cfm

36. Gerald Kelly. (1951, December). The duty to preserve life. *Theological Studies, 12*, p. 550.

37. Vatican Congregation for the Doctrine of the Faith. (1980, June 26). *Declaration on euthanasia*. Vatican City: Author.

38. Tom L. Beauchamp & James F. Childress. (2001). *Principles of biomedical ethics* (5th ed., p. 129) New York: Oxford University Press.

39. Patient's right to starve upheld. (1984, February 3). *The Washington Post*, p. A20.

40. Robert M. Veatch. (1977). *Case studies in medical ethics* (pp. 340–341). Cambridge, MA: Harvard University Press.

41. In re Quinlan, 70 NJ. 10, 355 A.2d 647 (1976).

42. Susan M. Wolf. (1990, January/February). Nancy Beth Cruzan: In no voice at all. *The Hastings Center Report, 20*(l), p. 39.

43. Cruzan v. Director, Missouri Department of Health et al. 110 S. Ct. 2841 (1990).

44. Malcolm Gladwell. (1990, December 27). Woman in right to die case succumbs. *The Washington Post*, p. A3.

45. Terri Schiavo's case is more complex than Nancy Cruzan's. Schiavo's diagnosis as being in PVS is disputed, and her husband and her parents are locked in a legal dispute about withdrawing life-sustaining hydration and nutrition. Florida's legislature and governor have intervened in the case, thus adding

a political dimension to an already highly emotional situation. At this writing Schiavo's fate is unknown.

46. Joanne Lynn & James E. Childress. (1983, October). Must patients always be given food and water? *The Hastings Center Report 13*(5), pp. 17–21; John J. Paris & Anne B. Fletcher. (1983, October). Infant Doe regulations and the absolute requirements to use nourishment and fluids for the dying infant. *Law, Medicine & Health Care, 11*, pp. 210–213.

47. American Hospital Association. (1986, March 15). *Withholding and withdrawing life-prolonging medical treatment.* Chicago: Author.

48. American Medical Association, Council on Ethical and Judicial Affairs. (1994). *Code of medical ethics: Current opinions with annotation* (pp. 36–38). Chicago: Author.

49. Michael E. Frederich. (2002, Fall). Artificial hydration and nutrition in the terminally ill. *AAHPM Bulletin, 4*(1), pp. 8–9, 13.

50. Robert J. Sullivan, Jr. (1993, April). Accepting death without artificial nutrition or hydration. *Journal of General Internal Medicine, 8*, p. 222.

51. *Ibid.*

52. Donald G. McNeil, Jr. (2003, July 1). First study on patients who fast to end lives: Survey says starving isn't painful or grisly. *The New York Times*, p. A19.

53. Child Abuse and Neglect Prevention and Treatment, 45 C.F.R. §1340.15(b)(2). (1999).

54. *Ibid.*

55. Child Abuse and Neglect Prevention and Treatment, 45 C.F.R. §1340.20 (Appendix to Part 1340—Interpretation of Guidelines Regarding 45 C.F.R. 1340.15.) (1999).

CHAPTER 11

PATIENT AUTONOMY AND THE PARADIGM OF PHYSICIAN-ASSISTED SUICIDE

n the United States, what is now called physician-assisted suicide (PAS) first became a prominent ethical and legal issue in 1990 when it was thrust into the public's consciousness by Jack Kevorkian, M.D. Though seldom discussed, it is widely understood that the preeminent role of the physician is to "comfort always," a role especially important when hope of benefit from further treatment has faded. This ethic has never included assisting in suicide, however. Sometimes, eliminating pain necessitated large amounts of morphine, but an unintended death in pursuit of comfort care raised few ethical (or legal) concerns. Doubtless, physicians and other caregivers (e.g., nurses) have sometimes heeded the pleas of pain-wracked patients to help them die, or solely from humanitarian instincts, they have occasionally performed involuntary, active euthanasia on a medically hopeless patient who could no longer communicate.

The Hippocratic tradition prohibits physicians from giving a deadly drug and considers it unethical for physicians to deliberately cause death, whether requested by the patient or for the noble purpose of pain relief. Patient wishes are given no weight. The Hippocratic ethic is reflected in legal prohibitions against homicide by physicians and the laws in many states that prohibit assisting in suicide.

PAS is one of three types of aid in dying or physician-assisted death. The three are sometimes incorrectly treated as synonymous. Strictly defined, PAS fits no types of euthanasia described in Chapter 10. It has characteristics of voluntary (patient desired), active (specific steps) euthanasia, but it differs in a critical aspect. PAS occurs when a physician provides the means and medical advice that enable someone to commit suicide. In some manifestations, the physician's assistance is such as to provide assurance that the suicide will be successful. In all manifestations of PAS, however, patients perform the act that directly causes their deaths. Broadly defined, it is a good death because it is intended to be pain free. It is not, however, euthanasia, as defined previously. Physical disability prevents some from engaging in an act that would cause death. They are candidates for voluntary, active euthanasia should it become legal. The mental competence of those wishing to be assisted in suicide or to be euthanized is always an issue.

LEGAL ASPECTS OF PHYSICIAN-ASSISTED SUICIDE IN THE UNITED STATES

Legalizing PAS was considered in initiatives on ballots in Washington State (1991) and California (1992). Both initiatives were rejected. In 1994, Oregon voters narrowly (52% to 48%) approved an initiative to enact PAS, the Death with Dignity Act. Court challenges delayed implementation. The legislature asked voters to repeal the law, a request that was soundly defeated (60% to 40%). PAS became available for terminally ill Oregonians in late 1997.

As of 2004, only Oregon has legalized PAS. In addition to Washington and California, unsuccessful attempts to pass PAS (or euthanasia) laws have been made in Michigan and Maine.[1] Similar legislation was considered in more than a dozen other states.[2] PAS is illegal by specific statute or common law precedent in almost all states. In 2003, statutes in 39 states criminalized assisted suicide; in 6 states the common law achieved the same purpose. Four states had neither statutory nor common law prohibitions against assisted suicide.[3] This legal context is resoundingly inconsistent with the polls that show, by a large majority, Americans favor physician help in ending the lives of people who are terminally ill (see the section titled "Issues for Health Services Managers")

In March 1996, the California-based federal 9th Circuit Court of Appeals ruled in *Washington v. Glucksberg* that the Washington State law making physician-assisted suicide a felony was a denial of due process of law under the 14th Amendment to the U.S. Constitution. Its reasoning relied heavily on the Supreme Court's abortion cases, which the circuit court found to have compelling similarities.[4] A month later, the New York-based federal 2nd Circuit Court of Appeals ruled in *Vacco v. Quill* that terminally ill people have the same right to hasten death by taking drugs as they do by refusing artificial life support, thus striking down a New York state law. Its ruling was based on the equal protection clause of the 14th Amendment.[5]

In 1997, the U.S. Supreme Court agreed to hear appeals of these two cases. A unanimous U.S. Supreme Court ruled in *Washington v. Glucksberg*[6] and *Vacco v. Quill*[7] that states may ban assisted suicide without violating either the due process or equal protection clauses of the 14th Amendment to the U.S. Constitution, respectively. The Court did not decide whether states could pass laws permitting assisted suicide. In a companion case the Court declined to review a lower court ruling in *Lee v. Harcleroad*,[8] holding that a group of terminally ill persons and their physicians had no standing to challenge the constitutionality of Oregon's PAS law because it posed no personal danger to them.[9] Thus, the issue of physician assistance in suicide remains firmly within the purview of the states.

The Case of "Dr. Death"

In 1990, 54-year-old Janet Adkins, who suffered from early-stage Alzheimer's disease, feared losing her memory and the ability to engage in normal activities. She sought the help of Dr. Jack Kevorkian, a retired pathologist, to assist her in committing suicide before her mental abilities became so impaired that she could no longer make a rational decision.[10] Kevorkian had gained national prominence earlier that year at a press conference in which he showed a device he had designed that enabled persons who wanted to die to self-administer toxic chemicals, after initial assistance from a physician. Kevorkian's help to Adkins was criticized as procedurally flawed, and Adkins's competence was questioned because of her diagnosis.[11] The case starkly focused the public's attention on the issue of active, voluntary euthanasia and the right to assisted suicide.

In several early assisted suicides, Kevorkian played an active role by starting a saline IV. The patient then initiated the flow of potassium chloride and barbiturates that caused death. Kevorkian's role changed as he continued to assist in suicides. After his medical license was revoked, Kevorkian, or "Dr. Death" as his critics called him, could no longer legally obtain the chemicals used previously. He began using carbon monoxide, which was breathed through a mask placed on the face of the patient, who then initiated the flow of gas. Kevorkian began videotaping conversations with "patients" held prior to assisting their suicide, in which they answered questions that documented their state of mind as well as their desire to die. By the end of 1996, Kevorkian had assisted in more than 40 suicides. All of his assisted suicides occurred in Michigan, which initially had no law banning it. Hastily passed legislation outlawing assisted suicide did not stop him and he continued to assist suicides.

The numerous criminal proceedings against Kevorkian for assisting in suicide were unsuccessful for various reasons: the Michigan court of appeals ruled that the ban on assisted suicides was passed illegally; judges dismissed charges against Kevorkian, ruling that assisted suicide is a constitutional right; and juries acquitted him.[12] Kevorkian was finally convicted of second-degree murder in 1998, a conviction substantially based on a videotape that he made showing him administering a lethal injection to a person with amyotrophic lateral sclerosis (ALS, or Lou Gehrig's disease). Kevorkian called it a mercy killing (euthanasia); prosecutors and a jury disagreed. He was sentenced to a term of 10–25 years in prison, where he continues efforts to gain his release. By his own count, Kevorkian assisted in at least 130 suicides.[13] Of 69 persons known to have died with Kevorkian's assistance or intervention, only 25% had been diagnosed as terminally ill.[14] Thus, the majority were suffering from early stages of degenerative disease, a fact that in itself raises significant ethical issues.

Kevorkian has been criticized on professional and ethical grounds, including assertions that he: did not know his "patients," was unqualified to diagnose or understand illnesses because he is a pathologist, had a conflict of interest because of his desire to publicize himself and his suicide machine, assisted persons who did not have terminal illness, and neither made little effort to nor was qualified to judge the competence of the persons he assisted. Kevorkian had hoped to establish an obitorium, a clinic where terminally ill persons wanting to commit suicide could be assisted to die.

One of Kevorkian's stated goals was to test the limits of patient autonomy. His primary defense was that the law criminalizing assisted suicide is an unconstitutional interference in a person's right to privacy. This defense used reasoning similar to that in *Roe v. Wade*, the U.S. Supreme Court decision that found a constitutional right to privacy protected a woman's decision to abort her pregnancy in the first trimester free from state interference. Assisted suicide presents an even stronger case for individual autonomy as expressed in the right to privacy because no other life (i.e., a fetus) is involved. Experts disagree on the constitutionality of assisted suicide, however.[15, 16] In mid-1995, the U.S. Supreme Court declined to review Kevorkian's appeals from his criminal conviction.[17]

The Oregon Experience

Oregon law permits physicians to prescribe but not administer medications to end life. To request a prescription for lethal medications, a person must be 18 years of age or older, a resident of Oregon, capable (able to make and communicate health care decisions), and diagnosed with a terminal disease that will lead to death within 6 months. Having met that threshold, a series of steps must be followed to receive the prescription:

- Patients must make two oral requests to their physician, separated by at least 15 days.

- Patients must provide a written request to their physician, signed in the presence of two witnesses.

- A prescribing physician and a consulting physician must confirm the diagnosis and prognosis.

- If either physician believes the person's judgment is impaired by a psychiatric or psychological disorder, the patient must be referred for a psychological examination.

- The prescribing physician must inform the patient of feasible alternatives to assisted suicide including comfort care, hospice care, and pain control.

- The prescribing physician must request, but may not require, the patient to notify their next-of-kin of the prescription request.[18]

The law was amended in 1999 to require that pharmacists be informed of the prescribed medication's ultimate use.[19] The physician may attend the patient when medication is taken but is not required to do so.[20] Physicians must report participation to the state health division; those who act in good faith within the law are protected from both professional discipline and legal liability.[21]

Results The first suicide under the Oregon law was reported in March 1998.[22] The Blue Cross and Blue Shield plans of Oregon began covering PAS in early 1998.[23] In late 1998, the Oregon Health Plan (which covers Medicaid patients) added PAS to end-of-life comfort care services such as pain medication and hospice care.[24] By the end of 2002, 129 Oregonians had been assisted in suicide.[25] At this writing, no nationwide trend for assisted suicide has developed.

Patient Characteristics Physicians reported that their patients who chose PAS were concerned about loss of autonomy, participation in activities that make life enjoyable, and losing control of bodily functions. Data comparing patients who used PAS with Oregonians who died from the same underlying cause are instructive. Younger patients were more likely to use PAS than older patients. Asians were more likely than non-Hispanic whites to use PAS. Divorced patients were twice as likely as married patients to use PAS. The likelihood of using PAS increased with educational attainment. Those with cancer and ALS were more likely to use PAS than individuals with other terminal conditions. Almost all had some form of insurance and 92% (in 2002) were enrolled in hospices.[26] Those who sought PAS under the Oregon statute tended to be better educated, insured, and often in hospice care, which should somewhat allay fears that the law will be used primarily by Oregonians who are poor, uneducated, mentally ill, or socially isolated. However, this may not assuage the fears of those who may already feel disadvantaged in society and thus vulnerable to potential abuse of PAS, including some ethnic groups and people with low incomes and low levels of education. Older adults may begin to believe that they have a unique level of risk because they are most likely to feel the effects of an express or implied utilitarian calculus. Chapter 14 addresses this issue in more detail.

Physician Characteristics   In 2002, 33 physicians wrote 58 prescriptions for lethal doses of medication. Prescribing physicians had been in practice a median of 18.5 years. Oncologists (45%), internists (29%), and family practitioners (24%) were most likely to write lethal prescriptions. Prescribing physicians were present for one third of the 38 deaths in 2002. No physicians were reported to the Oregon Board of Medical Examiners in 2002 for having acted in violation of the statutory requirements for PAS.[27]

Summary   In its annual report on PAS in 2002, Oregon's Department of Human Services noted that the availability of PAS may have led to improved end-of-life care using other modalities. The request for PAS offers an opportunity for physicians to explore patients' fears and wishes about end-of-life care and the options available. Reportedly, physicians have made greater efforts to learn more about pain medications for the terminally ill, to improve their recognition of psychiatric disorders, and to refer patients more frequently to hospice care.[28] Few complications have been reported from Oregon's assisted suicides, a result inconsistent with Netherlands's data (discussed in the next section). Complications reported in Oregon in 2002 were almost exclusively those of living as long as 2–14 hours after ingesting the lethal medication.[29]

One conclusion of the findings in Oregon is that physicians are using the law in a prudent and cautious manner. Other explanations are possible, however, including that there are too few data for a true picture to have emerged. The findings may also suggest a high level of tentativeness on the parts of both physicians and those who might seek assistance in suicide—tentativeness likely to diminish over time and as PAS becomes more common and more socially acceptable. Given the evolution of PAS in the Netherlands, this latter explanation has merit.

Opiates such as morphine are the drugs most often given to help patients die.[30] It is noteworthy that in 1998, Oregon led the nation in medical use of morphine, an increase of more than 70% since 1994, when voters approved the first assisted-suicide referendum.[31] Heavy use of morphine in Oregon may suggest a reliance on it for palliation. As noted, passage of the original law stimulated Oregon physicians to improve care of the dying.[32] Most major hospitals have established strong pain management programs to give patients an alternative to assisted suicide.[33]

PHYSICIAN-ASSISTED SUICIDE
AND EUTHANASIA IN THE NETHERLANDS

International comparisons are instructive. Assisted suicide has been available in parts of Switzerland since 1942; increasingly, that country is a destination for "suicide tourists."[34] In 2002, Belgium legalized voluntary euthanasia and assisted suicide with a law similar to that of the Netherlands.[35] In mid-2003, a year after passage of the original law, Belgian lawmakers proposed expanding euthanasia to children younger than 18 years of age.[36] PAS and euthanasia are being debated elsewhere in Europe, notably in Spain and France. A 2002 survey in France showed that 88% favor or would tolerate euthanasia.[37]

The vanguard of assisted dying, however, is the Netherlands, where euthanasia and PAS have been practiced since the 1980s, despite their illegality, and where 92% of the population supports euthanasia.[38] Before they were made legal in 1993, a 1990 government study found that 2% of deaths were caused by euthanasia and PAS.[39] It was found that in 1,000 other cases, a patient's life was ended without an explicit recent request to die.[40] The data also showed that in 1990, death was hastened for 16,850 patients, of whom 8,750 died by withholding or withdrawing treatment and 8,100 died by administering pain-killing drugs. Consent was obtained from only 3,100 of the 8,100 patients in the second group. Thus, the majority of patients from whom treatment had been withdrawn or withheld or who had died from administration of pain killing drugs (5,000) had not consented.[41] Data from a 1995 Dutch government study showed 3,600 deaths from assisted suicide and euthanasia, of which 900–1,000 were officially acknowledged to have been involuntary. Another 2,000 patients were given large doses of pain-killing drugs with the primary aim of ending their lives, but these were not classified as euthanasia.[42] These data show that even after voluntary euthanasia and PAS became legal, involuntary euthanasia continued, a practice that may have stimulated passage of another revision of the law in 2001.

The revision of the 1993 law that first legalized voluntary active euthanasia and PAS went into effect in 2002.[43] It expanded the categories of persons who may use euthanasia and PAS. Physicians who provide these "services" are required to use due care in terminating a life (euthanasia) or assisting in suicide. By performing the procedure in a medically appropriate manner, the crimes of euthanasia and assisted suicide are legally defined as medical treatments.

The statute specifically allows euthanasia for incompetent patients. Persons 16 years and older can make an advance written statement containing a request to terminate their life, which a physician may carry out. The written statement need not be made in conjunction with a specific medical condition and it could have been written years before, based upon views that may have changed. The physician can administer euthanasia based on the prior written statement.[44]

In addition, the law allows other categories of persons to request and receive euthanasia or assisted suicide: teenagers (with varying degrees of parents' or guardians' approval, depending on age [children as young as 16 may request termination of life in writing, which the physician can legally administer without parental or guardian approval {although they must be involved in the decision process}], children as young as 12 may request and receive euthanasia or assisted suicide [with agreement of parents or guardians]), and persons for whom the doctor "holds the conviction that the patient's suffering is lasting and unbearable."[45]

The 2002 Dutch law requires that specific criteria must be met if safeguards from criminal prosecution for physicians are to be available. The following concepts must be taken into consideration:

- *Voluntary*—The physician must be convinced that the patient has made a voluntary, persistent, and carefully considered request to die.

- *Suffering*—The physician must be convinced that the patient's suffering is unbearable and that there is no prospect of improvement of the patient's situation. (There is no requirement that the suffering must be physical or that the patient must be terminally ill.)[46]

- *Informed*—The physician has informed the patient about his or her medical situation and medical prospects.

- *Alternatives*—The physician, together with the patient, must be convinced that there is no reasonable alternative.

- *Consultation*—The physician has consulted at least one other physician with an independent viewpoint who must have seen the patient and given a written opinion on the due-care criteria [*sic*].

- *Due care and attention*—The physician must have assisted the patient to die with due medical care and attention.[47]

These criteria are similar to the 1993 law. Review of assisted deaths in the 2002 law is very different, however.

All oversight of euthanasia and assisted suicide is done after the patient's death by a regional review committee for termination of life on request and assisted suicide. The committees are comprised of a legal specialist, a physician, and an expert in philosophical issues, specifically with expertise as to the requisites for meaningful life. Significantly, the 2002 law shifts the burden of proof. No longer must the physician justify the need to terminate life. It is the prosecutor who must show that terminating a life failed to meet the requirement of due care. Prosecutors will only learn about termination of a life if information is sent to them by the regional committee. The law does not prohibit physicians from administering euthanasia to a nonresident.[48] It is hoped that the law will bring into the open euthanasia that has been hidden historically. New concerns about "hidden euthanasia" surfaced only a year after the 2002 law went into effect. Terminal sedation, for example, occurs when physicians give patients in severe pain quantities of morphine large enough to also hasten death. Because euthanasia is defined as the active termination of life on request, such overdoses are not reportable—it is not clear that the death was intended. The death is considered a natural death.[49]

Some argue that the Netherlands will in effect "be issuing retrospective licenses for consensual killing."[50] Legally sanctioning active euthanasia for various groups of "patients" (with varying degrees of consent from parents or guardians for certain of them) is a significant change and moves euthanasia from the exceptional to an accepted way of dealing with medical conditions beyond serious or terminal illness. Palliative care is one casualty of the Netherlands's history of PAS, and hospice care use there lags behind other countries.[51]

The technical aspects of PAS appear to be relatively simple. Data from the Netherlands suggest, however, that there are problems even when a physician is present. Problems include medications not working as expected, technical difficulties, or unexpected side effects. In 16% of cases in which patients tried to kill themselves using doctor-prescribed drugs, the medication did not work as expected. Furthermore, 7% of the time technical problems or unexpected side effects occurred. Physicians witnessing the attempted suicide felt compelled to intervene and ensure death in 18% of cases. Even when a doctor directly performed euthanasia, the researchers found that there were complications 3% of the time. In another 6% of attempts, patients took longer to die than expected or went into a drug-induced coma that was supposed to be fatal but from which they later awoke.[52] Thus, it appears that assisted suicide and euthanasia do not necessarily result in the easy and peaceful death that they promise and that they can add to the patient's misery and suffering.

The 1993 law may have only recognized existing practice—*de facto* became *de jure*. That a western European democracy was willing to acknowledge this development, however, raises important ethical questions. Seemingly begun as a way to enhance individual self-determination, the Dutch experience shows that active euthanasia is not limited to persons who request it. The continuing and troubling scenario of large numbers of persons involuntarily, actively euthanized highlights the slippery slope, defined by philosophers as one exception leading to other more easily accepted exceptions.

That there is no requirement for suffering to be physical or that the patient must be terminally ill suggests a significant new dimension for active euthanasia and assisted suicide—persons tired of living and choosing to end their lives. Persons who are in various states of aging, have a disability, or have health problems now face the prospect that they will have to justify their continued existence. Given that Dutch physicians historically have been willing to actively euthanize persons without their consent, the persons at risk fear that their lives will be ended without their consent.[53] This fear has caused many of those most vulnerable—individuals with disabilities and older adults—to carry cards specifying their desire to continue to stay alive.[54]

SUICIDE AND THE ORGANIZATION:
THE CASE OF ELIZABETH BOUVIA

In late 1983, a dramatic case began in California that highlights several of the concepts previously described in this chapter. Elizabeth Bouvia, who was 26 years old and had cerebral palsy, entered county-owned Riverside General Hospital and asked that the staff aid her in fasting until she died. Unable to move, she required assistance in all physical activities. She wanted the hospital to provide hygienic care and the drugs necessary to give her a painless death by starvation. A court injunction prevented the hospital from discharging her. To ensure adequate nutrition, hospital staff inserted a nasogastric tube, allegedly against her wishes. She asserted that she had reached a competent and rational decision, one her lawyer argued was protected by the constitutional right to privacy and self-determination. Her mental competence was confirmed by several psychiatrists.

California has criminal penalties against aiding and abetting a suicide. After a hearing on whether the hospital could be forced to assist Bouvia in her suicide, the court ruled that "despite her right to commit suicide, which is not illegal in California, she could not ask society in the person of the hospital staff to help her because she was not a terminal patient."[55] The court distinguished Bouvia from individuals with terminal illnesses. In January 1984, the California Supreme Court refused to hear her appeal.[56]

The decision permitted the hospital to force-feed Bouvia. She was discharged from Riverside General on April 7, 1984, and was hospitalized in Tijuana, Mexico.[57] It was reported that she had reconsidered her demand to die and would return to the United States for medical treatment. Her lawyer maintained that she still wished to die, despite the fact that she had been accepted for care somewhere in California on the condition that she not stop eating.[58]

After a year in the new institution and a subsequent stay of several months at an acute care hospital, where a morphine pump was installed for pain control, Bouvia was admitted to Los Angeles County-High Desert Hospital in late 1985. As at Riverside General Hospital, and against her wishes, the staff inserted a permanent feeding tube. Court action by Bouvia initially resulted in the court's refusal to order discontinuation of the forced feeding. On appeal, however, the case was remanded, with instructions to consider her request further. As a result, tube feeding was discontinued and Bouvia was discharged. Her attorney stated, "She's promised to continue to eat her liquid diet. I know she would welcome death . . . but she has renounced [suicide]."[59] In May 1986, Bouvia was hospitalized at Los Angeles County University of Southern California Medical Center, where she was treated for chronic pain.[60] In June 1986, the California Supreme Court affirmed a lower court decision allowing her to die by refusing force-feeding (at the time she was accepting a liquid diet). The hospital had argued that removing the tube would officially endorse suicide.[61] Since then, she has shunned publicity. Elizabeth Bouvia was reported alive in 2002.[62]

Ethical Issues and Legal Considerations

In addition to highlighting the problems of situations that do not involve terminal illness, the Bouvia case delineates the clash between organizational philosophy (here with both ethical and legal justification) and patient autonomy. Bouvia's problem was not that the health services organization where she was treated refused to discharge her; instead, it was difficult to find a facility that would admit her. Those that agreed to admit her insisted on doing everything they could to maintain or improve her physical condition—thus the force-feeding. Several state courts have specifically addressed this issue. A number of states have statutes that permit withholding or withdrawing tube feeding, but several prohibit such actions under certain circumstances.[63]

The Bouvia case suggests the limit of what patients can legally (and ethically) ask of health services organizations. As shown by the Bouvia case, the law determines what the organization and its managers can do and the obligation to obey the law is a minimum performance. The ethics reflected in the organization's philosophy determine the extent to which it uses a higher standard. The law is different in other states such as New York and New Jersey, and this difference reinforces the organization's need to be aware of state law and, more important, to address such issues prospectively.

If assistance in suicide becomes legal in more states and becomes more socially acceptable, health services organizations will have to face the ethical issues it raises. Nursing facilities, hospices, and acute care hospitals have patients with degenerative neurological diseases and those who are in persistent vegetative states or are terminally ill. It is unlikely that the traditional conscience clause exception will be overridden by laws that legalize assistance in suicide. The conscience clause protects personal and institutional providers who refuse to provide services they find morally repugnant. This reinforces the need for health services organizations to specifically address the issue of end-of-life treatment in their values statements. A long-term, clearly enunciated position lends credence to the organization's position. In developing their values statement, it is likely that most organizations will take into account patients' rights and reasonable expectations.

Perhaps the most important reason for traditional health services organizations to decline to provide assistance in suicide is that the members of the public may find it inconsistent that providers they trust to help them regain and maintain their health also assist in suicide. The public may begin to distrust such providers because the role the provider is playing at any one time may be unclear. This suggests that establishment of specialized facilities, as suggested by Kevorkian's obitorium, and even commercialization of assistance in suicide, are well within the realm of possibility.

ISSUES FOR HEALTH SERVICES MANAGERS

Public opinion polls in the United States consistently show a high and increasing level of support for legalizing and regulating PAS. Public opinion polls taken before and after the conviction of Jack Kevorkian in causing the death of a person with ALS showed that public support of PAS increased from 70% to 75%. Another survey found that 55% of those polled disagreed with Kevorkian's conviction.[64]

As noted, there are ethical distinctions between providing comfort care and pain control to allow a pain-free, dignified death and hastening death through active intervention. Kevorkian's actions never occurred in health services organizations, nor could an organization have legally assisted him. Even under Oregon law, the assistance provided is only that of a physician who writes a prescription. Kevorkian's "patients" were ambulatory and not the types normally hospitalized when a question of assistance in dying arose. They were assisted to die by various means and in settings, including a motel room and a van.

Nonetheless, the cited opinion poll findings suggest the importance of health services organizations prospectively addressing the issue of assisted suicide. In this effort, managers will be a vital resource. As moral agents and the organization's conscience, health services managers play a crucial role in identifying, reinforcing, modifying, and monitoring the organization's values. To be effective in these activities, the manager must have a well-defined personal ethic that is consistent with the organization's values and a clear understanding of its application in strategic and tactical management decision making. The importance of the manager's role in setting the ethical tone for the organization and leading by example cannot be overstated.

Economics of Physician-Assisted Suicide

Developments in Oregon suggest that third-party payers and managed care organizations will offer assistance in suicide as a covered benefit soon after it becomes legal. They may even urge enactment of such laws. Covering PAS, however, raises significant issues of duality of interests. Early death significantly reduces costs for the insurer, regardless of any reduction of suffering and discomfort for the insured.

Physicians who advocated for their patients and were not pressured to control costs or prioritize services tended to counterbalance efforts to limit services. Traditional relationships in the private sector are changing, however. This change will make more prominent the questions of aid in dying as arrangements that economically bind physicians and organizations, especially hospitals, become increasingly common. Networks and alliances are the logical extension, and the private sector is establishing them.

Psychological or economic oneness between physician and organization raise significant ethical issues, including the risk that patient interests will suffer. Economic incentives in traditional private, fee-for-service medicine reward too much care, and the physician's and organization's interest in voluntary or involuntary passive euthanasia is limited to questions of the futility, or hope of benefit, from continued treatment. Newer forms of payment and organizational arrangements will change the incentives for health services organizations, even as they become less able to meet the costs of services. Hospitals have already experienced a form of capitation in diagnosis-related groups (DRGs), which have the incentive to limit services. Cost shifting is increasingly difficult for health services organizations. Thus, they are either forced to reduce costs through greater productivity (achieving the same results with fewer resources) or by changing the content of care, easily done by providing aid in dying.

Fixed-sum payment schemes such as capitation or DRGs have the incentive to minimize the number and range of services, especially those that are more costly. Such incentives cause an inherent conflict of interest between providing services that might be in the patient's best interests and holding to a fixed monetary limit. The implications are the same for private insurers and government. Although government is likely to use euphemisms such as "quality of life" and insurers are likely to more overtly focus on costs, the issue is the same for both: How can costs be controlled? Certain services (especially costly ones) are likely to be withheld and services will be withdrawn from persons who are deemed to have a poor quality of life or prognosis (e.g., in cases of futile care). Here, the fact that earlier death is the ultimate cost reduction may provide an attractive economic alternative. Awareness that this duality of interests is present will enable the manager to monitor utilization data so that the potential for harm to patients is minimized. Systems in the United States in which capitation or global budgets are used may not take positive steps to end life but may simply deny certain types of care because they are uneconomic or have little effect on improving the quality of life. In such cases, Oregon's priority list of services for Medicaid beneficiaries, which is discussed in Chapter 13, is instructive.

Summary

Hospitals and nursing facilities commonly have patients who are in persistent vegetative state, bedridden with a terminal illness, or too ill for transfer elsewhere. What are their rights as compared with those of the organization? The importance of an organizational philosophy with specific attention to aid in dying is clear—again, because legally and ethically, the organization cannot be forced to participate in activities that compromise its ethic.

International comparisons may help predict evolution of the issues of assisted suicide and euthanasia in the United States. The Dutch experience clearly shows that 30 years of debate led to a slippery slope. The rules governing assistance in suicide and euthanasia became less demanding and ever broader in their application. There is no report of involvement of health services organizations, and no role was set out for them. PAS—illegally performed in Michigan, and legally performed in Oregon—did not involve health services organizations. It seems a small step to involve them, however. This concern was raised in Belgium as its euthanasia law was debated.[65] Given the seemingly inevitable erosion of safeguards protecting those whom caregivers may consider to have an inadequate quality of life, there will be heavy pressure on health services organizations to participate.

ISSUES FOR PHYSICIANS

A primary issue for many physicians is that their profession is being turned on its head. Traditionally, physicians have been guardians of life. Now they may be asked to assist in causing death. If physicians may legally euthanize their patients, the trust so important to the patient–physician relationship will end. Older adults, individuals with disabilities, and others with lives of perceived "diminished quality" will correctly fear that instead of helping them live, their doctors may hasten their deaths. To prove the assertion that physicians and nurses, like anyone, can become inured to what is essentially murder, one only need read media reports describing killing patients as common practice.[66] Although clearly extraordinary, the case of Dr. Harold Shipman, the general practice physician in Manchester who became England's most prolific serial killer, is chilling. Shipman, who early in his career received psychiatric and drug treatment after the death of his first victim, killed at least 215 of his patients during a 24-year medical career. Speculation as to why include easing the burden on the National Health Service (England's government-run health system) to wanting to play God. Of great concern is that Shipman could elude detection for so long by issuing death certificates attributing his patients' deaths to natural causes.[67]

Proposals in the United States that physicians provide aid in dying have been roundly condemned by organized medicine. This condemnation, however, may overstate physicians' views of opposition, and they may be much more willing to provide aid in dying than the Hippocratic tradition suggests. In the United States, a national survey taken in the late 1990s, when physician assistance in suicide was illegal everywhere, found that 6% of physicians responding who regularly cared for the dying had either given at least one lethal injection or written a prescription so patients could kill themselves. The survey also found that a third of doctors would write prescriptions for deadly doses and a quarter would give lethal injections if these activities were legal.[68] Similarly, in 1995, 12% of responding physicians in Washington state reported receiving one or more explicit requests from patients for PAS; 4% had received one or more requests for euthanasia.[69] State surveys reported in the mid-1990s found that a majority of physicians in Michigan (Dr. Jack Kevorkian's home state) and in Oregon favored legalization of assisted suicide, although a sizable minority (31%) in Oregon objected to legalization and participation on moral grounds.[70]

Data from a survey of Oregon physicians not opposed to PAS helps explain their concerns about assisting in suicide. Half feared that the attempt would fail and cause harm, half were not confident that their prognosis of 6 months to live was accurate, half were unsure which drug to prescribe, one third feared someone other than the patient would take the drug, one third were not confident they could recognize depression, and some did not want to become known as "suicide doctors."[71]

The willingness of physicians to perform euthanasia and PAS is reinforced by findings from the early 1990s that only 11% of Dutch physicians said that they would not participate in euthanasia or assisted suicide.[72] Given recent legal developments in the Netherlands and apparent widespread public support, however, even fewer are likely to be unwilling to provide aid in dying as of 2004.

The question of aid in dying raises significant moral questions and necessitates a thorough reexamination of the physician–patient relationship. To this point, physicians cannot be required to perform a procedure that they morally oppose. Our society's tradition of the overriding importance of personal conscience in such matters must govern. Perhaps thanatology, the study of death and dying, will be recognized as a new medical specialty.

CONCLUSION

As framed, the debate on decisions at the end of life focuses on negative rights. Freedom from unwanted health services is a negative ethical and legal right grounded in the right to freedom from unwanted interference. Simply stated, this is autonomy. Continued attention to the implications of technology for patient autonomy and the principle of nonmaleficence are necessary if the organization is to fulfill its mission in the context of its philosophy.

It is noteworthy that none of the legislation that allows physician assistance in suicide establishes a patient's positive right to assistance in dying. A physician willing to assist the patient must be found. As yet, physicians cannot be compelled to provide assistance in suicide. It is almost certain that if assistance in suicide or dying and active euthanasia become more accepted, the number of physicians willing to perform such acts will increase. The dehumanization of provider and patient will become ever more common, and the hardening of the human beings involved in it will make such actions commonplace, even lauded.

Demedicalizing assistance in suicide reduces ethical problems for physicians, but it raises ethical issues for society in general. German law, for example, effectively makes it illegal for physicians to assist in suicides. Neither suicide nor assisting in the suicide of persons who are capable of exercising control over their actions and have freely made a responsible choice to commit suicide are illegal, however, so unique views about suicide and assistance in suicide have developed in Germany. One expression of these views is the development of societies that are organized to assist members to commit suicide.[73]

The incentives resulting from cost constraints and the increasingly interlocking economic and psychological interests of physicians and organizations, whether or not under health care reform, ensures a reassessment of aid in dying. Numerous questions must be answered. Must physicians meet their patients' demands for aid in dying through active means? Is it reasonable (or wise) to ask those committed to preserving and extending life to become thanatologists? Do patients who cannot perform the acts necessary to commit suicide have a right to voluntary active euthanasia? For health services managers, does the organization have a role to aid in dying, regardless of how the current controversy is resolved? It is possible, however, that suicide, like abortion, will be defined by courts or legislatures as a privacy issue. If so, health services organizations and their managers will be forced to address assisted suicide solely from the perspective of its ethical implications. At minimum, health services managers are ethically obliged to ensure that in their organization, right to die does not become a duty to die.

NOTES

1. Carrie Gordon Earll. (2001, February 27). Status of physician-assisted suicide law. *CitizenLink Focus on Social Issues.* Retrieved November 4, 2003, from http://www.family.org/cforum/fosi/bioethics/euthanasia/a0028006.cfm

2. Elaine A. Lisko. (1998, March 5). *Oregon task force's guidelines for physician-assisted suicide are likely to have broad impact.* Retrieved November 4, 2003, from http://www.law.uh.edu/healthlawperspectives/Bioethics/980305Oregon .html

3. Longwood University. (2003, November 4). *Doctor-assisted suicide: A guide to web sites and the literature.* Retrieved March 17, 2004, from http://www. longwood.edu/library/suic.htm

4. Henry Weinstein. (1996, March 7). Appeals court in West strikes down prohibition against doctor-aided suicides. *The Washington Post,* p. A5.

5. Joan Biskupic. (1996, April 3). U.S. appeals court overturns New York assisted-suicide ban. *The Washington Post*, p. A1.

6. 521 U.S. 702 (1997).

7. 521 U.S. 793 (1997).

8. 522 U.S. 927, certiorari denied (1997).

9. Joan Biskupic. (1997, October 15). Oregon's assisted-suicide law lives on. *The Washington Post*, p. A3

10. Victor Cohn. (1990, June 12). An assisted suicide: Is it the first step toward euthanasia? *The Washington Post*, Health Section.

11. Nancy Gibbs. (1990, June 18). Dr. Death's suicide machine. *Time*, pp. 69–70.

12. Public Broadcasting Service. (1996, May). *Chronology of Dr. Jack Kevorkian's life and assisted suicide campaign*. Retrieved November 4, 2003, from http://www.pbs.org/wgbh/pages/frontline/kevorkian/chronology.html

13. Jack Kevorkian to remain in prison. (2003, October 2). *Wired News*. Retrieved November 4, 2003, from http://wireservice.wired.com/wired/story.asp?section=Breaking&storyId=787180

14. Howard Brody. (2001, January/February). Assisted suicide for those not terminally ill. *The Hastings Center Report, 31*(1), p. 7.

15. Yale Kamisar argued that assisted suicide is unconstitutional. See Yale Kamisar. (1993, May/June). Are laws against assisted suicide unconstitutional? *The Hastings Center Report, 23*(3), pp. 32–41.

16. Robert A. Sedler argued that assisted suicide is constitutional. See Robert A. Sedler. (1993, September/October). The Constitution and hastening inevitable death. *The Hastings Center Report, 23*(5), pp. 20–25.

17. Frank J. Murray. (1995, April 25). High court won't touch Michigan suicide aid ban. *The Washington Times*, p. A1.

18. Oregon Department of Human Services. (2003, August 30). *Fifth annual report on Oregon's Death with Dignity Act*. Retrieved March 22, 2004, from http://www.dhs.state.or.us/publichealth/chs/pas/year5/ar-index.cfm

19. *Ibid.*

20. Charles H. Baron. (1999, July). Assisted dying. *Trial, 35*(7), pp. 44, 46, 48–49.

21. Melinda A. Lee & Susan W. Tolle. (1996, January 15). Oregon's assisted suicide vote: The silver lining. *Annals of Internal Medicine, 124*(2), pp. 267–269.

22. William Booth. (1998, March 26). Woman commits doctor-assisted suicide. *The Washington Post*, p. A7.

23. Oregon health plans proceed with caution on suicide coverage. (1998, March 16). *AHA News, 34*(10), p. 5.

24. Assisted-suicide coverage could be expanded. (1998, November 2). *AHA News 34*(43), p. 6.

25. Oregon Department of Human Services, 2003.

26. *Ibid.*

27. *Ibid.*

28. *Ibid.*

29. *Ibid.*

30. Daniel Q. Haney. (1998, April 23). 6 percent of physicians in survey say they have assisted in patient suicides. *The Washington Post*, p. A9.

31. William Claiborne. (1998, April 29). An Oregon statute is blunting death's sting. *The Washington Post*, p. A1.
32. Linda Ganzini, Heidi Nelson, Melinda Lee, Dale F. Kraemer, Terri A. Schmidt, & Molly A. Delorit. (2001, May 9). Oregon physicians' attitudes about and experiences with end-of-life care since passage of the Oregon death with dignity act. *Journal of the American Medical Association, 285*(18), pp. 2363–2369.
33. Baron, 1999.
34. Alison Langley. (2003, February 4). "Suicide tourists" go to the Swiss for help in dying. *The New York Times*, p. A3.
35. Derek Humphry. (2003, March 9). A twentieth century chronology of voluntary euthanasia and physician-assisted suicide. *Euthanasia Research & Guidance Organization.* Retrieved January 1, 2004, from http://www.finalexit.org/chronframe.html
36. WorldNetDaily. (2003, June 21). Belgian lawmakers propose euthanasia for children. Retrieved November 17, 2003, from http://worldnetdaily.com/news/article.asp?ARTICLE_ID=33199
37. Delphine Soulas. (2003, October 27). Euthanasia debate renewed: Mercy killing of Frenchman forces society to re-examine right to die. *The Washington Times*, p. A14.
38. Charles Truehart. (1999, August 15). Holland prepares bill legalizing euthanasia. *The Washington Post*, p. A19.
39. Marlise Simons. (1993, February 10). Dutch parliament approves law permitting euthanasia. *The New York Times*, p. A10.
40. *Ibid.*
41. John Keown. (1991, November 5). Dutch slide down euthanasia's slippery slope. *The Wall Street Journal*, p. A18.
42. Herbert Hendin. (2003, July/August). The practice of euthanasia. *The Hastings Center Report, 33*(4), pp. 44–45.
43. International Task Force on Euthanasia and Assisted Suicide. (2003, November 4). *Holland's euthanasia law.* Retrieved December 5, 2003, from http://www.internationaltaskforce.org/hollaw.htm
44. *Ibid.*
45. *Ibid.*
46. *Ibid.*
47. Joris Vos, Ambassador, Embassy of the Netherlands. (2001, May 3). The Netherlands' euthanasia law explained [Letter to the editor]. *The Washington Times*, p. A18.
48. *Ibid.*
49. Keith B. Richburg. (2004, January 4). Death with dignity, or door to abuse? *The Washington Post*, p. A1.
50. James Meek. (1999, November 21). Dutch wrestle with morality of mercy killings: Parliament is expected to legalize euthanasia, doctor-assisted suicide. *The Washington Times*, p. C12.
51. Herbert Hendin, Chris Rutenfrans, & Zbigniew Zylicz. (1997, June 4). Physician-assisted suicide and euthanasia in the Netherlands. *Journal of the American Medical Association, 227*, pp. 1720–1722.
52. Assisted Suicide Takes a Hit. (2000, February 24). *The Washington Times*, p. A7.

53. Jenny Nolan. (2001). *Dutch legalize euthanasia and assisted suicide.* Retrieved November 14, 2003, from http://www.nrlc.org/news/2001/NRL05/dutch.html
54. Anne Allen. (2001, April 15). Euthanasia is threat to our freedom. *The Express on Sunday,* p. 1.
55. Jay Matthews. (1983, December 17). Judge rejects palsy victim's bid to starve. *The Washington Post,* p. A3.
56. California Supreme Court rejects appeal by Bouvia to starve. (1984, January 20). *The Washington Post,* p. A15.
57. Patient repeatedly calls off her effort to starve to death. (1985, April 24). *The New York Times,* p. B15.
58. The latest word. (1985, August). *The Hastings Center Report, 15*(4), p. 36.
59. Doctors stop force-feeding of quadriplegic who sued. (1986, April 18). *The Washington Post,* p. A12.
60. Bouvia moves to another CA hospital. (1986, May 30). *Hospital Week,* pp. 21–23.
61. Right to refuse forced feeding upheld in court. (1986, June 6). *The Washington Post,* p. A8.
62. Diane Coleman. (2002). *Assisted suicide: The ultimate discrimination.* Retrieved December 6, 2003, from http://www.disabilitylife.net/DL/AssistedSuicide.htm
63. Tinker Ready. (1989, December 18). Medical groups back plaintiffs in right-to-die case. *Healthweek,* 6–8.
64. Baron, 1999.
65. Elizabeth Bryant. (2001, August 13). Belgian left pushes vote on euthanasia law. *The Washington Times,* A12.
66. Maggie Gallagher. (2001, April 14). Dutch death. *The Washington Times,* A10.
67. Q&A: Harold Shipman. (2003, July 15). *Guardian Unlimited.* Retrieved December 5, 2003, from wysiwyg://104/http://www.guardian.co.uk/shipman/Story/0,2763,998536,00.htm
68. Haney, 1998.
69. Anthony L. Back, Jeffrey I. Wallace, Helene E. Starks, & Robert A. Pearlman. (1996, March 27). Physician-assisted suicide and euthanasia in Washington State: Patient requests and physician responses. *Journal of the American Medical Association, 275*(12), pp. 919–925.
70. Jerald G. Bachman, Kirsten H. Alcser, David J. Doukas, Richard L. Lichtenstein, Amy D. Coming, & Howard Brody. (1996, February 1). Attitudes of Michigan physicians and the public toward legalizing physician-assisted suicide and voluntary euthanasia. *The New England Journal of Medicine, 334*(5), pp. 303–309; Melinda A. Lee, Heidi D. Nelson, Virginia P. Tilden, Linda Ganzini, Terri A. Schmidt, & Susan W. Tolle. (1996, February 1). Legalizing assisted suicide: Views of physicians in Oregon. *The New England Journal of Medicine, 334*(5), pp. 310–315.
71. Hilary Evans. (1997, September). Pitfalls of physician-assisted suicide. *Physician's News Digest* [On line]. Retrieved November 4, 2003, from http://www.physiciansnews.com/commentary/997wp.html
72. *Ibid.*
73. Margaret P. Battin. (1992, March/April). Assisted suicide: Can we learn from Germany? *The Hastings Center Report, 22*(2), pp. 44–51.

SECTION V

EMERGING ETHICAL ISSUES

There have been numerous changes in the management of health services organizations since the early 1970s. Change is the future and seems to be occurring at an accelerating pace. New managerial challenges mean greater demands on organizational philosophies and cultures and on the manager's personal ethic. Managers with an ill-defined personal ethic will feel adrift in a world that seems to have few solid foundations.

Chapter 12 examines marketing and managed care in competitive environments, Chapter 13 focuses on resource allocation, and Chapter 14 considers the social responsibility of health services organizations. These areas have become much more important, and their ethical implications require special attention.

The competitive environment has convinced health services mangers that marketing their organizations and programs is essential to their survival. Marketing is not new to them; however, applying it in ways that are more commercial and entrepreneurial is. Many managers question the ethical implications, especially if they manage not-for-profit organizations.

Managed care has emerged as a primary means of organizing and financing health services delivery. Like marketing, managed care is not new to health services, but its prevalence, coupled with quality and cost pressures, raise complex ethical issues that will challenge management.

Health services managers cannot but be aware of the increasingly ominous struggle for resources occurring at all levels of society. The health services organization is a microcosm of this struggle. Given their importance in providing critical services to society, health services organizations and their managers play a central role as arbiters of resource allocation. The ethical implications are enormous.

CHAPTER 12

ETHICS IN MARKETING
AND MANAGED CARE

Although the elements of marketing—product, place, promotion, and pricing—have been applied to health services with apparent ease, the purposes and the context of health services differ from the typical business enterprise.

In the 1920s, President Calvin Coolidge noted that the business of America is business. This statement remains accurate. The United States continues to be a bastion of democratic capitalism. Unique among its businesses is the health services industry. Health services differ from other enterprises in purpose, type of service provided, orientation, and motives. Unlike most other enterprises, health services providers may be affiliated with a specific religion and may have not-for-profit tax status. Health services organizations are also unique in that they are intimately involved with several professions and provide services that comprise significant emotional and psychological dimensions. Health services organizations are social enterprises with an economic dimension rather than economic enterprises with a social dimension.

Unlike the marketing of traditional business enterprise, which seeks to create demand for its goods and services, health services marketing seeks to meet a demand, perhaps unrealized, for its services. The distinction between business enterprise and health services has become less clear since the 1980s. Health services organizations have engaged in marketing for many years. Any type of community outreach was an implicit form of marketing. Historically, marketing occurred in several ways, including community health days, disease screenings, well-baby clinics, and press releases. The milieu of the competitive marketplace, however, requires that marketing become systematic, focused, and much more aggressive.

NEED VERSUS DEMAND

Opinions vary when the role of marketing is assessed: Is demand being created or is it being met? Important to answering this question is disagreement about which types of health services demand are meritorious, a value-laden concept in itself. Few persons would disagree that it is important to create consumer demand for hypertension or colorectal cancer screenings. The desirability of such efforts is tempered by calculating costs and benefits. Depending on the population and the disease, screening may be unacceptably expensive when measured by the number of true positives found and the morbidity and mortality prevented. Screening may be done even when it is not cost-effective for reasons of political correctness or to further a feeling of well-being in a population.

Both price and nonprice competition may increase demand. Competition in the business sector is generally deemed to be desirable. Its desirability is less clear in health services, primarily because of the duplication of services and the costs of competing for physicians, staff, and patients. Despite acceptance of competition, disagreement as to whether the demand created is appropriate continues.

In addition, conditions requiring medical intervention may be treated with different therapies. Coronary artery bypass surgery or angioplasty for individuals who have had mild heart attacks is an example of an expensive therapy that patients may be able to avoid. One study found that patients given the most elaborate tests and treatments were two or three times more likely to suffer a second heart attack or die within 30 days than were those diagnosed and treated with noninvasive therapies, such as exercise stress tests and drugs that dissolved blood clots. It has been estimated that 400,000–600,000 Americans could avoid angioplasty each year at a cost of $20,000–$25,000 per procedure.[1] Potential savings are enormous.

Similar controversies regarding treatment have surrounded other diagnoses, such as that of prostate cancer. Following early detection using the prostate-specific antigen test, the standard therapy is to treat all malignant prostate tumors aggressively with surgery or with a 7-week course of radiation therapy. As a result, men who would neither die from nor likely even notice small prostate tumors endure treatment that often invites complications, such as incontinence, impotence, injury, and, sometimes, death. The watchful waiting, or expectant management, approach has been proposed as a less detrimental alternative. Both entail closely monitoring the progression of a small, slow-growing tumor and initiating treatment only when necessary. Such an approach is appropriate for men who may not live another 10 years, such as those older than age 75 or those with severe heart disease or diabetes. Cost and quality-of-life differences are obvious.[2]

More subjective situations contrast with the objective need to intervene when coronary artery disease is present. Cosmetic surgery is often cited as an example of an "unnecessary" medical service. It is claimed that face lifts, tummy tucks, and silicone implants waste medical resources—regardless of payment source—and that these resources should be available for other health uses. This is a subjective definition of need. Reasonable persons could reach different conclusions as to what patients need and how or whether the demand that arises from that need should be met by the health care system. Perhaps activities such as cosmetic surgery should not be defined as health services but as consumer services similar to hair styling, exercise and yoga classes, laser vision correction, and bodybuilding, some of which use elements of the health care system.

Epidemiologic studies should be used to develop data about populations. These data reveal the incidence and prevalence of diseases as well as psychological and physical concerns of the population that may fall outside the more traditional definitions of disease. The real problem in terms of assessing need and demand arises when those judging such data apply their personal value systems to determine the problem's importance. These judgments cause the process to be less-than-objective, whether it affects decisions in determining what to study or what is to be done with the results. In turn, these decisions affect the choice of regimens and decisions about whether to treat.

The debate about need is most heated when the ethics of marketing are included. This is especially true when marketing is to be used to affect demand or to encourage persons to seek elective procedures. Physical or psychological conditions about which an individual is either unaware or unwilling to seek treatment represent potential demand for medical services. Conditions for which no help is sought because of financial barriers also represent potential demand; examples include dental care, hammer toes, hemorrhoids, cataracts, and psychiatric services.

Troubling in this debate is the suggestion that meeting potential demand is unethical. The constitution of the World Health Organization defines health as "a state of complete physical, mental, and social well-being and not merely the absence of disease or infirmity."[3] This broad definition includes all efforts to improve physical, mental, and social well-being as beneficial. It is instructive to consider wellness (prevention) activities. The possibilities for organizational involvement are almost limitless because every facet of life could be affected to improve general health and prevent medical problems. Beyond wellness activities are questions of how to treat demand for services that may seem foolish to some observers. Should people be denied cosmetic surgery simply because other people judge such procedures to be trivial or because what they seek to correct is not life threatening? Such infringements on individual autonomy are currently greater than the public will accept.

It is not clear how and by whom need and demand are to be judged. Despite the presence of the occasional hypochondriac or Munchausen's syndrome patient, demand for services should be accepted as rational. In looking at demand for medical services, it is most useful to focus attention on "typical" patients. When typical patients hear about new medical problems or treatment and diagnostic possibilities, they respond rationally. The "worried well" are persons who are not clinically ill but are appropriately concerned about their health and the quality of their lives. Their decisions about elective procedures are personal cost–benefit analyses. It is when publicly funded programs use cost–benefit analyses to make macroallocation decisions that services formerly provided may become unavailable. Oregon's example of prioritizing health services in its Medicaid program is thus instructive and rational when political decisions make resources adequate (see p. 304).

Responsible Marketing

How does the health services organization market to patients and potential patients in a way consistent with its ethical obligation to avoid creating unnecessary demand while meeting its obligation to seek and serve those who might be in need? In its Management Advisory on Ethical Conduct for Health Care Institutions, the American Hospital Association (AHA) includes a statement on advertising, a major element of marketing. Advertising may be used to advance the organization's goals and objectives and support its mission. Advertising is used to educate the public, report to the community, increase awareness of services, increase support for the organization, and recruit employees. The Management Advisory states,

> Health care advertising should be truthful, fair, accurate, complete, and sensitive to the health care needs of the public. False or misleading statements, or statements that might lead the uninformed to draw false conclusions about the health care facility, its competitors, or other health care providers are unacceptable and unethical.[4]

The AHA statement on advertising sets a proper tone for an important element of responsible marketing. If profits and return on investment are the primary reasons for their existence, organizations will take a very different view of what responsible marketing is, as well as what is appropriate competition. This is the difference between giving people whatever they want and tempering desires and potential demand with some effort to judge value and usefulness. This view of the patient involves elements of paternalism, but it should be consistent with the organization's mission statement.

Demarketing to Avoid Bankruptcy

Chief executive officer (CEO) Chris Hines had finally gotten down far enough in the stack of papers on her desk to get to last month's emergency department (ED) activity report. She had already digested the grim news about the continued financial hemorrhage affecting Community Hospital. The current deficit was $500,000—and it was only the fourth month of the fiscal year. Because Community Hospital served largely inner city patients, many of whom were uninsured or whose care was paid by a chronically underfunded Medicaid program, there seemed to be little hope that the financial situation would improve.

Hines knew that more than 40% of Community Hospital's admissions come through the ED and that about half of those admissions arrived by taxi, private automobile, or on foot. The other half arrived via the city-owned ambulance service. Hines had tried to implement a plan to increase elective admissions, and thus improve the payer mix, by encouraging her attending physicians to admit their private patients to Community. Her effort failed. Next, Hines tried to work with city officials to implement a new ambulance routing system that would give Community a chance to improve its financial condition. Unsympathetic city officials refused to help.

Hines knew that Community Hospital's endowment would carry the hospital for approximately 3 more years but that the hospital would have to close if it was not breaking even by then. Because the city was uncooperative, Hines concluded that the key to survival lay with reducing the number of uninsured and Medicaid patients admitted through the ED.

Hines spoke with several marketing consultants, one of whom offered to do pro bono work for Community Hospital. He seized upon the idea of "demarketing" the ED. He reasoned that it was the fine reputation enjoyed by Community Hospital's ED that was largely responsible for the 50% of ED patients who arrived other than by city ambulance. He listed the following ways the ED could be made less attractive to potential patients: reducing ED staffing to a minimum; closing the parking lot near the ED; reducing housekeeping services so that the physical plant would be dirty and unkempt; deferring nonsafety-related maintenance; changing triage policies, procedures, and staffing to increase waiting time for nonemergency patients; using staff who were most likely to be rude and inconsiderate; and encouraging rumors that closure of the ED was imminent.

The consultant knew that there might be repercussions beyond the ED, but Community was desperate, and he believed extreme action was necessary.

In analyzing this case, one must first ask whether there were other steps Hines and her managers could have taken to improve the financial condition of Community Hospital. Examples include closing the ED rather than demarketing it (a more honest solution); undertaking other, more remunerative medical care activities to offset the ED losses; or opening less costly primary care clinics to care for the worried well and other nonemergency medical problems coming into the ED.

Assuming, however, that such options were unavailable, the demarketing strategy raises two ethical issues. First, the steps contemplated are likely to negatively affect the quality of care in the ED. Beyond staffing and the physical aspects directly affected, the psychological impacts on ED staff, with a probable ripple effect on inpatient care, will negatively influence morale and ultimately the quality of care. Such actions violate the principles of beneficence and nonmaleficence and the virtues of caring and honesty.

A second ethical principle is justice. People in the community are caught between the city bureaucracy and the efforts of Community Hospital to remain financially viable. They may have little choice but to endure the indignities and reduction in quality of service resulting from the demarketing strategy. Deliberately adding insult to injury should give all concerned a great deal of discomfort. A dimension of justice and the virtue of fidelity deplore the unfairness associated with forcing ED staff to work under such conditions. They will bear the brunt of angry patients and the dilapidated, depressing environment of the ED.

The fact that the declining financial condition of Community Hospital might have resulted in many of the same changes in the ED eventually does not justify deliberately undertaking them in the manner contemplated. Desperate managers may consider desperate acts, but such actions cannot be morally justified.

FUTURE OF COMPETITION

A political science theory suggests that over time enemies begin to take on one another's attributes. This concern deeply troubles the not-for-profit sector of the health services system, which views itself as holding and furthering values different from those in the for-profit sector. They fear that competition for market share and the focus on financial considerations and economic survival will cause them to lose sight of their humanitarian and charitable motives.

In this regard, payment systems are especially significant. The advent of reimbursement using diagnosis-related groups for hospitalized Medicare beneficiaries was the opening round of what is proving to be a continuing reassessment of payment schemes. Competition and cost-cutting are furthering the shift from fee-for-service to various forms of fixed payment. Physician and organizational providers are becoming aligned in relationships that add a significant amount of complexity to traditional ethical problems and raise several new ones. Physicians are beginning to push back against the various pressures on them, however. Many are limiting the number of Medicare and Medicaid patients in their practices, refusing to accept assignment from managed care and managed care organization (MCO) fee schedules, and establishing boutique practices exclusively for fee-for-services patients. Hospitals have less flexibility, but market conditions may allow them to negotiate better reimbursement schedules with MCOs.[5]

Some writers suggest that the pressures of fixed-fee reimbursement will lead to an adversarial relationship between patients and health services organizations (and perhaps physicians) and that patients' interests will be overrun by the demands of efficiency and economic survival. Such results are possible under any payment system or ownership and will occur whenever caregivers and managers lose sight of their reason for being. Doing more with less is not at variance with efforts to operationalize the principles of respect for persons, beneficence, nonmaleficence, and justice and various of the virtues. It remains for all who organize, plan, and deliver health services to keep these values in mind.

COMPETITION AND HUMAN RESOURCES POLICY

Highly competitive suburban and metropolitan markets bring with them a whole new set of ethical issues, especially as they arise in hiring practices.

Hiring the Competition

The two nursing facilities in town are highly competitive. This competition has caused each to oppose the other's certificates of need applications to the point of suing one another. The chief operating officers (COOs) of the nursing facilities have been friends since before they joined their respective nursing facilities. They play golf monthly. When the COO of one nursing facility is fired because of political intrigue on the board of directors, the other COO offers to hire him as a consultant.

Professional codes of ethics do not cover such circumstances. The fired COO is privy to proprietary information that could give the other nursing facility an unfair competitive advantage. In theory, it is possible that the fired COO could consult on matters that would not require him to reveal or use proprietary information. Given the organizations' history, however, this is unlikely. The ethically superior answer is not to hire the former competing manager. Short of that, it may be possible to avoid using the competitor's proprietary information, something that could be determined only by the specifics of what is to be done by the newly minted consultant.

Does a fired manager have any duty to a former employer? Managers have an ethical duty to keep proprietary information confidential after they sever relations with an employer. This duty of confidentiality continues until events have overtaken the confidential information. If there were no duty of confidentiality, organizations could be held hostage by former employees and managers would be among the first to agree that this is an undesirable situation from both managerial and professional perspectives.

MANAGED CARE

Simply put, managed care is an organized effort to control the costs of health services through a variety of means. The primary ethical issue that arises in managed care is the duality of interests that leads to conflicts of interest. The potential for conflicts of interest is inherent in managed care because the goals, purposes, and objectives of management and personnel may be at variance with the interests of enrollees. The tension between the MCO and its enrollees and potential enrollees occurs as early as initial marketing, when benefits packages and market segments are identified. The duality of interests that may become conflicts of interest are unavoidable, but their presence and consequent negative effects can be minimized if they are recognized by clinicians and managers. Enrollees are increasingly aware of this duality of interests.

The possibility that conflicts of interest will arise is exacerbated because many not-for-profit MCOs seek to establish and maintain a perception that they are more public-service oriented and on a higher moral plane than their for-profit competitors. Historically, not-for-profit health plans and health maintenance organizations (HMOs) have enjoyed a perception that they are a "purer" delivery system, one untainted by profit motive and one through which members gain access to high-quality medical services at reasonable cost. That perception is changing because of financial scandals in charitable organizations, disclosures of very generous compensation paid to their executives, and highly publicized denials of services to enrollees. Nonetheless, the historical perception generally remains. To the extent that marketing ignores or purposely excludes high-risk groups ("cream skimming"), there may be variance between historic and current missions. The duality of interests present when no relationship exists between providers and those toward whom marketing is directed can lead to conflicts of interest.

Adverse Selection and Marketing Managed Care

The marketing strategy must consider whether to minimize significant clinical strengths that provider components may possess. If the MCO is or is perceived to be a leader in treating complex or high-cost medical conditions, adverse selection is likely, and the MCO will be inundated with persons requiring that treatment. If higher quality results in higher costs, the MCO falls into a vicious cycle. An MCO's reputation for high-quality results encourages more high-risk persons who need expensive care to join. Straining against this adverse selection may cause quality to decline for other enrollees, or the MCO may be forced to restrict benefits or increase premiums. Thus, to survive, MCO marketers may have to minimize references to superb care of specific types and focus instead on developing a reputation that the MCO delivers general medical services of high quality but without centers of excellence.

I Want to See Dr. Nightengale

Dr. Nightengale is a pediatrician with HMO, Inc., located in a medium-size city. She has had no specialty training beyond her residency, but she has developed into an adept diagnostician, often diagnosing cases that baffle her colleagues.

At the last open enrollment, management noted that an unexpectedly large number of families with young children enrolled. As is typical, HMO, Inc., limits in-area, out-of-plan services and restricts referrals to subspecialists. Dr. Nightengale uses subspecialists more often than her colleagues, but she achieves excellent results. The new member survey showed that for many families, the presence of excellent pediatric care was an important factor in making their decision to join HMO, Inc. A few named Dr. Nightengale specifically.

Management expressed fears that such perceptions might cause significant adverse selection. Management even suggested that to protect the organization's financial position, a special review of Dr. Nightengale's use of subspecialists should be undertaken. Some thought this was an overreaction. They
agreed on a wait-and-see approach. If there were problems, they would talk
to her.

Another example of adverse selection occurred in treating individuals who
were HIV positive. An HMO in the Washington, D.C., area has achieved
a deserved reputation for providing high-quality care to this group. Dissem-
inated throughout the community, this knowledge has caused high-risk
individuals to disproportionately enroll. The HMO has not compiled data
showing higher costs for enrollees with HIV. However, it is generally
agreed that hospitalization and high-cost drug therapies as HIV progresses
to frank AIDS will make care expensive, although less expensive sources
of care are increasingly available. Sicker enrollees require more care, which
places an MCO with disproportionate numbers of such persons at financial
risk and, in terms of survival, at a competitive disadvantage.

Service Utilization in Managed Care Organizations

Managers, staff, and clinicians in the MCO bureaucracy seek to maximize
position, power, income, and rewards with the least disruption of the
organization's homeostasis. Achieving these goals, especially maximizing
income, may minimize service, whether or not that is consistent with the
contract between MCO and payer. The bureaucratic response may even
be at variance with the MCO's long-term survival needs. To regain or
retain their health, enrollees want to pay as little as necessary but obtain
all needed services—at the least they want value for their premium. When
enrollees use services efficiently and stay well at minimum cost, MCO and
enrollee goals are congruent. The situation is rarely that simple, however.

A primary source of differing interests is in the utilization of services.
Enrollees may be divided into two groups: light and moderate users of
services and heavy users. The MCO's interests and the interests of light
and moderate users are generally congruent; to be competitive, the MCO
must control heavy users. Even moderate users are potential financial
threats to MCOs in a competitive environment, and to cut costs, the MCO
may seek to transform them into light users. The likelihood that conflicts
of interest will arise is clear.

How do the differing interests, as shown by incongruent goals of
MCO and enrollee, become conflicts of interest? The MCO's marketing

will stress access to primary and specialty services and minimize limits on services. Enrollees may be constrained by limited hours, services, and having too few clinical staff to meet demand, thus purposely creating queues. Waits for appointments will reduce operating costs, especially for the 85% of medical complaints that are self-limiting. Enrollees are unlikely to endorse a deliberate strategy of deferring treatment, regardless of its clinical and economic soundness. MCOs have an escape valve for these pressures by providing advice nurse consultation and treating walk-ins during office hours. The furor resulting when the CEO of a large East Coast HMO stated publicly that the HMO used a deliberate policy of allowing queues, noting their value in reducing demand for certain services (especially self-limiting conditions), was a lesson to all MCO managers. Such policies may cause disenrollment in the long term but are effective in the short term.

Physician Incentives and Disincentives

For the enrollee, the more subtle and potentially more serious constraints imposed by MCOs are directed at affiliated physicians. A duality of interests is present between MCO and enrollee and between physician and enrollee. The Hippocratic oath requires physicians to act in the patient's best interests. The AMA's Principles of Medical Ethics state, "A physician shall be dedicated to providing competent medical care, with compassion and respect for human dignity" and "A physician shall . . . be honest in all professional interactions. . . . "[6] These guidelines suggest that patients' interests are primary as physicians connected to MCOs choose the level and content of care.

The physician is the fiduciary in the physician–patient relationship. It is perverse that a relationship necessitating such trust is influenced at all by financial incentives. Given that neutral financial incentives are likely to be impossible, it must be asked which type of payment best protects the interests of patients. Here, minimizing the interference of third parties must be the primary criterion, and the relationship that best achieves this result is fee-for-service practice. Because physicians are paid more for doing more, however, fee-for-service medicine has the incentive of overtreatment, with some increased risk to patients. On balance, however, the choices that patients make regarding third-party carriers, if any, and physicians continue the direct connection of traditional medicine and provide the best possibility of maintaining the trust so essential to this fiduciary relationship. It is unrealistic to expect physicians alone to resist the pressures of financial incentives—they need the assistance of their patients.

MCOs, however, determine the context that facilitates or inhibits physician responses. Initially, there is a self-selection bias when physicians choose in what setting and with whom they will contract. Physicians who cannot accept the rules imposed by an MCO will look elsewhere, although choices in this regard are increasingly limited. Once a physician joins an MCO, management can use a range of actions to modify or direct behavior, including financial incentives and disincentives, treatment protocols, prior authorization of services, peer pressure such as that achieved by disseminating practice profiles and comparisons with peers and best practices, nonrenewal, and dismissal. MCOs can limit referrals, especially outside the MCO; strictly control hospitalizations; establish quotas on the number of enrollees who must be seen, as in a staff-model HMO; and use a system of peer review. Peer pressure plays an important role in most constraints. Constraints are positive when they encourage judicious but appropriate use of resources. This may partly account for use of fewer ancillary services and hospital days by MCOs than fee-for-service providers.

Financial incentives and disincentives are high-risk propositions in terms of conflicts of interest, and among these, physician-at-risk or capitated payments are among the most problematic. Bonuses may be based on the use of ancillary services, referrals, and hospitalizations and may be incentives or disincentives. The effect of a potential bonus is insidious in that clinical decision making may be affected subconsciously or in ways not fully appreciated, even by the physician. Patients are almost always ignorant of such incentives or relationships. A further problem with bonuses is that staff begin to view them as a usual and expected part of their compensation, and failing to pay them is likely to result in lower morale or other, more negative consequences.

When do constraints become excessive and deny members needed services? When do constraints violate the principles of nonmaleficence and beneficence? Such questions are not easily answered because they are a function of the MCO's willingness, prompted by its managers acting as virtuous moral agents and the organization's conscience, to institute the safeguards that balance competitiveness and financial factors with furthering the interests of enrollees. Even when the virtues of compassion and caring are expressed by managers (and clinical) decision makers, media hyperbole and the political process may override clinical judgment, as when laws were passed to require 24-hour hospital stays for normal childbirth deliveries.

Other Constraints in Managed Care Organizations

In addition to physician-oriented constraints, other types of constraints are found in the organization and management of MCOs. By employing a complicated process (e.g., significant committee involvement and several levels of review), the MCO may be slow to approve use of new procedures, techniques, or equipment that raise costs. Such complexities are found more often in not-for-profit than in investor-owned MCOs. The more complex processes in not-for-profit MCOs may result from a greater degree of democracy and not from deliberate efforts to diminish access. The effect may be the same, however. For-profit MCOs tend to use a narrower management pyramid that gives the CEO more authority and greater efficiency.

MCOs may forgo purchasing high-technology equipment, or they may contract with physicians and hospitals without such equipment. For example, the higher operating costs of teaching hospitals place them at a competitive disadvantage, which means they are less likely to have contracts with MCOs. Such strategies lower costs. If lower costs enhance financial integrity and guarantee the continued availability of services to enrollees, all parties' interests are congruent. A conflict arises, however, between enrollees who might have benefited from access to the technology.

Controls on access, such as using primary care physicians as gatekeepers or case managers, limiting out-of-plan services, and specifying dollar limits on referrals and consultations, help MCOs curtail costs. Those in competitive environments, however, must show that enrollees who need services get them (or at least create such a perception) lest they lose market share. In addition, indirect and retrospective controls on access occur through use of utilization review, which is conducted on resource consumption patterns of various types of services by physicians, with special focus on those that are high cost. Controls risk malpractice suits and negative publicity if limiting access and utilization are perceived as resulting in poor outcomes.

Dissatisfaction regarding access to treatment was reflected in a study of nonelderly sick enrollees. Those in managed care were almost twice as likely (22% versus 13%) to state that they experienced major or minor problems obtaining treatment they or their physicians thought was necessary. The managed care group experienced greater difficulty (21% versus 15%) than the fee-for-service group in seeing a specialist in the past year when one was needed.[7] Data such as these support widespread anecdotal impressions that there is a cost–quality trade-off in managed care. In addition, the media regularly reports horror stories describing alleged denials of (usually specialty) care to enrollees who suffer significant morbidity or death as a result. The issue of payment source and availability of services has not been lost on patients. Fee-for-service indemnity patients had higher levels of trust in their physicians than did patients whose physicians were in salaried, capitated, or fee-for-service managed care settings.[8] The ethical obligations of MCOs, whether for-profit or not-for-profit, are seen much differently by some commentators.[9]

Minimizing Conflicts of Interest and Other Conflicts

How do MCOs and their managers prevent or minimize conflicts of interest? An indispensable first step is a willingness to acknowledge that a duality of interests is inherent in the relationships between MCOs and enrollees, physicians and the MCO, and physicians and enrollees. Awareness permits avoidance or minimization. It is also obvious that third parties have legitimate interests in physician–patient encounters, but as third-party demands for information and control increase, "physicians must reassert their own moral authority and that of their patients."[10] Without the active cooperation of health services managers, such a task is likely to be impossible.

A system of checks and balances is also needed. One solution includes an ombudsman or customer relations specialist to assist enrollees. In addition, there should be due process procedures for persons who wish to have a decision reviewed. Federally qualified HMOs must have an effective grievance procedure for enrollees. This requirement provides some protection. To be useful, however, enrollees must know that a problem has occurred; lack of knowledge is especially problematic when subtle quality-of-care issues arise. Enrollees are protected if they are able to participate effectively and if management is enlightened and the education and personal characteristics of staff involved are adequate.

MCOs may use the managing physician or gatekeeper concept to limit services provided to enrollees. Such roles are certain to cause conflicts between physicians' ethical obligations to foster the best interests of their patients and the economic expectations and constraints imposed on them by the MCO.[11] Internal audits of MCO utilization data or comparisons with external data from similar MCOs enable management to determine whether utilization is in an acceptable range. Comparisons such as these alert managers to problems in the delivery of services that may result from a duality of interests. Awareness of the way in which conflicts of interest arise will help prevent them or minimize their effect. Such activities are essential if managers are to meet their ethical obligations to enrollees.

Mixing the employed medical staff of an MCO with voluntary fee-for-service physicians raises several difficult questions.

Practice Pattern Problems Persist

Cedars-Sinai is a 400-bed community hospital located in a large East Coast metropolitan area. It has a reputation as a high-quality, low-cost provider. The medical staff at Cedars-Sinai comprise board-certified physicians who are overwhelmingly solo practitioners or part of two- or three-physician practices. No single- or multispecialty group practices are affiliated with Cedars-Sinai. Medical staff matters are handled cautiously and conservatively by hospital governance and administration.

In 1987, a large West Coast HMO established a presence and grew rapidly. Because of its fine reputation, Cedars-Sinai has become a leading provider of services for the HMO, and many of the HMO's physician-employees have admitting privileges. Almost 20% of Cedars-Sinai's inpatient days come from HMO enrollees.

Following a review of the HMO's utilization patterns, a West Coast consultant noted the large difference in hospital days per 1,000 enrollees between East and West Coast branches of the HMO. The HMO's clinical director was asked to assess how many days of care and, consequently, how many premium dollars could be saved by progressing toward the West Coast utilization level.

Word of this study came to the attention of Cedars-Sinai's CEO, who was immediately alarmed by the implications. She knew that reducing lengths of stay in any significant way by moving utilization patterns toward the West Coast experience would send shock waves through the majority of the members of her medical staff—the voluntary, fee-for-service physicians who already believed that the HMO's physicians were underutilizing services. One consequence of such a disparity in patient–day utilization patterns could be a decision by her medical stuff leadership not to reappoint the HMO's physician-employees to the medical staff because her voluntary medical staff would judge that the lengths of stay were inappropriately short and risked patient morbidity and mortality.

The CEO faces a true ethical dilemma: She has a duty of loyalty (fiduciary obligation) to the organization, but she also has a duty of beneficence to patients treated in the hospital and to potential patients in the community. Medical staff conflict will negatively affect the hospital's financial situation.

Yet, decreasing lengths of stay consistent with quality of care, patient safety, and patient satisfaction is desirable from the standpoint of patients and payers and meets the hospital's social responsibility as well. An evolutionary push toward shorter lengths of stay may meet the needs of both groups, although neither is likely to consider it desirable.

Long-Term Cost Savings of Managed Care

As this book publishes, the easy cost savings from managed care have been realized; the lower rate of health services inflation during the 1990s partly reflects this finding. The low-hanging fruit has been picked. Primarily, the savings resulted from lower payments to providers, with other payers subsidizing the deep discounts demanded and received by MCOs. Absent cross-subsidies, managed care could not have received the pricing it did and thus could not have shown the savings. For example, during the 1990s, U.S. Healthcare, a large HMO, doubled its profit margin in 2 years by cutting fees paid to doctors and hospitals 12%–20%, not by enhancing productivity or quality.[12]

A 1995 Congressional Budget Office (CBO) report stated that "the most efficient health maintenance organizations cut patients' use of health services by 19.6% while maintaining levels of care roughly comparable to other types of health plans."[13] This statement is contradictory, but its accuracy hinges on how services and care were defined. The CBO identified two caveats. The first was that the finding applied only to staff- and group-model HMOs—those that employ physicians; similar savings were not found in independent practice association-model HMOs, a type that is popular among enrollees. The second caveat was that even if all insured people enrolled in staff and group model HMOs, health care costs would not decrease 19.6% because administrative costs, pricing decisions, and doctor and hospital fees would also be factors. The study also questioned whether the successes of prepaid care among relatively younger, healthier individuals, who tend to choose HMOs, can be replicated among sicker patients, who tend to choose fee-for-service insurance. A major unknown is the amount that enrollees spent out of pocket for health services their plans did not cover, such as access to specialty referrals.

Managed competition was the cornerstone of the Clinton health plan in 1993. In that context, *managed* was a euphemism for government regulation and control. Given that basic benefits packages were mandated and that providers would have been highly regulated, savings might have occurred, but only in the short term. Significant economic costs would have been borne by providers, and there would have been large noneco-nomic costs to users, especially in the long term. In addition, the inevitable expenditure caps, as in the British National Health System or in Canada's global budgets, would have invariably led to less access for referrals and high-technology procedures.

In the late 1990s and early in the third millennium, MCOs increased premiums significantly; increases as high as 13% are expected in 2004. Net income is projected to increase by 16% to $6 billion on revenue of about $225 billion in 2004.[14] If the projections hold, this will mean a profit margin of less than 3%—hardly excessive on turnover of $225 billion.

Short of capitation, the ability of MCOs to reduce or even control costs in the future will depend on how well they can begin "managing care." Financial incentives and disincentives to enrollees are likely to be important in managing care. Clinical practice guidelines, disease manage-ment, utilization control, and financial incentives and disincentives for physicians and health services organizations were interim steps in the evolution of managed care—itself a likely way station in the progression to direct contracting between employers or other groups and health services providers, thus eliminating the middle man.[15]

Ultimately, however, *managed care* must become *managed lives*. Health care costs are best controlled by reducing health risks, which inevitably means affecting lifestyles. Lifestyle initiatives may be economic, such as charging higher premiums for people with unhealthy habits; medical, such as early detection of disease or disenrolling noncompliant enrollees; or legal, such as providers or MCOs lobbying for passage of laws that promote healthful activities or limit those that are unhealthy.[16] In its latter stages, this evolution will bring us an Orwellian relationship with MCOs. Even then, delaying death from preventable diseases will only bring more people to slow, long-term deaths from chronic diseases, especially those of neuro-logical etiology. Total costs to the health services system are unlikely to decrease.

CONCLUSION

The competitive environment in the field of health services brought with it the perception that marketing was essential. Almost universally during the 1980s, health services organizations engaged in marketing, at least at the level of building name recognition. For the not-for-profit organization especially, the question of whether to market raised a host of ethical issues that began with the basic question of the propriety of marketing itself and extended to issues such as creating demand and distinguishing among various types of demand.

Physicians are reacting to the constraints of third-party payers and managed care in one of two ways. More than a third admit to having deceived insurance companies to help patients by exaggerating an illness's severity so patients can stay in the hospital longer or billing for incorrect diagnoses and reporting nonexistent symptoms. Over half of physicians approve of such deceitful practices.[17] That physicians believe it is necessary to deceive third-party payers and risk civil and criminal penalties suggests major problems in that system of payment. The second reaction to third-party constraints is that physicians are refusing to participate. They are cutting their ties with insurers and asking patients to pay for their services directly and then request reimbursement from the insurer. This has put patients in the middle and has forced payers to review their policies and relationships with physicians.[18] Some physicians simply decide to retire early or leave clinical practice entirely.[19] These problems cry out for solutions.

Hospitals struggling with mountains of uncompensated care see offering better reimbursed services as a way to offset losses. "No margin, no mission" has become such an oft-repeated justification that it is almost cliché. More fiscally sound hospitals must ask themselves whether they are meeting a general duty under the principle of justice to offer unprofitable but necessary services that benefit the wider community.

As with all activities undertaken by the health services organization, philosophy and mission statements provide an ethical context for marketing. Managers should apply virtues of honesty, candor, trustworthiness, and compassion in the organization's marketing. The principle of justice suggests that careful attention must be paid to the groups and medical conditions at which marketing is focused. Non–MCO health services organizations have the same ethical problems.

It behooves health services managers to read beyond the headlines and to be especially skeptical of claims that certain remedies are universal cures. Research findings must also be questioned, especially when studies from small samples or small universes are generalized to a population. Painting with a broad brush should alert everyone. As in life, when something sounds too good to be true, it probably is.

Institutional ethics committees (IECs) should prospectively and retrospectively assess the ethical issues raised in competition, marketing, and managed care. They should review the ethical implications of competition as it affects their patients, organization, and community. Marketing initiatives and their results should be understood from an ethical perspective, especially in terms of creating demand and the honesty and promise keeping involved. IECs can be valuable in monitoring care and outcomes to provide assurance that patients in managed care as well as in other payment categories receive the same, high-quality levels of care.

NOTES

1. Researchers: Risky heart attack therapy often unneeded. (1998, June 17). *CNNInteractive*. Retrieved January 12, 2004, from http://www.cnn.com/ HEALTH/9806/17/mild.heart.attacks

2. P.J. Skerrett. (1994, August/ September). Screening for prostate cancer. *Technology Review*, *97*(6), pp. 16–17.

3. John J. Hanlon & George E. Pickett. (1990). *Public health: Administration and practice* (9th ed., p. 4). St. Louis: Times Mirror/Mosby College Publications.

4. AHA Management Advisory. (1992). *Ethical conduct for health care institutions*. Retrieved December 6, 2003, from http://www.hospitalconnect.com/aha/ resource_center/resource/resource_ethics.html

5. Peter Wehrwein. (1998, June). The big squeeze. *Managed Care Magazine* [On line]. Retrieved January 2, 2004, from http://www.managedcaremag.com/ archives/9806/9806.squeeze.shtml

6. American Medical Association. (2003). *Newly adopted principles of medical ethics, June 2001*. Retrieved August 18, 2003, from http://www.ama-assn.org/ama/ pub/category/4256.html

7. Sick patients not fond of managed care plans. (1995, October). *Medical Ethics Advisor*, p. 133—citing findings of a study conducted by the Harvard University School of Public Health.

8. Halina Brukner. (2001, February 15). Only human? The effect of financial productivity incentives on physicians' use of preventive care measures. *The American Journal of Medicine 110*(3), pp. 226–228.

9. Allen Buchanan. (1998, August). Managed care: Rationing without justice, but not unjustly. *Journal of Health Politics, Policy and Law*, *23*(4), pp. 616–634.

10. Warren L. Holleman, David C. Edwards, & Christine C. Matson. (1994, Summer). Obligations of physicians to patients and third-party payers. *The Journal of Clinical Ethics*, *5*(2), p. 120.

11. Edmund D. Pellegrino. (1994, Fall). Managed care and managed competition: Some ethical reflections. *Calyx*, *4*(4), p. 3.

12. Steven Findlay. (1994, October). The managed care dilemma. *Business and Health*, p. 66.

13. Spencer Rich. (1995, March 19). Study finds savings in some HMOs. *The Washington Post*, p. A5.

14. Evan Pondel. (2003, October 22). HMO profits rising again; premium increases may fuel 16% gain. *The Daily News of Los Angeles* [as cited on the web site of The Foundation of Consumer & Taxpayer rights]. Retrieved January 2, 2004, from http://www.consumerwatchdog.org/healthcare/nw/ nw003770.php3

15. Wehrwein, 1998.

16. E. Haavi Morreim. (1995, November/December). Lifestyles of the risky and infamous: From managed care to managed lives. *The Hastings Center Report*, *25*, pp. 5–6.

17. Doctors say they deceive insurers to help patients. (2000, April 12). *The Washington Post*, p. A11; Ellen Goodman. (2000, April 15). Medical civil disobedience. *The Washington Post*, p. A21. When third-party payers find physicians mischaracterizing services, they change the rules. In turn physicians, become more clever at finding ways to provide the services their patients need. This is a war of escalation between payers and physicians that leads from one deception to another.

18. Julie Appleby. (2000, July 20). Frustrated doctors rebel against insurers. *USA Today*, p. 1B.

19. Yuki Noguchi. (2003, December 23). No heart for the business: A cardiologist learns that fixing broken hearts is a tough way to make a living these days. *The Washington Post*, p. F1.

CHAPTER 13

ETHICS IN RESOURCE ALLOCATION

Ethical issues are integral to resource allocation decisions. Whether resource allocation affects populations or groups (macroallocation) or individuals (microallocation), it involves making choices. Decisions are based on explicit or implicit criteria. Some managers use subjective criteria such as social worth, usefulness to society, and need; others use more objective criteria such as selection through a lottery or queue or ability to pay once medical need has been determined. Values and philosophical statements about individuals and society underlie both, although these are usually implicit and may be only vaguely understood by decision makers.

Various methods and guidelines are used by decision makers in allocating resources. Often, decisions made by governments are based on economic motives or political effect. Like governments, health services organizations involve managers and clinicians in making macroallocation decisions. Microallocation in health services means making decisions about clinical treatment for individuals and involves nonclinician managers to a lesser extent. Important aspects of microallocation decision making are a physician's willingness to refer, patient geographic and economic access to services and technologies, and patient desire for treatment. Decisions at the microlevel are often guided (in a sense, prejudged) by macroallocation decisions that the organization (or government) has made. Carefully husbanding resources is an important dimension of both macro- and microallocation decisions. Emphasis in the latter has led to efforts to minimize use of clinical resources when there is no reasonable hope of benefit.

As noted in Chapter 1, utilitarians judge the morality of an act by assessing the results produced and determining which course of action results in the greatest good for the greatest number. Economists and managers use this approach in their cost–benefit analyses. Applying criteria of utility is only a partial answer, however. This narrow approach ignores considerations of human need, fairness, and justice, all of which health services managers find important.

MACROALLOCATION

Specific theories have been developed to suggest how macroallocation does or should occur. The concept of a right to health care is prominent in several theories. An extreme view is hyperegalitarianism, which asserts that all treatments must be available to all persons needing them. Its corollary is that treatments not available to all should be available to none. This theory is an extreme expression of respect for persons and mandates that society recognize everyone's inherent right to equal health services. Providing different levels of treatment implies that some persons are, in effect, given less respect than others. Equal respect means receiving equal health care services, consistent with need. If this criterion cannot be met, the treatment should be available to none.

At the other end of the continuum are those who assert that health services are a privilege, not a right guaranteed by society. This hyperindividualistic position holds that health services providers, such as physicians, have no moral obligation to render services. In providing services, they act out of free will and humanitarian instinct. Hyperindividualists argue that if there were a right to health care, providers would be obliged to render services. An obligation (duty) to render services diminishes the freedom and dignity of providers and fails to recognize their inherent value and worth as human beings, thus violating the respect they are owed.

Between these extremes is the position that society has a duty to assist in developing, encouraging, and even providing health services. Fried argued that routine basic services ought to be available to all, a position known as the "decent minimum."[1] Beyond the decent minimum, this concept allows persons to purchase additional service as resources and interest permit. Contrast this approach with the Oregon Health Plan, which offers a decent minimum to Medicaid recipients. It prioritizes health services and pays for them to the extent the legislative assembly-approved budget allows, thus rationing services. It implicitly uses hyperegalitarianism which, proponents argue, means sacrifice for some Medicaid recipients but equal, if limited, access for all.

Generally, exotic high-technology services are limited because of location, cost, and referrals and are available on a different basis. Political decision making limits such services in publicly funded programs. Governing bodies and managers of health services organizations face similar questions in macroallocation decisions. Typically beneficence, fidelity (promise keeping), and justice are applied as supplemented by various of the virtues.

Ultimately, such values result in answers to questions of who gets what, when, where, and how. These questions are found in many issues, such as whether to build a new outpatient department, when to purchase a magnetic resonance imager, and how to allocate staff. Answering these questions requires careful attention to economic considerations. Financial well-being enables the organization to undertake its mission, a common aspect of which is serving the socially and economically disadvantaged.

The organization's mission and values provide the context for macro-allocation decisions. General criteria that may be applied include 1) the needs of external (the service area), interface (physicians), and internal (staff and volunteers) stakeholders (but primarily the first) and 2) the goal of improving or providing high-quality services at a competitive price. Cost–benefit analyses are useful in measuring the desirability of projects, but these should be part of the general screening of projects. It is very likely that several proposed macroallocation proposals (e.g., programs, equipment, physical plant) will receive recommendations to proceed. It is from this list that organizational values and mission are applied for a final selection.

The Feasibility of Brain Electrical Activity Mapping

Brain electrical activity mapping (BEAM) is a relatively new technology used to image the brain. It significantly improves the ability to localize an abnormality. Responding to demands for the procedure from staff radiologists and local neurologists and to reports in the literature on its usefulness, City Hospital decided to investigate the possibility of acquiring access to BEAM. Options included leasing, purchasing, and approaching nearby County Hospital about sharing its recently acquired BEAM machine.

A factor in the decision was uncertainty as to how changes in reimbursement would affect hospital revenues. Questions about reimbursement and a potential major expenditure of capital funds caused the chairman of the board to ask the chief executive officer to form a committee to evaluate options, including forgoing access to BEAM. This assessment would be used to make a final decision between BEAM and a proposed addition to the intensive care unit (ICU), a project that is strongly supported by the surgical staff and already has been delayed twice.

The board wanted to delay the decision on BEAM until the reimbursement implications were understood, but several attending physicians stated that BEAM testing is critical to their practices. They said they prefer the nursing staff at City but felt that they will be forced to admit certain patients to County in order to use BEAM. A rumor surfaced among the medical staff that several prominent members were considering forming a consortium to purchase and operate BEAM and other diagnostic equipment in a professional office complex under construction.[2]

What are the important aspects of this case? First, the new technology will improve the quality of care. Second, its availability will affect the organization's financial situation—operating costs for BEAM are high, typically exceeding capital costs in a few years. Financial considerations are complicated by reimbursement issues. Third, the physicians are divided about the expenditure, and this adds to the complexity of medical staff politics. Fourth, BEAM is expensive technology, which makes the decision even more important and difficult.

The obvious starting point in solving this problem is to review the organizational philosophy and vision and mission statements. If City Hospital's mission is to serve special populations or needs, both BEAM and an ICU addition may use resources in a manner consistent with that mission. Are there even better uses for the resources? The various issues are not easily resolved, but internal decision processes, such as an ethics committee, can be of assistance. The expected context for decision making will be the organizational philosophy, as reflected in the strategic plan, which was described in Chapter 3. The technological imperative is present not only in delivering services to individual patients but also in macroallocation decisions.

In another example, senior management of a for-profit hospital system decided to spend $3.8 million for a piece of statuary while denying payment for heart transplants; this is a macroallocation decision with profound affects on service availability (microallocation). The statue was used to decorate the corporate offices.[3] No one expects the corporate offices of a multibillion dollar organization to have sheetrock walls and bare floors; it would seem, however, that the virtue of temperance ought to guide one's decisions in such situations.

MICROALLOCATION

One usually thinks of microallocation decisions in terms of exotic lifesaving treatment. All scarce resources require allocation, however, and scarcity may be a function of time and circumstances.

Who Gets the Penicillin?

In 1943, penicillin was new and in short supply among U.S. armed forces in North Africa. Competitors for its use were two groups of soldiers suffering from infections that would respond to it: those with venereal disease and those with battle wounds. The chief surgical consultant advised that priority be given to the wounded; the theatre medical commander directed that priority be given to soldiers with venereal disease, arguing that soldiers cured of venereal disease could be restored to fighting trim more rapidly and that left untreated, such men represented a threat of spreading the infection. The decision to use the penicillin on soldiers with venereal disease was a pragmatic judgment consistent with the morality of utility in a situation where objectives—achieving maximum fighting power as rapidly as possible—were narrowly defined.[4]

Exclusively treating men infected with venereal disease is the morally correct choice only if the utilitarian criterion of returning the greatest number of troops to the line as quickly as possible is applied. This decision is made without judging either the relative worth of the soldiers in need of treatment or the way in which they came to require it.

Foreign transplant recipients obtaining human organs from American donors suggests another dimension of microallocation decisions. These patients tend to come from countries in which technological impediments or religious and social customs prevent organ harvesting. They pay out of pocket rather than out of private or public sources and thus are favored by transplant centers. In addition, they are generally willing to accept organs that may be less fresh or are not optimal tissue matches. Transplanting American organs into non-Americans raises legitimate concerns about priorities in a system in which American patients wait for organs while non-Americans receive them.

Theories of allocating exotic lifesaving treatment to individual patients have been developed by James Childress and Nicholas Rescher.[5] They address the problem of how decisions about who gets what should be made. Childress rejected the use of subjective criteria, such as worth to society, because such comparisons demean the potential recipient and run counter to a belief in the inherent dignity of each human being. His position is Kantian because it stresses respect for persons and its derivative, autonomy. He argued that a system that views all persons requiring treatment as equals recognizes inherent human worth. According to Childress, once medical criteria determine the need for and the appropriateness of therapy, opportunities for exotic lifesaving treatment should be available on a first-come, first-served basis or alternatively, through some random selection process, such as a lottery.

A world-class ethicist, the late Paul Ramsey, agreed with Childress as to the desirability of a lottery or a policy of first-come, first-served that ignores the subjective judgments one finds in other, criteria-oriented schemes. At the same time, Ramsey found nondiscriminatory, predetermined, and announced rules based on statistical medical probabilities to be acceptable. This view would, for example, permit groups such as the very young and the very old to be excluded from kidney dialysis programs.[6]

Rescher's schema has two tiers. The first tier is devoted to basic screening and applies to groups of potential patients. It consists of factors such as constituency served, benefit to science, and likelihood of success by type of treatment or recipient. The second tier deals with individuals. It judges medical factors (e.g., relative likelihood of success, life expectancy) and social aspects, such as family role, potential future contributions, and past services rendered. Rescher stated that if all factors are equal, a random selection process should be used for the final choice. The social aspects caused Rescher the most difficulty because they rely heavily on value judgments. However, he considered it irrational to make choices subject to chance, even if medical criteria are objective.

Each of these microallocation theories has advantages and disadvantages, both moral and pragmatic. Each theory develops a formal or semiformal process that permits users to address issues and problems in an organized manner. Although these approaches may produce a decision that satisfies everyone, the theories offer the advantage of an identified system that at least provides frameworks within which to make decisions. Given that medical criteria are met, a person's chances of being selected for exotic lifesaving treatment may be unpredictable (Childress), partially predictable (Ramsey), or almost totally predictable (Rescher). The basis for selection may hinge on largely subjective criteria (Rescher) or may be solely a matter of chance, and in that sense eminently fair to all who need the treatment (Childress) or all who meet the criteria for medical statistical probabilities (Ramsey).

Choices

Randy Glenn had just fallen asleep when the telephone rang. It was the night supervisor at the comprehensive care center and hospital of which Glenn was the chief executive officer. The supervisor was quite agitated and had trouble getting her words out. It took a few minutes for the message to become clear. One of Glenn's nightmares had come true: The four-bed ICU was full and an emergency case had just arrived.

The night supervisor explained that the new patient had been injured in a car accident. She had been stabilized in the emergency department but neither air medevac nor mobile ICU ambulance services were available. It was certain that she would not survive transfer by any other means. She needed to be admitted to the ICU within 2 hours.

The night supervisor then quickly described the patients currently occupying ICU beds:

- Patient A: 60 year-old woman, comatose, stroke victim who required respirator support, 27 days in the ICU; uncertain prognosis; retired; no family; city resident

- Patient B: 9-year-old boy with Down syndrome, acute respiratory infection; 4 days in ICU; family in adjacent city

- Patient C: 36-year-old man who had undergone an emergency appendectomy, developed severe wound infection and probable septicemia; source of infection unknown; requires ICU care for blood pressure instability secondary to sepsis; bachelor, mother lives in city

- Patient D: 12-year-old girl undergoing chemotherapy for leukemia with an experimental drug; had been in remission three times; monitoring of experimental protocol and potential reaction to drug requires ICU care; family in city

- New Patient: 24-year-old woman; college honor student in physics, scholarship winner; pregnant, engaged; no family known

The supervisor ended the telephone call by asking Glenn, "What should I do?" Indeed, what to do, thought Glenn, who suddenly wished the institutional ethics committee had been more active. Glenn pondered the alternatives as the garage door opened and the 10-minute trip to the hospital began.[7]

This example is the classic "last bed in the ICU" dilemma. Under Childress's and Ramsey's criteria, if all patients meet the medical criteria for ICU care, the new patient would be left to receive the best care she could obtain outside of the ICU. Applying Rescher's criteria, the prognosis (likelihood of success) for one of the current patients is not as good as the prognosis for the new patient. Thus, one of the current patients should be removed from the ICU. None of the models permits patients unable to obtain ICU care to be abandoned and left to fend for themselves. In all models, they would receive the best alternative care the facility could offer.

Public awareness of how choices are made may or may not enhance the public's view that health services organizations and the system act justly. Public scrutiny, however, will focus greater attention on decision criteria, the decision process, and the fairness of their application. Kantian principles of respect for persons and of not using persons as ends are reflected in Childress's approach, which stresses autonomy. Rescher's approach includes a mix of Kantian and utilitarian views and, most important, emphasizes justice, as described in Chapter 1. Some health services organizations make resource allocation decisions using formal ethical criteria—the preferred method. As with all macroallocation decisions, these criteria must be developed within the context of the organizational philosophy and vision and mission statements.

Near-Futile Treatment

Some situations have all of the elements of futility save one—the patient is not terminally ill. Sidney Miller's birth is such a case. Sidney was expected to die shortly after birth; aggressive intervention kept her alive, albeit with significant disabilities. In many respects, cases such as Sidney's are the most difficult of all. The literature has yet to use the concept of near-futile treatment, but it is appropriately distinguished from futile treatment. The Sidney Miller case should be borne in mind and distinguished from the discussion of futile treatment below.

Sidney Miller[8]

In 2003, Sidney Miller was 12 years of age. In 1991, she was a 23-week-old premature infant delivered to Karla and Mark Miller at The Woman's Hospital of Texas in Houston. At birth, the attending obstetrician-gynecologist told the Millers that the infant was unlikely to survive. The parents determined that Sidney should receive comfort care in the form of food, water, and warmth. She would survive or not on her own.

Other physicians recommended an experimental procedure that would likely result in brain damage or severe disability. Again, the parents chose comfort care. Hospital administrators overrode the Millers's decision and told them that an unwritten hospital policy and the "law" required that they resuscitate infants who weigh more than 500 grams (1.1 pounds).

The experimental treatment was undertaken. Sidney survived. Her cognitive age is 3 months, she has cerebral palsy, and she cannot walk or talk. Sidney will require lifelong care.

The Millers sued. In 1998, a Texas jury awarded them $60.4 million against Columbia/HCA, the owners of The Woman's Hospital of Texas in Houston.

In 2000, a Texas court of appeals overturned the jury verdict citing the state's advance medical directives law: "parents are only allowed to withhold or withdraw life-sustaining medical treatment from a child where the child's condition has been certified in writing by a physician to be terminal." The appeals court did not address the countless other decisions to continue aggressive treatment of Sidney during 7 months of hospitalization.

In mid-2003, the Texas Supreme Court agreed with the appeals court. The Millers will receive nothing.

Ethical Issues in the Miller Case   The ethical issues of Sidney Miller's case are clouded by questions of applicable law. The federal Child Abuse Prevention and Treatment Act Amendments of 1984 (PL 98-457) allow physicians to decline to treat a newborn when the infant is chronically and irreversibly comatose, when treating would prolong dying or not correct all life-threatening conditions, or when treatment would be virtually futile and inhumane. The Texas court of appeals made no reference to the federal law, citing instead state law requiring that a physician certify in writing that the infant's condition is terminal. Apparently, such a determination had not been made.

Ethicists are in broad agreement that withholding and withdrawing life-sustaining treatment are morally indistinguishable. The psychology of these two actions is different. Withdrawing life-sustaining treatment seems to cause death, and family and caregivers may find it difficult to recognize that the underlying medical condition or the disease process causes death, not the act of withdrawing life-sustaining treatment. When it is clear that continuing to treat is futile (no hope of benefit) it may be easier for those involved and decision makers to feel comfortable in discontinuing it. Paradoxically, Mrs. Miller could have had a legal abortion, even while in labor, had she chosen to do so.

It unclear whether the hospital actually had a written policy (or policies) regarding the role of parents in cases like this. The principle of justice (fairness) makes it clear that the hospital's policy (or policies), if existent, regarding aggressive resuscitation and a trial period on a ventilator should have been communicated to the Millers before labor started. This information would have allowed them to make an informed choice and might have caused them to seek medical services elsewhere.

Sidney was hospitalized for 7 months, with costs of care totaling millions of dollars. Whether paid from private or public sources, one must raise the question of macroallocation of resources in this and similar cases. Perhaps it is time to reconsider expenditures that have such limited positive results. In the case of premature infants, however, this debate must factor in the high levels of uncertainty in making accurate prognoses.

FUTILITY THEORY

Modern technology allows clinicians to support life far into the dying process. Applying technology when there is a probability or even hope of benefit raises few ethical issues. Treatment continued beyond hope of benefit suggests futility. Applying the futility concept has been described as a unilateral do-not-resuscitate (DNR) order, a decision made by physicians using a physiologic definition.[9] At its root, futility theory focuses on the absence of benefit from continued treatment. Quality of life is not expressly considered, although it cannot be ignored as a psychological factor that may be implicitly considered by physicians. It is the issue of demands for treatment that clinicians consider to offer no hope of benefit that futility guidelines address. Extraordinary, almost miraculous cases haunt decision makers and cloud futility theory and guidelines. These are cases in which patients improve months or even years after reasonable hope of benefit from life-sustaining treatment should have ended. Sometimes, the improvement is dramatic.[10, 11]

Futile treatment invariably raises questions of resource consumption and economics. A skeptic might ask whether economics are really the driving force. Similar questions have been raised about advance medical directives (AMDs), which are touted as giving patients control but almost always limit services. Some futile treatment policies specifically address resource consumption and the moral obligation of the health services organization to use its resources judiciously.

Background

In many ways futility theory is old wine in new bottles. Its origins lie in the distinction between ordinary and extraordinary care, which is reviewed here. *Ordinary care* is all medicines, treatments, and operations that offer reasonable hope of benefit and that can be obtained without excessive expense, pain, or other inconvenience. *Extraordinary care* is all medicines, treatments, and operations that cannot be obtained or used without excessive expense, pain, or inconvenience, or that, if used, would not offer a reasonable hope of benefit. This definition makes it ethical to withhold any medicine, treatment, or operation that offers no reasonable hope of benefit or that cannot be obtained or used without excessive expense, pain, or inconvenience. A common mistake is to define ordinary as usual or customary treatment; this results in statements such as "Ill persons must always be given food and water because this is ordinary (i.e., usual and customary) care."

Futility theory has quantitative and qualitative aspects. The *quantitative* aspect is concerned with the probability of success if a treatment were attempted or continued. Probability of success means that the treatment can be successfully performed and achieve its intended purpose. So, for example, tube feeding will maintain the life of a patient in a persistent vegetative state (PVS), but it will not restore cognition. This highlights the importance of viewing care as a continuum, not an isolated event.

Qualitative assumes a successful treatment that achieves its intended purpose but asks whether the result is such that the treatment ought to be undertaken. The quantitative determination is made by clinical experts. The qualitative determination (judgment) can be made only by the patient or, as necessary, the patient's surrogate. The concept of futility limits the qualitative decision.

There are three basic variations of circumstances that raise questions of futile treatment. The first is that patients demand services that offer no hope of benefit. Lacking data, this situation may be an urban myth or incorrect perception. AMDs are generally used to limit medical intervention, although they can also demand services that clinicians later deem futile.

A second type of futile treatment occurs when organizations insist on providing treatment that surrogates have determined offer no hope of benefit and should end. The cases of Karen Ann Quinlan and Nancy Beth Cruzan illustrate such policies (especially Cruzan, whose continued treatment was required by state law). The Quinlan and Cruzan cases suggest that futility policies are better directed toward legislators, organizations, and staff than toward patients and families.

The third type occurs when treatment is continued because surrogate decision makers demand it. An example is the case of Helga Wanglie, a Minneapolis woman in PVS whose husband demanded that all efforts be made to keep her alive, despite a prognosis that doing so offered no hope of benefit. A second example is that of Baby K, an infant with anencephaly whose mother refused to authorize a DNR order and insisted that all treatment continue.

Baby K

The legal case captioned *In the Matter of Baby K** began in 1992, when a baby girl with anencephaly was born at Fairfax Hospital in northern

---

*The identities of the mother and child were sealed by the court and were not revealed until after the U.S. Supreme Court refused to review the federal appeals court decision.

Virginia. This case raises several ethical issues; the focus here is on resource allocation and the organization's obligations when futile treatment is demanded.

This case is distinguished from others involving infants with anencephaly in that the mother demanded that everything be done for Baby K. In the realm of ethics, decisions about infants with anencephaly raise questions of futile treatment. In the realm of politics, such emotionally charged situations are almost beyond public debate; politicians will undoubtedly flee any discussion of them.

Anencephaly is a rare congenital anomaly in which the cerebral cortex of the brain has not developed and the top of the skull and scalp are absent. It is estimated that 1,000–2,000 infants with anencephaly are born annually in the United States. Most die within hours or days of birth, with or without intervention. Some are born with better-developed brain stems and live weeks or months. Rarely do infants with anencephaly live more than a few months. Baby K was an exception and lived 2 years, with the need for intermittent aggressive intervention.

Clinical Aspects   Baby K's anencephaly had been diagnosed prenatally. The mother, Ms. H, continued the pregnancy despite the recommendations of her obstetrician and a neonatologist that terminating the pregnancy was best. Baby K's father was not married to her mother and was not involved in her care nor in decision making regarding her. He did, however, support efforts to have a DNR order written.

Baby K was delivered by cesarean section. She was born permanently unconscious and could not see, hear, or otherwise interact with her environment. Brain stem functions were limited to feeding and respiratory reflexes and she reflexively responded to sound or touch. Mechanical ventilation was begun at birth, but it served no therapeutic or palliative purpose because the underlying anencephaly was untreatable.

Ethical and Legal Aspects   The physicians urged the mother to authorize a DNR order, but she refused and would not authorize discontinuation of the ventilator. Ms. H and Baby K's physicians met with a specially appointed three-person panel of the hospital ethics committee, two of whom were physicians (a family practitioner and a psychiatrist). The third member was a minister. The three-person panel "concluded that Baby K's ventilator treatment should end because 'such care was futile' and decided to 'wait a reasonable time for the family to help the caregiver terminate aggressive therapy.'"[12] If the mother refused to follow the advice, the panel recommended that the hospital seek a legal solution. Ms. H rejected the panel's recommendation. The extent to which ethical issues were discussed is unclear. The panel met multiple times, and the entire ethics committee discussed the case on more than one occasion. The roles of both were seen as advisory, not as achieving a certain result or acting as an advocate for any position.

Baby K was successfully weaned from the ventilator. After disagreement about treatment, Fairfax Hospital sought to move her to another hospital, but hospitals with pediatric intensive care units declined. Six weeks after the birth, Ms. H allowed Baby K to be transferred to a nursing facility on the condition that Baby K could be readmitted to the hospital if respiratory problems recurred. Baby K was brought to the hospital in respiratory distress several times after the transfer. Between acute episodes, Baby K remained at the nursing facility and did not require life-sustaining treatment except for occasional use of a ventilator.

Trial Court   To protect itself legally, Fairfax Hospital sought a declaratory judgment in federal district court that it would not violate the Emergency Medical Treatment and Active Labor Act (EMTALA) of 1986 (PL 99-272), the Rehabilitation Act of 1973 (PL 93-112), or the Americans with Disabilities Act (ADA) of 1990 (PL 101-336) by refusing to administer life-sustaining treatment to an infant with anencephaly. The EMTALA requires that emergency departments (ED) in hospitals that receive Medicare funds must treat all who arrive at the ED with emergency medical conditions and continue treatment until the person can be transferred safely. The Rehabilitation Act and the ADA prohibit discrimination because of handicap or disability, respectively.

The hospital conceded that respiratory distress is an emergency condition but argued that the EMTALA should be interpreted to include an exception for treatment deemed "futile" or "inhumane" by hospital physicians. The trial judge found no such exception in the EMTALA; regardless, he reasoned, the exception would not apply to Baby K because her breathing could be restored and therefore mechanical ventilation could not be considered futile or inhumane. The trial court also found Baby K's condition was a handicap and a disability and that the hospital could not legally refuse treatment (per Section 504 of the Rehabilitation Act and the ADA, respectively). Denying care to Baby K would constitute discrimination. The trial court ruled further that as a general matter of law, absent a finding of neglect or abuse, parents have a constitutionally protected right under the 14th Amendment's due process clause to raise children as they see fit and to make decisions about medical treatment for them. The judge concluded that when parents disagree, the courts should support the parent who decides in favor of life. The attorney appointed by the court as guardian *ad litem* (guardian for the purposes of a legal proceeding) for Baby K agreed with the hospital. Fairfax Hospital appealed the trial court decision.

Appeals Court   In a 2 to 1 decision, the 4th U.S. Circuit Court of Appeals affirmed the trial court decision. It ruled that the EMTALA requires hospitals receiving Medicare funds to provide care in life-threatening situations, regardless of the patients' conditions. The appeals court determined that because the hospital has a duty to render medically stabilizing treatment under the EMTALA, there was no need to determine the hospital's obligations under other federal statutes or the laws of Virginia.

The majority agreed with the hospital that the standard of care for infants with anencephaly is to provide only warmth, hydration, and nutrition. Nevertheless, it held that the statutory language was unambiguous and included no such limitation. The majority declined to legislate from the bench:

> It is beyond the limits of our judicial function to address the moral or ethical propriety of providing emergency stabilizing medical treatment to anencephalic infants. We are bound to interpret federal statutes in accordance with their language and any expressed congressional intent.[13]

The dissenting judge argued that the EMTALA was enacted to prevent patients from being dumped for economic reasons, that dumping was not an issue for Baby K, and that therefore the statute should not apply. Baby K's respiratory failures related to anencephaly; her necessary care should be viewed as a continuum in which no medical treatment can improve her condition of permanent unconsciousness.

Aftermath   Various groups filed *amici curiae* (friends of the court) legal briefs in the appeal. The American Academy of Pediatrics and the Society of Critical Care Medicine supported the hospital. The Virginia Department for Rights of Virginians with Disabilities provided legal assistance to Ms. H and argued that Baby K had a right to treatment. In 1994, the U.S. Supreme Court refused to review the case and the appeals court decision was allowed to stand.

A statement released by Fairfax Hospital in 1993 before the appeals court decision stated,

> We believe that continuing to provide extraordinary measures to pro-long the dying process is medically and ethically inappropriate, and not in the best interests of this infant. . . . The hospital and its physicians remain ready to provide appropriate medical care, which in this case includes nutrition, hydration, and warmth.[14]

Baby K had a grim prognosis but lived far longer than other infants with her condition. She died in April 1995, 2 years after her birth. Private insurance and Medicaid covered her medical bills of almost $500,000, approximately one half of which was the cost of hospital services. Hospital officials' denial that economics motivated their legal action is supported by the fact that all hospital services had been paid.[15] The challenge for health services organizations in cases such as Baby K will be to meld the concerns of family, caregivers, and organization in a way that eliminates or minimizes futile and inhumane treatment while meeting federal and state laws, organizational values, and the personal ethics of those persons involved.

Analysis   Anencephaly had been diagnosed months before Baby K's birth. If the physicians believed mechanical ventilation was medically inappropriate, this should have been made clear to Ms. H at that time. She should have been encouraged to find alternative sources of physician and hospital care, which may have been impossible through her health plan. It is certain, however, that had Ms. H refused to follow the physicians' recommendation or had she been unable to find a physician and a hospital to provide the care she wanted, Fairfax Hospital and its physicians would have had little choice but to continue treating Baby K. Further efforts might have convinced Ms. H that her decision was wrong.

If mechanical ventilation were to be used, the goal of the intervention (e.g., confirmation of the diagnosis) should have been specified and respiratory support should have continued only until that goal was reached or found to be unattainable. Ms. H might have reneged on an agreement to discontinue respiratory support, however, which would have put the physicians and hospital back where they started.

Hospital administration and legal counsel seem to have overreacted. They should have supported the physicians in their application of existing medical standards and encouraged further discussions with Ms. H through

the ethics committee and its special panel. Such efforts could have continued even after Baby K was discharged to the nursing facility. By going to
court, they turned an issue of medical practice and medical ethics into a
legal issue. Having once undertaken legal proceedings the hospital effectively lost control of the situation—highly undesirable by any measure.
Court proceedings are always difficult, expensive, unpredictable, and
energy and emotionally intensive. The publicity surrounding such cases
is often a public relations nightmare, regardless of the result.

The appeals court decision rejected the argument that the medical
standard of care should be used implicitly to guide interpretation of the
EMTALA. This substantially limits the discretion of providers in terms
of the circumstances that justify withholding or withdrawing care where
patients have not or cannot express their wishes regarding life-sustaining
treatment. Meeting the standard of care may protect physicians and hospitals from malpractice actions, which are governed by state law, but it does
not protect them from liability under federal law.

The extent to which the ethics committee or its special panel sought
to solve the problem from an ethical standpoint is unclear. Apparently,
the focus was advising as to medical practice and legal strategy. The result
confirms this focus, which runs counter to good practice. Organizations
and their ethics committees must reflect the values of their organizational
philosophy when they prospectively address ethical issues such as futile
treatment. Specific cases are analyzed in this context. This analysis provides
the basis for advising participants and maintaining the integrity of the
hospital's philosophy.

Rarely do ethics committees make decisions, but their evaluative,
educative, and consultative roles are well known. In terms of the educative
and consultative roles, all efforts should have been made to continue a
dialogue with Ms. H until a resolution acceptable to both sides was reached.
Here, however, they advised only on the question of futility and how
clinical decisions should be addressed. Such a role is too passive.

In addition, one must question whether it was wise to focus on the
medical dimensions of the case by appointing physicians as two of the
three members of the special panel. Ms. H must have been knowledgeable
about the clinical (scientific) aspects of anencephaly, but she chose to
ignore them. This decision suggests the need to focus on the psychosocial
dimensions, a task likely best undertaken by nonphysicians. The role of
the member of the clergy and whether Ms. H was of his faith are unknown.

Because the ethics subcommittee and Baby K's mother were at logger-
heads, mediation could have been attempted as a way to resolve the dispute.
A mediator is a neutral person who works with the parties to develop an

acceptable solution, which may be a compromise. In such situations, keeping the parties talking is essential to success.

Summary   The U.S. Supreme Court may consider a similar case in the future and reverse the decision in Baby K. In the meantime, Congress can amend the EMTALA as well as other federal legislation to allow treatment to be withheld or withdrawn when it is deemed futile or inhumane by caregivers. Such exceptions are found in the Child Abuse Amendments of 1984 (PL 98-457), which were enacted to prevent denial of treatment to infants with disabilities. The problem for Congress is that within a political context, it will be virtually impossible to deny parents the right to demand treatment even when it is deemed futile or inhumane by caregivers.

Futile Treatment Guidelines

Increasingly, health services organizations, especially acute care hospitals, have futile treatment guidelines or policies. Developing and adopting them have been stimulated by the perception that patients and their surrogates demand treatment that clinicians have determined has little, if any, likelihood of benefiting the patient. The concept of consent and autonomy drive the initial phases of decision making for patients able to participate. They should be provided with the information necessary to make an informed choice about treatment or nontreatment options. Patients bear the brunt of continued treatment, a fact that likely makes them more willing than surrogate decision makers to limit what is done. Patients and surrogates sometimes have unrealistic goals or expectations of what medical science can do. When patients' decisions (or demands) will not result in efficacious medical treatment or will only prolong suffering and the dying process, clinicians have a moral obligation to withhold or withdraw treatment. Typically, guidelines regarding withholding or withdrawing life-sustaining treatment require agreement of both attending and consulting physicians that the treatment is futile.

Decisions about appropriateness of continued medical treatment are made within the context of the purposes of medical care:

> There is . . . general agreement that the goals of standard medical treatment are to cure, restore, improve or maintain some level of a person's ability to think, feel, and interact with others and the environment. Medical interventions that have little likelihood of achieving any of these treatment goals can be considered futile.[16]

The futility guidelines for Trinity Health, a nationwide, faith-based health care system, begin by positing the religious context for the guidelines, describing the role of the patient in decision making and the importance of professional integrity of caregivers, as well as the need for stewardship of resources. The guidelines continue by defining medically futile treatment and providing examples.[17] Trinity Health defines medically futile treatment as any treatment which, within a reasonable degree of medical probability, has little likelihood of

- Having any positive physiological effect on the patient's condition; or
- Reversing the patient's imminent dying; or
- Restoring the patient's ability to function as a person, i.e., his/her cognitive, affective and interactive functions[18]

Several aspects of these futility guidelines are notable: 1) the criteria are stated in the alternative (e.g., if reversing imminent dying is likely by applying a treatment, that treatment is not futile); 2) there is no consideration of "quality of life," either as judged by the patient or someone else; and 3) there is no specific attention to the economic dimensions of the treatment being rendered.

Examples of futile treatment given the Trinity Health guidelines include continued ventilator support for a patient who meets brain death criteria, CPR for a patient with end-stage cancer that has metastasized or a patient with multiple organ failure, and aggressive therapies for a PVS or permanently comatose patient. The guidelines also outline a process for making decisions about medical futility. Steps include the following:[19]

1. Judgment that a treatment is futile is made by agreement of the attending physician, medical consultants, and caregiving team.
2. The attending physician informs the competent patient or surrogate, as appropriate, that the treatment judged medically futile will not be started or will be stopped, if already underway. Assurance will be given that comfort care will be provided.
3. If the competent patient or surrogate (as appropriate) agrees, appropriate orders will be written in the chart.
4. Lacking agreement, the ethics committee is consulted. The ethics committee determines that the guidelines' criteria have been met and assists with communication and negotiation between the parties involved.
5. Judgments about futile treatment involving incompetent patients without a surrogate will be reviewed by the ethics committee. If it concurs the attending physician will document the process in the chart and write appropriate orders.

6. If, after the ethics committee concurs with the attending physician that a treatment is medically futile, a competent patient or surrogate, as appropriate, refuses to agree, a mediator will be used to try to resolve the dispute.

7. If the patient or surrogate chooses to remain in the facility or if they remain because no alternative facility can be found the medically futile treatment will: a. not be started, b. (be) started or continued for a goal-specific or time-limited trial as the result of mediation, or, c. if started, will be discontinued.

The guidelines end by providing direction for situations in which physicians and caregivers disagree regarding potentially futile treatments. Here, the ethics committee is a significant part of the process. Emphasis is also placed on the need for ongoing dialogue with patients or surrogates. Using a mediator, who is by definition a neutral third party, presents important possibilities in resolving intractable disagreement. Because both sides must agree to a solution, Number 7c in the preceding guidelines presents the most likely and best possibility for a compromise result.

Futile treatment guidelines or policies should emphasize that physicians have no moral (or legal) obligation to provide treatment that they judge to be inappropriate. Physicians' professional integrity is compromised and they fail to meet their duty to their patients if they provide treatment that is of no benefit or offers no hope of benefit. Physicians fail, too, in their ethical obligation to make effective use of resources if they are consumed by patients for whom they offer neither benefit nor hope of benefit.

Most states allow physicians and hospitals to decline to provide care based on reasons of conscience. Almost all states have enacted statutes that give physicians and hospitals latitude in refusing to provide care that is determined to be futile at the end of life. Thirty-eight states permit both institutions and individual providers to refuse to comply with the instructions of a health care agent; six states permit only individual providers to refuse to comply. For example, California's noncompliance provision for physicians and hospitals applies if a requested treatment "requires medically ineffective health care or health care contrary to generally accepted health care standards applicable to the health care provider or institution."[20] Despite such laws, however, it is doubtful that either physicians or hospitals will refuse to provide treatment that they deem to be futile, except after a considerable period of continued treatment and when the prognosis is unequivocal. The potential is too great for accusations from the public and media that passive, involuntary euthanasia is occurring or that patients are being treated cruelly. Reaction to highly publicized futile treatment cases show significant levels of ignorance among the public. In this milieu, enforcing futile treatment guidelines could cause a public relations nightmare. Health services organizations must have guidelines or a policy on futile treatment, nonetheless.

The presence of guidelines will encourage physicians to take steps to withhold or withdraw futile treatment. Thus encouraged, their frank discussions with patients or surrogates may yield results in terms of withholding or withdrawing futile treatment. By informing patients or surrogates of their moral objection to continuing treatment because it is medically inappropriate and harmful physicians may gain assent without invoking the organization's guidelines. The "transfer out" option is unlikely to be viable and is more useful as a way to convince patients or surrogates of how seriously physicians view the problem. In practical terms patients may be too ill to transfer or no facility is willing to take them. Transferring out becomes virtually impossible if all hospitals in a region agree to a common set of futile treatment guidelines, as for example in Knoxville, Tennessee, and Houston, Texas. Thus, after a reasonable time in which no alternative source of care is found the facility must face the task of acting to withhold or withdraw futile treatment.

The concept of futile treatment is not without its critics, however, as shown in the following case.[21]

Knowing Whether or When to Stop

An 18-year-old woman suffered severe brain injuries in a car accident in 1987. After a few weeks in a coma, she opened her eyes, but was totally nonresponsive for 15 months. Then, nurses noticed a hopeful sign when she twice seemed to obey their orders to move her leg or to close her eyes. These responses were rare, but 2 months later her physicians administered drugs to improve alertness and her condition slowly improved. Over time, she learned to answer multiple-choice questions and calculate simple math problems using eye blinks. At one point, she wrote, "Mom, I love you."

Three years after the accident, she was communicating regularly with eye blinks and could move her arms somewhat. After 5 years, she could mouth words and short phrases. Although her attention span was limited to 15 minutes, she liked to be pampered and took pleasure in teasing her nurses. Her favorite joke was pretending not to know their identities.

Her mother was overjoyed; she reveled in each small bit of progress. The young woman was sent home 5 years and 2 months after the injury, totally dependent on others. Her rehabilitation had cost well over $1 million.[22]

This tragic case raises squarely the issue of futile treatment. By emerging from PVS, this patient had a rare, almost miraculous outcome. Care was continued at her family's demand.

Implications

Futility theory goes well beyond the contemporary concept of autonomy. Patient autonomy is a negative right, the right to be free from unwanted treatment—to be able to say no. Futility theory limits what is asserted as a positive right, the right to demand treatment—even when there is no medical benefit to receiving it. From an ethical standpoint, it is generally agreed that no positive rights exist.

Futility theory seeks to deal with the issues of extraordinary, disproportionate, and burdensome care. The decision maker is the physician. The preceding sample guidelines stated that there is a need to educate and inform the patient. The patient and/or family need not concur with the decision, however. Futility theory is very different from the shared decision making in what is considered the ideal, nonpaternalistic physician–patient relationship. In fact, the problem that futility theory purports to address may be only partly attributable to patient demands. Research documents many shortcomings in the care of patients who are seriously ill and dying, especially the effectiveness of patient–physician communication.

The findings of the Study to Understand Prognoses and Preferences for Outcomes and Risks of Treatments (SUPPORT) research are compelling:

> [The] Study to Understand Prognoses and Preferences for Outcomes and Risks of Treatments patients were seriously ill, and their dying proved to be predictable, yet discussion and decisions substantially in advance of death were uncommon. Nearly half of all DNR orders were written in the last 2 days of life. The final hospitalization for half of patients included more than 8 days in generally undesirable states: in an ICU, receiving mechanical ventilation, or comatose. Families reported that half of the patients who were able to communicate in their last few days spent most of the time in moderate or severe pain.[23]

These results occurred in the intervention phase of the SUPPORT study, despite the presence of nurses whose task was to improve communication and encourage the patient and family to engage in an informed and collaborative decision-making process with a well-informed physician. The authors concluded that additional proactive and forceful measures may be needed. It was estimated that patients meeting SUPPORT criteria account for approximately 400,000 hospital admissions per year in the United States. Such findings seem to uphold the seemingly harsh approach in the previously listed futility guidelines, but there is reason for caution.

In a corollary to the first phase of SUPPORT, investigators examined the impact of prognosis-based futility guidelines on survival and hospital length of stay on a cohort of adults with serious illness. They calculated the hospital days that would not be used if, on the third day, life-sustaining treatment had been stopped or not initiated for patients with an estimated 2-month survival chance of 1% or less. They found that only 10.8% of hospital days would have been forgone and concluded that only modest savings would have resulted.[24]

If large numbers of patients demand futile treatment, such guidelines will have several important effects: voluntary passive euthanasia (i.e., patient and/or surrogates have consented) will exist in theory but will be rarely necessary. Involuntary passive euthanasia (i.e., patient and/or surrogates have not consented) will increase dramatically. Futile treatment guidelines may cause physicians to feel less obligated to talk to their patients and surrogates.

An apparent contradiction exists between science and the quality of life suggested in the previously noted definition of futile treatment. This contradiction raises the question of whether a paternalistic quality of life decision is masquerading as scientific, objective decision making. If so, futile treatment guidelines are a large step back for patient autonomy—a return to the physician paternalism of the Hippocratic tradition.

Another possible result is that the right to die may become a duty to die. Do futile treatment policies put health services organizations and providers on a slippery slope? Will the policies become broader and increasingly focused on the quality of life that clinicians determine would be acceptable to the patient? These questions can be answered only in retrospect, in itself not a cheery prospect.

Supplements to Futile Treatment Guidelines

Absent data showing that patients and surrogates commonly demand treatment that caregivers consider futile, it is possible that futility guidelines are solving a nonproblem. In addition, the SUPPORT investigators' findings as to economic impact should be explored further.

If the problem exists, however, the first alternative solution is the status quo—patients and/or surrogates must agree to discontinue treatment after physicians determine it is futile. An adjunct to this alternative is to enhance the communication skills of physicians and other caregivers. It may be that patients and surrogates inadequately understand the prognosis. Health professionals such as nurses and social services staff may be used more effectively, for example. The task should not be left only to physicians and ethics committees since both are likely to be much more daunting to patients and surrogates.

Increasing availability of objective predictions of survival or probability of good result, such as the Acute Physiological and Chronic Health Evaluation (APACHE) system, can be used to assist decision makers (patients and/or surrogates) in understanding the best course of action. APACHE was developed at The George Washington University Medical Center in 1981. APACHE II, introduced in 1985, was a simplified approach that used 12 acute physiological variables, age, and chronic health status to predict the probable outcomes of treatment. Further refinements produced APACHE III in 1990.[25] Systems such as APACHE are helpful in efficiently using critical care resources, such as intensive care units (ICUs). Patients who are too well or too sick should not be admitted to an ICU; the former have no need for the technology available there, and the latter will die despite all therapeutic efforts.[26] Scoring systems that quantify the probability that critically ill patients will survive give patients, surrogates, and physicians an important supplement for their decision making.

A second alternative solution that is more long range is to change the presumption about treatment. It is presumed that appropriate treatment is to be provided absent express directives to the contrary. This presumption, reflecting Baconian theory about science conquering nature, has been reinforced by the law. Recognizing that medicine has limits requires a return to the Hippocratic tradition.[27] The presumption should be that when terminal illness or PVS has been diagnosed, treatment will be provided only if it is probable that the patient will benefit from it.

A third alternative solution is to develop and apply a community standard. Although this approach is not easy, all health services organizations have the ability to develop its operational aspects. Here, the idea is to protect the commons—or its contemporary manifestation, communitarianism, a concept championed by Amitai Etzioni. Communitarianism involves recognizing resource limits and cooperatively working within them.

CONCLUSION

Questions of resource allocation are common to all health services organizations. Both macro- and microallocation issues are becoming more important as economic constraints increase, and it is crucial that the organizational philosophy and vision and mission statements guide these decisions. This guidance requires a level of precision and specificity lacking in many organizations. This deficit must be overcome.

Hospitals with large amounts of uncompensated care may offer better reimbursed services to offset losses. Fiscally sound health services organizations must ask whether they are meeting their obligations under the principle of justice to offer unprofitable but needed services that benefit the wider community. They also must ask whether they are meeting a duty of general beneficence to use surpluses to assist persons requiring services.

Futile treatment guidelines are becoming common. Before developing them, the extent of the problem should be determined. Other remedies, such as more effective education on AMDs and improving the processes of getting them on the medical record, may be more effective. The most important use for futile treatment guidelines may be to provide moral and administrative support for physicians, whose clinical practice will benefit from defining and understanding futile treatment. In turn, the guidelines may be used to convince patients or surrogates that treatment without hope of benefit should be withheld or withdrawn.

NOTES

1. Charles Fried. (1976, February). Equality and rights in medical care. *The Hastings Center Report, 6*, pp. 29–34.
2. From Beaufort B. Longest, Jr., Jonathon S. Rakich, & Kurt Darr. (2000). Health care technology. In *Managing health services organizations and systems* (4th. ed., p. 303). Baltimore: Health Professions Press; adapted by permission.
3. Milt Freudenheim. (2003, May 23). Art, commerce and a heart transplant denied. *The New York Times*, C1.
4. From Jonathon S. Rakich, Beaufort B. Longest, Jr., & Kurt Darr. (1985). *Managing health services organizations* (2nd ed., pp. 139–140). Philadelphia: W.B. Saunders; adapted by permission.
5. James E Childress. (1970, Winter). Who shall live when not all can live? *Soundings: An Interdisciplinary Journal, 53*(4), 339–355; Nicholas Rescher, (1969, April). The allocation of exotic medical lifesaving therapy. *Ethics, 79*(3), 173–186.
6. Paul Ramsey. (1970). *The patient as person* (p. 252). New Haven, CT: Yale University Press.
7. From Beaufort B. Longest, Jr., Jonathon S. Rakich, & Kurt Darr. (2000). Ethics. In *Managing health services organizations and systems* (4th., pp. 676–677). Baltimore: Health Professions Press; adapted by permission.

8. Sources for the Sidney Miller case: Kris Axtman. (2003, March 27). Baby case tests rights of parents. *The Christian Science Monitor* [On line]. Retrieved March 24, 2004, from http://www.csmonitor.com/2003/0327/p01s01-usju.htm; Vida Foubister. (2001, February 5). Texas court overturns ruling on resuscitation of premature baby. *American Medical News* [On line]. Retrieved May 6, 2004, from http://www.ama-assn.org/amednews/2001/02/05/prsb0205.htm; Traci Neal. (2002). Who has the right to decide when to save the sickest babies? *Hartford Advocate* [On line] (no date).Retrieved May 6, 2004, from http://old.hartfordadvocate.com/articles/pullingtheplug.html; and Anthony J. Sebok. (2002, December 2). When a hospital ignores parents' request to let their newborn die, is it a tort? *FindLaw.*

9. David B. Waisel & Robert D. Truog. (1995, February 15). The cardiopulmonary resuscitation-not-indicated order: Futility revisited. *Annals of Internal Medicine, 122*(4), 304–308.

10. Man in coma awakes, believes Reagan is still president. (2003, July 10). *The Washington Times*, p. A10.

11. Wesley J. Smith. (2001, July 23)."Futile care" and its friends. *Weekly Standard.* Retrieved May 3, 2004, from http://www.weeklystandard.com/Utilities/printer_preview.asp?idArticle=230&R=9E37234FA; Wesley J. Smith. (2002, December). Futile care theory and medical fascism: The duty to die. *FrontPage Magazine* [On line]. Retrieved March 24, 2004, from http://216.247.220.66/archives/miscellaneous/futile.htm

12. *In the Matter of Baby "K."* 832 F. Supp. 1022 (E.D. Va. July 1, 1993).

13. *In the Matter of Baby "K."* 16 F. 3d 590 (4th Cir., February 10, 1994).

14. Bill Miller & Marylou Tousignant. (1993, September 25). Mother fights hospital to keep infant alive. *The Washington Post*, p. A14.

15. Marylou Tousignant & Bill Miller. (1995, April 7). Death of "Baby K" leaves a legacy of legal precedents. *The Washington Post*, p. B3.

16. Trinity Health. (2001, December). *Q&A: Guidelines on medically futile treatment.* Novi, MI: Author.

17. Trinity Health. (2001, December). *Trinity Health Guidelines on Medically Futile Treatment.* Novi, MI: Author.

18. *Ibid.*

19. *Ibid.*

20. Veda Foubister. (2000, August 14). California law facilitates advance directives for end-of-life medical care. *American Medical News* [On line]. Retrieved November 14, 2003, from http://www.ama-assn.org/amednews/2000/08/14/prsb0814.htm

21. Nancy Valko. (2003). Futility policies and the duty to die. *Voices* [On line]. Retrieved March 24, 2004, from http://www.wf-f.org/03-1-Futility.html

22. Nancy L. Childs & Walt N. Mercer. (1996). Brief report: Late improvement in consciousness after post-traumatic vegetative state. *The New England Journal of Medicine, 334*(l), pp. 24–25; "Permanent" coma can be misnomer, Texas case shows. (1996, January 4). *The Washington Post*, p. A16.

23. The SUPPORT Principal Investigators. (1995, November 22/29). A controlled trial to improve care for seriously-ill hospitalized patients: The study

to understand prognoses and preferences for outcomes and risks of treatments (SUPPORT). *Journal of the American Medical Association, 274*(20), p. 1595.

24. Joan M. Teno, Donald Murphy, Joanne Lynn, Anna Tosteson, Norman Desbiens, Alfred E Connors, Jr., Mary Beth Hamel, Albert Wu, Russell Phillips, Neil Wenger, Frank Harrell, Jr., & William A. Knaus for the SUPPORT Investigators. (1994, November). Prognosis-based guidelines: Does anyone win? *Journal of the American Gerontological Society, 42*, pp. 1202–1207.

25. SATELLIFE. (2002, December 28). *Critical care medicine: Introduction* (pp. 3–4). Retrieved January 9, 2004, from http://www.healthnet.org.np/resource/thesis/anes/Introduction.PDF

26. SATELLIFE. (2002, December 28). *Critical care medicine: Literature review* (p. 1). Retrieved January 9, 2004, from http://www.healthnet.org.np/thesis/anes/Review.PDF

27. Nancy S. Jecker. (1991, May/June). Knowing when to stop: The limits of medicine. *The Hastings Center Report*, pp. 5–8.

CHAPTER 14

SOCIAL RESPONSIBILITY

Three dimensions of the social responsibility of health services organizations are examined in this chapter; they are framed in terms of service versus financial performance. One dimension is protecting and enhancing organization assets while maximizing community benefit. A second is the moral obligation of health services organizations to provide services appropriate to a patient's needs, with no hint of decision making based on nonrelevant factors such as age, payment status, race, or sex. The third dimension of social responsibility considered is the organization's obligation to protect the commonweal—in terms of both private resources and public ones such as Medicare and Medicaid.

COMMUNITY BENEFIT

Controlling costs and improving efficiency are matters of great concern to administrative staff. They ultimately benefit the community and should be a focus for clinicians.

Different Settings, Different Costs

In late 1991, Metropolitan Hospital undertook successful negotiations for a 50–50 joint venture with a six-physician group of gastroenterologists to establish a freestanding endoscopy center. This agreement was a natural outgrowth of a long-term affiliation with the same single-specialty group whose members had been on the active staff at Metropolitan for more than 10 years. Two thirds of the endoscopies at Metropolitan were performed by these six physicians.

Alice Macalin, a member of Metropolitan's staff, manages the center as well as inpatient endoscopy services at Metropolitan. Cost data were collected from the time the center became operational. These data showed that supply costs at the center were almost 35% lower than for endoscopies performed in the hospital. Initially, it was thought that the higher acuity level of patients undergoing endoscopy at the hospital increased costs significantly, but investigation showed this had only a marginal effect.

Macalin noted significant differences in attitudes among the physicians, depending on where they were working. As center director, Macalin is often approached by the physicians with cost-savings ideas, such as switching to reusables for certain supplies. The physicians took it upon themselves to ask technologists to remind them of the cost of expensive disposables before they opened the package. In addition, they tracked one another to determine who might be overusing supplies or using expensive supplies when less expensive alternatives could have been used. On their own, the physicians discussed what might be done to increase operational efficiency at the center, and they devised a scheduling change to better fill down time.

Little of this interest in cost reduction transferred to the hospital. When practicing at Metropolitan, the physicians are not deliberately wasteful, but they are noticeably less interested in developing or initiating cost savings. Macalin had hoped that the patterns from the center would transfer automatically to the hospital, but after almost a year this had occurred only marginally and cost differences continued to be significant. She knew something should be done, but what?

Waste is an ethical issue. Obviously, the financial implications of even shared ownership make the physicians much more interested in improving efficiency at the center. Changing physicians' attitudes about the use of resources is a major challenge for managers and is reflected in efforts to tie physicians into the economic health of the organization through such arrangements as physician–hospital organizations. Macalin could attempt to force changes, but doing so would risk both physician antipathy and apathy. Gross transfers of expectations and patterns from the center to the hospital may be interpreted by physicians as interfering with professional judgment and decision making because the patients are hospitalized when endoscopies are performed in Metropolitan. Education and working patiently with the physicians to gain their understanding of the applicability and transferability of efficiency from the center to the hospital are essential activities for Macalin as she exhibits the virtue of thrift.

Improving efficiency benefits (general duty of beneficence) the community by reducing costs, thus making health services more affordable and accessible. In addition to reducing waste, health services organizations have a moral obligation to collect debts owed to them. Not-for-profit organizations are expected to provide uncompensated care—services that provide community benefit—to retain their special tax status. Yet, they should, and arguably must, take reasonable steps to collect monies legally owed to them. Part of a health services organization's fiduciary obligation to its service area is to maintain its financial status. Aggressive debt collection raises ethical issues, however, even if the law allows the actions being taken by the organization.

Pursuit[1]

Memorial Hospital is a 250-bed, not-for-profit organization. It is financially successful but has chronic problems with accounts receivable (AR) and writes off more bad debt each year than comparable-size not-for-profit hospitals. Memorial hired a financial consultant who told them to become much more aggressive in collecting patient debts. The consultant recommended filing lawsuits against debtors, garnishing patients' wages, and seizing their income tax refunds. When the new tactics were explained, some senior managers demurred. Ultimately, however, the chief executive officer (CEO) and chief financial officer (CFO) decided to use the legal but extreme methods that had been recommended.

As an ultimate expression of collection efforts, debtors who missed court appearances were arrested pursuant to an order issued by the presiding judge. These orders resulted from a court's authority to punish those who fail to appear as directed.* Some debtors were jailed briefly, until bail was posted. The collection efforts caused bankruptcy for others.

When the media became aware of Memorial's debt collection policy, critical stories were published. One astute reporter noted that the uninsured were being asked to pay charges rather than the discounted rates paid by payers who had contracts with the hospital. Charges are typically several times the discounted rates.

Memorial's CEO and CFO were very pleased with the reduction in the amount and aging of AR, but governing body members began asking questions about the collections practice of one another and of the CEO.

The case describes an ethical dilemma for health services organizations. The oft-repeated mantra "no margin, no mission" fits here. One must ask whether hospitals are meeting their duty of fidelity to their service area, patients, and staff if they fail to make significant efforts to collect what is owed them. In addition, organizations have vendors to whom timely payment must be made lest essential goods and services become unavailable. Hospitals further defend such practices by noting that they must collect

---

*Various jurisdictions call them *body attachments, civil arrest warrants, bench warrants,* or *writs of capias.* Technically, they are not punishment for the debt but for flouting the court's authority.

the debts they are owed because costs are increasing even as reimbursement from third-party payers declines. It must be asked whether practices such as body attachments treat the debtor (and former patient) with dignity and respect. The patient owes respect to the organization and its needs, as well, and the organization may have been unable to get the debtor's attention any other way. Certainly, the bad press diminishes the organization's reputation and community standing. Positive for the organization, however, is that public knowledge about extreme collection practices will cause self-selection—patients unwilling or unable to pay for services will go elsewhere. Thus, the hospital's financial situation is improved, even as access may be lessened.

Hospitals' financial problems are exacerbated by the millions of persons who are uninsured. The Congressional Budget Office reported that the Survey of Income and Program Participation estimated that the number of nonelderly individuals without health insurance in 1998 ranged from 21.3 million (uninsured for the entire year), to 40.5 million (uninsured at a specific point in time during the year), to 56.8 (uninsured at any time during the year).[2] Notably, the burden of the uninsured falls disproportionately on hospitals by region and even within a region. In 1998 and 1999, uninsured rates generally were highest in the South and West and lowest in the Midwest and Northeast. Among the states, New Mexico had the highest rate at 26.6 %, Minnesota the lowest at 9.6 %. More populous states such as Florida and New York tended to have higher rates of uninsured individuals.[3] Similarly, major metropolitan areas have disproportionate numbers of persons who are uninsured and cannot pay for health care.

We've Earned It, We'll Keep It!

Freeland Hospital is a not-for-profit, general acute care hospital located in an affluent suburban neighborhood. Its Medicare census is less than 20%, and it receives less than 1% of its revenues from Medicaid. Uncollectibles are less than 3%. Freeland Hospital's current financial situation is sound.

Sherwood Shurman had been the CEO of Freeland for almost 20 years and is justifiably proud of the changes and improvements that he has achieved during his tenure. One improvement has been to establish the Freeland Hospital Foundation, Inc., which receives charitable donations as well as excess of income over expense from the operations of Freeland Hospital. In only 10 years, the Foundation has accumulated $12 million; $2 million were used to acquire equipment.

Occasionally, board members question whether the hospital is sufficiently socially conscious. The most common suggestion is that Freeland ought to establish an outpatient clinic in the inner city, where access to primary care is limited. Shurman has assiduously avoided acting on these informal recommendations.

Shurman hired a marketing director, Maureen O'Riley, and asked her to identify new initiatives for Freeland. O'Riley's market research resulted in a plan that included programs for respite care, addiction treatment, and rehabilitation medicine. O'Riley noted that there are no competing programs in their service area and that expected demand will be covered by private-pay patients or nongovernmental third-party payers, at least the former of whom are likely to pay charges. Shurman was enthusiastic about the suggestions and asked the board to review the proposal.

Shurman was shocked when the plan met significant resistance. No member of the board disputed the well-documented need and the potential demand for the proposed programs. Instead, they were troubled by the prospect of generating additional revenues and adding them to the endowment. Several members indicated that they would support the new programs only if a large part of any surplus was used to assist the city's underserved areas. Others mentioned social consciousness; one even used the word guilt to describe her feelings about having so much while others had so little. The proposal was tabled.

Shurman was angry as he left the board meeting but took care not to allow others to see his state of mind. After a few minutes' reflection on the meeting, he asked to meet with his chief operating officer, Maria Sanchez. Shurman told Sanchez what had happened and asked her to solicit any equipment requests submitted by the medical staff and to ensure that they were in his office by week's end. He told Sanchez to dust off the plans that had been developed several years earlier to build a staff education wing and the more recent request from the oncology department for an expanded unit. As Sanchez left, Shurman thought to himself that he would be damned if he would see his hard work and fiscal success wasted on a harebrained scheme to provide primary care to a population that was the city's responsibility.

Freeland Hospital is wealthy and likely to become wealthier. Some members of the board recognize a broader social responsibility for the hospital, whereas Shurman has a narrower view of Freeland's role. The questions raised by the board should have been addressed in the hospital's philosophy and vision and mission statements, and these documents should be reviewed for guidance—or amended. If no attention has been given to Freeland's broader social responsibility, this fundamental issue must be addressed before decisions are made about the marketing plan and the recommended programs. It is folly to proceed without a clear direction and a consensus to pursue this responsibility.

The service area concept is Shurman's strongest reason for opposing the board's interest in aiding the city's underserved. The inner city appears to be out of Freeland's service area. Is it just to take resources from Freeland's service area and redirect them to individuals elsewhere, however compelling the reason? This view suggests that Freeland should reduce its surpluses and simultaneously benefit its service area by reducing charges. This action would directly benefit those whom it serves. Alternatively, Freeland could identify health needs that are not adequately insured or are not likely to be highly sought by private payers but are important nonetheless. Examples of such needs include mental health programs and various types of counseling services.

Shurman's attitude seems extraordinarily parochial, whereas the board's attitude may be too altruistic. A wide middle ground exists that could accommodate both. It is reasonable to study what role Freeland could play in meeting the health needs of the wider community, whether or not it is in Freeland's service area. Additional information may make the answer apparent.

Historical attitudes about competition, lack of profit motive, and not-for-profit status have both helped and hindered the health services system. The absence of economic incentives has contributed to health services organizations feeling good about themselves because they were doing good rather than concentrating on performing well and efficiently.

A health services organization loses public confidence if it appears not to be working in the community's best health services interests. The conflict is between protecting its financial integrity—an ethical obligation of the organization linked to its role of providing services to the community—and serving individual patients.

EQUAL NEED, UNEQUAL TREATMENT

It may be fruitless to set a goal of achieving the same services for all persons with the same medical need. The numbers and types of variables involved are staggering. For example, access is limited by geography, availability and capability of providers, individual desire to receive services, a subculture's attitudes about health, physicians' ability or willingness to treat or refer, insurance status, financial circumstances, mental state, and dozens of other attributes of individuals and the health services system. The problems of equity (fairness) are legion and are probably unresolvable, regardless of how health services are organized, provided, or financed. Even systems with universal access have disparities in use or access because of system expenditures for services and technology, socioeconomic class, geography, and physicians' willingness to refer patients. Given the number of factors and the certainty that variability in service access and use are inevitable, it is nonetheless important that providers seek to identify these types of problems and make reasonable efforts to eliminate them or minimize their effects. Disparities begin as far upstream as the funding of research where, for example, the National Cancer Institute (part of the National Institutes of Health) spent less than 1% of its $2.9 billion budget on end-of-life research and training in 1999.[4]

Ageism appears to be present in parts of the health services system. For example, although older adults are at greater risk of dying from heart disorders, cancer, and influenza/pneumonia, there is evidence that they do not get the most aggressive forms of treatment and diagnostic and preventive care, which is standard for younger patients. The disparity seems to be based on the perception that older adults either cannot tolerate more aggressive treatments or do not want them, neither of which is necessarily true. There is also evidence that physicians are less likely to suggest that these individuals participate in screenings for various cancers or receive influenza vaccinations.[5] Other disparities are present at the end of life, with statistics showing that African Americans comprise 14% of the U.S. population but only 7% of hospice patients, even though they have a higher cancer incidence and higher mortality rates than Caucasians.[6] In addition to variation in hospice use by ethnicity, there is wide geographic variation in the use of the Medicare hospice benefit by older individuals.[7]

Research at five teaching hospitals found disparities in using cardiopulmonary resuscitation (CPR). CPR was more likely to be used for men, younger patients, African Americans, patients whose reported preferences were for CPR, and those who had higher physician estimates for 2-month survival. Rates also vary significantly by geographic location and diagnosis.[8]

A sample of 1.56 million nursing facility residents found that African Americans are approximately one third as likely as Caucasians to have living wills and one fifth as likely to have do-not-resuscitate (DNR) orders. Hispanics are approximately one third as likely as Caucasians to have DNR orders but just as likely to have living wills. The researchers concluded that the presence of advance care plans is related to race, even after controlling for health and other demographic factors.[9]

Another dimension of DNR orders is whether they are written equitably for patients with different diseases but similar prognoses. In 1995, the results of a study reported that DNR orders are written more often for older patients, women, and patients with dementia or incontinence and less often for patients who are African American, have Medicaid insurance, or are in rural hospitals.[10] Similar disparities were found in an earlier study in which DNR orders were much more likely to be written for patients with AIDS or inoperable lung cancer than for patients with other diseases with equally poor prognoses, such as cirrhosis or heart failure.[11]

General concerns have been raised regarding the unequal treatment of individuals who are dying:

> Ample evidence exists that the process of dying is less than optimal. Too many dying patients suffer unnecessary physical symptoms such as pain, dyspnoea, nausea, and vomiting; too many suffer untreated depression, anxiety, and hopelessness; and too many feel they have lost their dignity. It is the perception that dying is a painful process filled with unnecessary suffering and indignity that fuels campaigns—and public support—for legalizing euthanasia and physician-assisted suicide.[12]

Reforms suggested include training physicians, nurses, and other health providers to communicate better with dying patients; improving management of pain, anorexia, insomnia, fatigue, and other physical symptoms; appropriately diagnosing and treating depression; referring dying patients to hospice care earlier; improving palliation; and facilitating dying at home.[13] Patients who have DNR orders apparently receive no less contact from staff and visitors than those who do not have DNR orders, however.[14]

Variation in types and amounts of care also occurs by region of the country. It is well known that the rates at which various surgical and medical treatments are used vary widely by region, state, and even county. Apparently, these variations are a function of how physicians practice medicine. Not unexpected, then, is wide variation in the use (prevalence) of tube feeding by state. A study of patients 65 years of age and older who had severe cognitive impairments, including total dependence in eating, and who resided in nursing facilities in nine states showed wide variation in use of tube feeding. Prevalence ranged from a low of 7.5% in Maine to a high of 40.1% in Mississippi, with the other seven states falling in between. Differences in state law may have contributed to some of the variation, but the authors concluded that after accounting for clinical and demographic variables, there are true differences in the prevalence of tube feedings in the nine states studied. In addition, there are differences in use of tube feeding by race, with Caucasian residents being less than half as likely as other ethnic groups to receive this treatment.[15] Sometimes, availability of services results from a payment system that makes it impossible for providers to survive financially. One example is the attribution of hospital closures to inadequate payment from managed care and other contracting practices, thus reducing access to both emergency department (ED) and general hospital services. Between 1991 and 2001, nearly one in five hospitals with EDs closed.[16]

Between the extremes of hyperegalitarianiasm and hypermeritocracy is the position that society has a duty to assist in developing, encouraging, and even providing health services. Fried argued that routine basic services ought to be available to all, a position known as *the decent minimum*.[17] More exotic high-technology services are limited by factors such as location, cost, and referrals and must be available on a different basis. Where to draw this line is a political decision and depends on society's willingness to provide the resources needed.

Hospital EDs go on ambulance reroute (i.e., the EDs close) when they are filled to capacity and cannot safely accept more patients. The need for reroute is communicated to the centers that dispatch ambulances, and the ambulances are directed elsewhere. It is common for busy EDs to go on reroute, as illustrated in the following example.

The Emergency Department

University Hospital, a private, partially investor-owned academic health center hospital, is located in a major East Coast metropolitan area. Its ED is the city's busiest. Two years ago, closure of the city-owned hospital eliminated the major source of services for persons who are uninsured and cannot pay for health care. The city established a fund to pay private providers such as University Hospital for the uncompensated care it provided to city residents.

The city-owned ambulance service has a policy to take patients to the closest available ED that can provide the services the patient needs. Ambulance dispatchers are informed when an ED is at capacity, and ambulances are rerouted to other EDs. The decision to close an ED is made by the ED director.

University's ED director determined that her ED was at capacity and told a staff member to call the ambulance dispatch center to request temporary reroute of patients. The call was made, but communication failed at the dispatch center. When an emergency medical technician (EMT) radioed to tell University's ED that they were bringing in a patient, the ED director asked what the patient's medical problem was and from where she was being brought. The EMT told her the patient was from the inner city. The ED director then told the EMT that University's ED was on reroute. The EMT decided that the reason he was told that University's ED was on reroute was because the patient was coming from the inner city, was likely a minority, and was probably uninsured. This belief caused several EMTs to file a complaint with the city health department. An investigation followed.

The investigation found that the ED was on reroute when the EMT called and that the decision was made consistent with city guidelines. This case suggests problems of general perception, a perception of bias, and miscommunication. The EMTs' conclusion that the decision was made on non-medical grounds suggests a preexisting poor relationship with University Hospital. Improving that relationship should receive early attention from the hospital and the EMTs. The EMTs' perception of biased decision making can only be improved over time; by the hospital's determining its source; and, if there is substance behind the perception, by the hospital's making the necessary changes to prevent that perception from continuing. Even if substance is lacking, the hospital does not want perception to drive reality. In either event, it will take a long-term effort on University's part to improve relations with the EMTs.

It has been argued that rationing is the only way to bring fairness to the health care system. This position is supported by identifying the extraordinarily high cost of early "last-chance therapies," such as totally implantable artificial hearts; left ventricular assist devices; and Herceptin, a drug to treat metastatic breast cancer.[18] More ultra-expensive therapies are likely to follow. Any system that guarantees a decent minimum of primary care and specialty services is unlikely to be able to afford to pay for ultra-expensive services that might be available and demanded by all. The concept of meritocracy—those with greater disposable income may buy more services if they choose—is generally acceptable to all but the most dedicated hyperegalitarians.

The microallocation decisions that health services providers make constantly result in rationing. The last bed in the ICU is an often-cited, classic example. Yet, there are many others, most of which more subtle and less easily identified—for example, allocation of donor organs, blood products in short supply, and even general medical-surgical beds. Micro-allocation decisions that have the effect of rationing occur as well.[19]

THE COMMONWEAL

American Hospital Association (AHA) data show that in 2002, hospitals provided $22.3 billion in uncompensated care.[20] This was a substantial increase from $16 billion in 1995, which was an 8.8% increase from 1992.[21] *Uncompensated care* has been defined as the total of charity care and bad debt valued at the cost to the hospital of the services provided. Some health services organizations define *uncompensated care* more broadly and include costs in excess of payments received for Medicare and Medicaid services.[22] Hospitals' uncompensated care averages 6% of total costs. Major publicly owned teaching hospitals and urban government hospitals typically have an uncompensated care rate two to three times as high.[23] The concern during the 1990s that hospitals would reduce uncompensated care to counter payment shortfalls from Medicare and Medicaid, as well as price discounts negotiated by managed care plans, did not materialize.[24] Hospitals' commitment to treating those unable to pay continues largely unabated.

During the 1990s, a number of not-for-profit hospitals were converted to investor-owned (for-profit) status, a development that seems related to declining economic performance of the not-for-profits. From 1991 to 1997, there were 431 conversions. The uncompensated care provided by the converted entities decreased from 5.3% to 4.7%, approximately equal to a $400,000 reduction in per hospital spending. The decline was more substantial in public facilities that converted to investor-owned status, with reductions from 5.2% to 2.5% of total expenses, or approximately $800,000 less per hospital per year. Overall, changing from not-for-profit to investor-owned status resulted in a reduction of about 13% in uncompensated care.[25] The study did not attribute the need for or decision behind conversion to a specific problem. There is concern that wholesale conversions of not-for-profit hospitals to investor-owned ones will eliminate major sources of services to persons who are uninsured and cannot pay for health care.

Comparisons of not-for-profit and investor-owned hospitals offer insights into uncompensated care. Analyzing 1993 data, a study of 116 Tennessee hospitals, approximately one third of which were investor-owned, showed that as a percentage of expenses, not-for-profit hospitals provided more uncompensated care than did investor-owned hospitals. On average, however, differences were not large. The median for all Tennessee hospitals was 8.4%; the median for not-for-profit and investor-owned hospitals was 8.9% and 8.1%, respectively. Notably, the value of taxes paid by investor-owned hospitals was not included in calculating direct and indirect contributions to programs such as Medicare and Medicaid. Taxes included federal and state income taxes and sales, property, and local business taxes.[26] Findings similar to those in Tennessee were reported by the Medicare Payment Advisory Commission: Investor-owned and not-for-profit hospitals provided substantially the same amount of uncompensated care in 1999 as a percentage of costs, 4.2% and 4.6%, respectively.[27]

The tax variable was considered in a study undertaken by the Virginia Health Services Cost Review Council, an independent state data commission. Using 1993 data, it ranked 88 acute care hospitals in Virginia via 18 productivity and efficiency variables. A variable used to measure community benefits provided by each hospital proved controversial. *Community support* was defined as the percentage of a hospital's total expenses for charity care, bad debt, and all taxes. Including taxes put for-profit hospitals ahead of most not-for-profit hospitals. A Virginia Hospital Association analysis, which excluded two state-supported university hospitals, found that 13 for-profit hospitals used 14% of their operating expenses for community support as compared with the 73 not-for-profit hospitals, which spent 7.7%. In commenting on the data, members of the investor-owned sector argued that taxes should be included because they support local communities, as well as Medicaid and Medicare. Conversely, members of the not-for-profit sector asserted that including taxes is misleading because most taxes are state and federal income taxes, which may or may not be used for local health care programs.[28]

Data from California hospitals, who provided uncompensated care totaling $1.5 billion in 2000, provides another perspective on the problem. When using the expanded definition of uncompensated care (i.e., including the costs in excess of payments for Medicare and Medicaid services), however, the total jumps to $5.3 billion. Not-for-profit hospitals provided 61% of uncompensated care. Government-owned hospitals provided twice as much uncompensated care per bed as not-for-profit hospitals, and thrice as much as investor-owned hospitals.[29]

Such studies are often marred by methodological problems; the definitive study may never be done. It is clear, however, that caution must be used in attributing motives and results solely to ownership. Since 1983, the AHA has not provided data on uncompensated care that distinguish not-for-profit and investor-owned hospitals.

The tragic case of Jesica Santillan riveted the public's attention in early 2003. It has elements of both resource allocation and social responsibility, but is discussed here because it highlights important issues of social responsibility and the obligation of U.S. health services providers to treat illegal aliens.

Jesica Santillan[30]

Jesica Santillan was 17 years old when she died. She had been born near Guadalajara, Mexico, with congenital cardiac insufficiency. Her family smuggled her into the U.S. to obtain the heart/lung transplant she needed to stay alive. Jesica was placed on the transplant list at Duke University Hospital. North Carolinian Mack Mahony, who had become a family friend, helped raise the $500,000 needed to pay for the transplant.

The United Network of Organ Sharing (UNOS) manages a nationwide organ matching system under a contract with the federal government. Its criteria allow 5% of organs transplanted at any hospital to be used for illegal aliens or foreign nationals.

Although Jesica was on the transplant list, she was not on the list of potential recipients for the heart and lungs that were available—she was not a match. Nonetheless, the transplant coordinator and Jesica's doctor discussed giving the available organs to her. Neither realized that she was not on the list as being a match.

Jesica received the mismatched heart-lung transplant on February 7, 2003. It was soon apparent that her body was rejecting the organs. A correctly matched heart and lungs were transplanted, but her condition worsened. Jesica was declared brain dead at 1:25 P.M. on February 23. Life support was stopped at 5:00 P.M.

North Carolina law defines someone who is brain dead as no longer having life to support. Thus, life support may be ended without obtaining consent.

The Santillan family objected to the decision to discontinue life support. Mack Mahony asked for time to obtain a second opinion as to Jesica's condition. No extension of time was given, however.

This is an emotionally wrenching story of a young woman fighting for life. Despite her critical medical condition, there was every reason to believe she could have been saved. The following elements of the situation involve ethical issues: medical error(s), microallocation decision by Duke University Hospital in the first transplant, microallocation by Duke University Hospital in the second transplant (preferential treatment, low probability of success), a non–U.S. citizen receiving scarce organs, and macroallocation by UNOS.

Crossing the ethical-legal boundary is that of the medical errors committed by staff at Duke University Hospital. The medical errors here did not involve the surgeons' technique or other treatment. Rather, they resulted from the failure of the processes that supported the transplant activity—processes developed and maintained by management. The hospital and its staff failed to meet their ethical duties of nonmaleficence and beneficence in the care provided to Jesica.

The ethical principle of justice is found in two microallocation decisions made at Duke University Hospital. The first has to do with the decision to allow an illegal alien to receive the transplant, regardless of the availability of funds and organs. Perhaps fresh in the minds of Duke's clinicians and administrators was the experience involving the Cleveland Clinic which, in similar circumstances, initially refused to provide a liver transplant to an illegal alien. It bowed to political pressure from an Hispanic city councilman, however, and provided the treatment. The principle of justice also arises in the microallocation decision Duke University Hospital made when it transplanted a second (correctly matched) set of heart and lungs. Questions about preferential treatment abound in that one patient received a second set of organs, which were transplanted despite a very low probability of success.

Finally, there is the issue of macroallocation of organs to non–U.S. citizens, which is even more questionable for illegal aliens. Given the scarcity of transplantable organs, it seems morally unjust that non–U.S. citizens receive any at all. Non–U.S. citizens contribute no organs to the pool of organs available for transplantation. Indeed, anecdotal evidence suggests that many noncitizens come from cultures where organ donation is religiously or socially unacceptable. It is noteworthy that the Santillans declined to donate any of Jesica's organs.[31] The Santillan case strongly suggests that UNOS reconsider its position on allocation of organs to non–U.S. citizens—especially illegal aliens, who bring with them the double problem of an enlarged service area and, typically, lack of resources to pay the costs of care.

How Can We Afford This?

A 63-year-old woman slipped into an irreversible coma after having two heart attacks. Three years later she was still a patient in an acute care hospital. Her aggregate unpaid bill totaled $750,000 after private insurance coverage lapsed. The insurer argued that the patient was receiving only custodial care, and therefore it would not pay for acute care. According to state law, the patient could be transferred to another facility only if she were declared mentally incompetent. Hospital efforts to achieve this through court action caused much adverse publicity in the community. Ultimately, the hospital failed to achieve its goal of moving the woman out of the facility, and she died there.

The organization and its managers faced an ethical dilemma—their ongoing relationship with a patient who no longer needed acute care. The principles of beneficence and nonmaleficence and the virtues of caring and compassion prevented them from abandoning the patient, but the uncompensated costs of her care increasingly conflicted with the hospital's obligation to maintain its financial integrity, which was necessary to serving the community. Thus, managers failed to meet the virtues of loyalty and thrift. This large, financially healthy hospital could absorb the losses attributable to this patient, but the issue of resource allocation remains, nonetheless. The cost of a microallocation decision—continued treatment for someone unable to benefit from hospital care—could have overwhelmed the ability of other hospitals to provide services to the community (macroallocation).

It seems trite to characterize this case as a public relations failure, but the hospital might have gained community understanding had it been more forthright and communicative in describing the problem and the dilemma it faced as it sought to move the woman into a suitable alternative facility. Working to change the law so that mental status is but one criterion used in making such decisions is important for the future and should be undertaken by the trade association.

Noncompliant patients pose a special problem in microallocation decisions. Typically, they have chronic health problems that need continuing, periodic treatment, such as renal dialysis that treats end-stage renal disease. These patients may be noncompliant in terms of following a dietary and medication regimen or submitting to treatment as scheduled, or they may engage in behavior that makes it difficult or impossible for staff to treat them. The organization is morally obligated to facilitate treatment for all patients needing its services, but those with significant behavior problems or who are noncompliant with the treatment regimen should be discharged from the program, with proper attention to legal requirements.

A new dimension to the policy issue of uncompensated care is raised when non–U.S. citizens are taken to United States hospitals for treatment. Mexican ambulances are using unguarded border crossings to bring illegal aliens to U.S. hospitals, after the patients were denied care in Mexican hospitals because they could not pay. U.S. hospitals must provide services because of the Emergency Medical Treatment and Active Labor Act (EMTALA) of 1986 (42 USC § 1395dd.), which makes no distinction between citizens and illegal aliens. Adding significantly to costs is providing helicopter transport from border hospitals to inland medical centers when more sophisticated treatment is needed. It has been estimated that hospitals along the Mexican border have lost more than $200 million in unreimbursed costs for treating illegal aliens, and the losses show no signs of abating. Some verge on bankruptcy; others have been forced to close their EDs. The result is compromised access for legal immigrants and U.S. citizens. A study found that 77 hospitals along the Mexican border with California, Arizona, New Mexico, and Texas face a medical emergency.

The federal government has been unwilling to address the problem and has left it to state and local governments to solve; mostly the burden has fallen on the hospitals themselves.[32] The injustice of this situation and its negative impact on the legal immigrants and U.S. citizens served by these hospitals are patent. The federal government is charged with maintaining the integrity of the nation's borders. It has, however, been unwilling to stop or pay for the abuses described. Given present attitudes, the problem is irresolvable. Absent effective action, the hospitals will spiral into further decline and eventual closure—to the detriment of those they were meant to serve.

CONCLUSION

This chapter examined some of the issues attendant to the social responsibility of health services organizations, primarily hospitals. Although organizations have an ethical obligation to husband resources, there are ethical limits, for instance, to how aggressively they should collect monies owed them. Also, sharp business practices should be avoided because they are inconsistent with various virtues and the principle of respect for persons. The virtues are fully consistent with the organization's efforts to protect and enhance its assets while maximizing patient and community benefit.

Through their managers, health services organizations are morally obliged to provide services that meet the patient's needs without considering nonrelevant factors such as age, payment status, race, or sex. Persistent variations in provisions of medical services appear to be more a function of how physicians practice medicine than deliberate expressions of bias. What is identified as ageism may be as much an expression of the culture's emphasis on youth as it is a bias against older adults. Ethically unacceptable, however, are implicit judgments about poor quality of life. Health services managers must identify and eliminate any hint of systemic or personal bias in medical decision making and delivery of services.

Protecting the commonweal—the sum of private and public resources—is a more ethereal responsibility. Much of what can or should be done is beyond the control of health services managers. Nonetheless, wasteful programs, regardless of funding source, and those of lesser clinical quality or that unnecessarily put the public at risk must be eliminated. Husbanding resources is an ethical obligation for managers, because all resources, regardless of ownership, are part of the commonweal.

NOTES

1. Lucette Lagnado. (2003, October 30). Hospitals try extreme measures to collect their overdue debts. *The Wall Street Journal*, p. A1.

2. Congressional Budget Office. (2003, May). *How many people lack health insurance and for how long?* Washington, DC: Author.

3. *Health insurance: Characteristics and trends in the uninsured population: Hearings before the Senate Committee on Finance*, 107th Congress (2001, March 13) (testimony of Kathryn G. Allen, Director, Health Care—Medicaid and Private Health Insurance Issues, General Accounting Office).

4. Susan Okie. (2001, June 20). Better cancer care urged: Focus on cure hurts treatment of symptoms, study finds. *The Washington Post*, p. A14.

5. Joyce Howard Price. (2003, December 1). Seniors medical care poses bias question. *The Washington Times*, p. A1.

6. The National Journal Group. (2001, June 21). Palliative care: Report urges increased research, focus. *American Health Line*.

7. Beth A. Virnig, Sara Kind, Marshall McBean, & Elliott Fisher. (2000, September). Geographic variation in hospice use prior to death. *Journal of the American Geriatrics Society, 48*(9), pp. 1117–1125.

8. Sarah J. Goodlin, Zhenshao Zhong, Joanne Lynn, Joan M. Teno, Julie P. Fago, Normal Desbiens, Alfred F. Connors, Jr., Neil S. Wenger, & Russell S. Phillips. (1999, December 22). Factors associated with use of cardiopulmonary resuscitation in seriously ill hospitalized adults. *Journal of the American Medical Association, 282*(24), 2333–2339.

9. Howard B. Degenholtz, Robert A. Arnold, Alan Meisel, & Judith R. Lave. (2002, February). Persistence of racial disparities in advance care plan documents among nursing home residents. *Journal of the American Geriatrics Society 50*(2), pp. 378–381.

10. Neil S. Wenger, Marjorie L. Pearson, Katherine A. Desmond, Ellen R. Harrison, Lisa V. Rubenstein, William H. Rogers, & Katherine L. Kahn. (1995, October 23). Epidemiology of do-not-resuscitate orders: Disparity by age, diagnosis, gender, race, and functional impairment. *Archives of Internal Medicine, 155*, pp. 2056–2062.

11. Robert M. Wachter, John M. Luce, Norman Hearst, & Bernard Lo. (1989, September). Decisions about resuscitation: Inequities among patients with different diseases but similar prognoses. *Annals of Internal Medicine, 3*(6), pp. 525–532.

12. Ezekiel J. Emanuel. (2001, June 9). Euthanasia: Where the Netherlands leads will the world follow? No. Legalisation is a diversion from improving care for the dying. *British Medical Journal, 322*(7299), pp. 1376–1377.

13. *Ibid.*

14. Very sick patients left all alone, Georgetown study finds. (2001, December 3). *American Medical News* [On line]. Retrieved November 14, 2003, from http://www.ama-assn.org/amednews/2001/12/03/prbf1203.htm

15. Judith C. Ahronheim, Michael Mulvihill, Carol Sieger, Pil Park, & Brant E. Fries. (2001, February). State practice variations in the use of tube feedings

for nursing home residents with severe cognitive impairment. *Journal of the American Geriatrics Society, 49*(2), pp. 148–152.

16. Maureen Glabman. (2003, June). Managed care makes it tough for some hospitals to stay afloat. *Managed Care Magazine* [On line]. Retrieved January 2, 2004, from http://www.managedcaremag.com/archives/0306/0306.er.html

17. Charles Fried. (1976, February). Equality and rights in medical care. *The Hastings Center Report, 6*, pp. 29–34.

18. Leonard M. Fleck. (2002, March/April). Rationing: Don't give up. *The Hastings Center Report 32*(2), pp. 35–36.

19. Greta Anand. (2003, September 12). The big secret in health care: Rationing is here. *The Wall Street Journal*, p. A1.

20. Mary Ann Costello. (2004, February 18). Nation's hospitals provided $22.3 billion in uncompensated care in 2002. *AHA News Now*, p. 1.

21. David Burda. (1995, May 8). Hospitals' care for poor rises slowly. *Modern Healthcare, 25*(19), p. 30.

22. Health First. (2003.) *What are not-for-profit/community-minded hospitals? What it means to your community.* Retrieved January 12, 2004, from http://www.health-first.org/company_info/not_for_profit.cfm

23. National Association of Public Hospitals and Health Systems. (2001, February). *What is a safety net hospital?* Retrieved January 10, 2004, from http://www.naph.org/Content/NavigationMenu/About_Our_Members/Frequently_Asked_Questions1/FAQpdf5.pdf

24. David Burda. (1995, May 8). Hospitals' care for poor rises slowly. *Modern Healthcare, 25*(19), p. 30.

25. UC Davis Health System. (2000, November 17). *Uncompensated care spending declines with for-profit conversions.* Retrieved January 4, 2004, from http://www.ucdmc.ucdavis.edu/update/archives/Nov_17_00/uncompensated.htm

26. David Burda. (1995, April 24). Tennessee for-profits lag in care for poor. *Modern Healthcare, 25*(17), pp. 70, 72, 74.

27. *Statement of the Federation of American Hospitals: Hospitals' non-profit status: Federal Trade Commission and Department of Justice hearings on health care and competition law and policy* (2003, April 10) (testimony of Eugene Anthony Fay).

28. David Burda. (1995, May 8). For-profits, not-for-profits reignite battle. *Modern Healthcare, 25*(19), pp. 28, 30.

29. Sarah Yang. (2003, October 27). New briefs find relatively few hospitals providing bulk of charity care in the state. *UC BerkeleyNews* [On line]. Retrieved January 6, 2004, from http://www.berkeley.edu/news/media/releases/2003/10/27_charity.shtml

30. Sources for the Jesica Santillan case: Angela Heywood Bible & Sarah Avery. (2003, February 24). *At odds over Jesica's last hours.* Retrieved May 4, 2004, from http://organtx.org/ethics/mismatch.htm; Donna Gregory. (2003, February 23). Santillan family planning lawsuit. *MSNBC News* [On line; no longer available]; Michelle Malkin. (2003, March 18). Illegal alien health care has crippling effects on citizens. *Insight on the News.* Retrieved May 4, 2004, from http://www.findarticles.com/cf_0/m1571/7_19/98923512/p1/article.jhtml

31. Teenage victim of botched transplant dies after 2nd one. (2003, February 23). Associated Press, as reported in the *Dubuque Telegraph Herald.*
32. Jerry Seper. (2002, December 12). Mexican medics take sick to U.S.: Americans left to pick up tab. *The Washington Times*, p. A1.

ORGANIZATIONAL PHILOSOPHIES AND MISSION STATEMENTS

MISSION, VISION, AND
VALUES STATEMENT OF SUTTER HEALTH

Mission

We enhance the health and well-being of people in the communities we serve, through a not-for-profit commitment to compassion and excellence in health care services.

Vision

Sutter Health will be a recognized leader in transforming health care to meet the needs of the 21st Century. At both the local and regional levels we will be:

- The preferred provider to our patients and customers

- The best place to work and practice

- A role model of community citizenship

Values

Caring and Compassion

Excellence and Quality

Teamwork

Honesty and Integrity

Community

From Sutter Health. (n.d.). *About us: Our mission*. Retrieved August 21, 2003, from http://www.sutterhealth.org/about/mission

MISSION, CORE VALUES, AND
VISION STATEMENT OF TRINITY HEALTH

Mission

We serve together in Trinity Health, in the spirit of the Gospel, to heal body, mind and spirit, to improve the health of our communities and to steward the resources entrusted to us.

Core Values

Respect   We value and esteem every human person because each and every one is created by God, in the image of God. Everyone, regardless of title or position, income, education or status, race, religion or ethnicity has a dignity that is sacred. We treasure and hold human life sacred from its simplest beginnings until its end. (Gen. 1:26; Luke 9:47-48; John 10:10)

Social Justice   In this age of globalization and instant communication, we more quickly recognize our common humanity. We recognize as well the great gaps in economy, health, education and development among the peoples of this earth. Social justice commits us to the common good so that all may have their basic needs met. We recognize health and access to healthcare as a basic human right and seek to provide and advocate for it. (Wisdom 9:2f; Isaiah 32:16-18)

Compassion   People come to us when they are in need and in distress. In the spirit of Jesus, we recognize their need and seek to respond to it. We reach out to them in their pain and suffering and care for them in body, mind and spirit. The ability to feel and to respond to the suffering of others is an essential value in our ministry of healthcare, no matter where we serve. We recognize also that those we cannot cure we can still love, care for and be with in their suffering. (Mark 1:40f; Mark 10:51; Luke 4:40; Luke 10:30-37; Romans 12:15; I Cor. 13:4-7)

Care of the Poor and Underserved   God hears the cry of the poor and so, with respect and compassion, we seek out the poor and underserved as a special focus of our healthcare ministry. It is those without resources of their own who need us most. We seek to care not only for their immediate needs but also to change the structures that keep them in unhealthy environments and inhumane conditions. Through our ministry of health care and our persistent advocacy, we seek to serve the poor and underserved of our communities. We too hear the cry of the poor and underserved. (Acts 4:32-35; James 2:15)

Excellence   The scriptures look to the day when there will be a new heaven and a new earth, when creation will be made perfect. Our vision is no less. In all we do, we reach for more—greater respect, fuller justice, deeper compassion, better care, less poverty. We are impatient to do better and hold ourselves accountable for continuous improvement in the services we offer. (Matthew 25:14-23; II Corinthians 9:6; Revelations 21:1)

Vision Statement

Trinity Health, a mission-centered Catholic system, is the recognized leader in excellent care and service. We are a trusted partner in all relationships. We advocate for those in need.

From Trinity Health. (2004). *Who we are.* Retrieved April 13, 2004, from http://www.trinity-health.org/who/mission.shtml; reprinted by permission.

VISION, MISSION, AND CORE PRINCIPLES OF THE GEORGE WASHINGTON UNIVERSITY MEDICAL CENTER

The George Washington University is dedicated to furthering human well-being and values a dynamic, student-focused community stimulated by cultural and intellectual diversity and built upon a foundation of integrity, creativity and openness to the exploration of new ideas. The University commits itself to excellence in the creation, dissemination and application of knowledge and the promotion of lifelong learning from both global and integrative perspectives.

Vision

Within the larger mission of the University, the vision of The George Washington University Medical Center is to be a preeminent academic health institution, dedicated to improving the health and well-being of our local community, our country and beyond. The Medical Center will achieve this goal through commitment to excellence and innovation in education and to research that expands the frontiers of science and knowledge.

Mission

As a leader in education and research, The George Washington University Medical Center strives to set standards of excellence by:

- Valuing a diverse and dynamic community that encourages life-long learning

- Striving for, refining and defining quality in all endeavors

- Providing exemplary and innovative teaching programs that produce astute, highly competent and compassionate health professionals and scientists trained and prepared for the future

- Generating and expanding health knowledge through superior research programs

- Enhancing the delivery of compassionate and high-quality healthcare through our education and research activities

- Improving the health and well-being of our local, national and international communities

The Medical Center implements this mission by building on our history and heritage, remaining true to our core principles and responding to the changing context of contemporary education, technological innovations, advancing research, public health, policy and community needs.

Core Principles

We will achieve our mission through our commitment to the following principles:

- Altruism
- Collaboration
- Communication
- Compassion
- Excellence
- Innovation
- Integrity
- Respect

From The George Washington University Medical Center. (2003). *GWUMC vision and mission.* Retrieved April 13, 2004, from http://www.gwumc.edu/mcinfo/aboutgwumc/vision.html; reprinted by permission.

MISSION, VISION, AND
VALUES OF SIBLEY MEMORIAL HOSPITAL

Mission

Our mission is to provide quality health services and facilities for the community, to promote wellness, to relieve suffering, and to restore health as swiftly, safely and humanely as it can be done, consistent with the best service we can give, at the highest value for all concerned.

Vision

Our vision is to provide superior healthcare service and value, with the goal of improving the health and well being of our community. We plan to continuously improve that service by using scientific methods, teamwork, and knowledge of best practices and customer expectations. Our vision guides us to work continuously to improve our services.

Values

Our values provide guidelines and parameters for the decisions that we make as we work to improve our processes and respond to our patients and other customers needs:

- Personalized and compassionate service

- Excellence and continually improving quality

- Teamwork

- Job satisfaction

- Professionalism

- Wise use of resources to provide value

- Innovation

- Trust and respect

- Up-to-date technology

- A clean, attractive, quiet, safe environment

- Honesty, integrity, flexibility and selflessness

From Sibley Memorial Hospital. (2002). *Employment at Sibley: Mission, vision, values.* Retrieved April 13, 2004, from http://www.SIBLEY.ORG/employment/emphil.tmpl

356

MISSION, PRIMARY VALUE, AND CORE PRINCIPLES OF MAYO CLINIC

Mayo's Mission

Mayo will provide the best care to every patient everyday through integrated clinical practice, education and research.

Primary Value

The needs of the patient come first.

Core Principles

Practice: Practice medicine as an integrated team of compassionate, multidisciplinary physicians, scientists and allied health professionals who are focused on the needs of patients from our communities, regions, the nation and the world.

Education: Educate physicians, scientists and allied health professionals and be a dependable source of health information for our patients and the public.

Research: Conduct basic and clinical research programs to improve patient care and to benefit society.

Mutual respect: Treat everyone in our diverse community with respect and dignity.

Commitment to quality: Continuously improve all processes that support patient care, education and research.

Work atmosphere: Foster teamwork, personal responsibility, integrity, innovation, trust and communication within the context of a physician-led institution.

Societal commitment: Benefit humanity through patient care, education and research. Support the communities in which we live and work. Serve appropriately patients in difficult financial circumstances.

Finances: Allocate resources within the context of a system rather than its individual entities. Operate in a manner intended not to create wealth but to provide a financial return sufficient for present and future needs.

From Mayo Clinic. (n.d.). *Mayo's mission.* Retrieved August 21, 2003, from http://www.mayoclinic.org/about/missionvalues.html

357

MISSION, PRINCIPLES OF SERVICE, CORE VALUES, AND FOUNDATIONAL BELIEF OF SUNRISE SENIOR LIVING

These are what motivate us. They are what guide and focus our team members from day-to-day at any one of our nearly 350 senior living communities.

Our Mission

To champion quality of life for all seniors

Our Principles of Service

Preserving Dignity   We value the life experiences of every senior and give each the respect they deserve.

Nurturing the Spirit   We care for the whole person—mind, body and spirit.

Celebrating Individuality   We recognize that every one of our residents is a unique senior.

Enabling Freedom of Choice   We empower seniors to live as they wish by offering choices.

Encouraging Independence   We encourage resident's right to self-reliance in whatever ways possible.

Involving Family and Friends   Friends and family are always welcome, and their involvement is wholeheartedly encouraged.

Our Core Values

Passion

Joy in service

Stewardship

Respect

Trust

Our Foundational Belief

Belief in the sacred value of human life.

From Sunrise Senior Living. (2003). *Principles of service and core values.* Retrieved April 13, 2004, from http://www.sunrise-al.com/difference/PrinciplesOfService.do

ETHICAL CODES

THE AMERICAN COLLEGE OF
HEALTHCARE EXECUTIVES (ACHE) CODE OF ETHICS

Preamble

The purpose of the *Code of Ethics* of the American College of Healthcare Executives is to serve as a standard of conduct for affiliates. It contains standards of ethical behavior for healthcare executives in their professional relationships. These relationships include colleagues, patients or others served; members of the healthcare executive's organization and other organizations, the community, and society as a whole.

The *Code of Ethics* also incorporates standards of ethical behavior governing personal behavior, particularly when that conduct directly relates to the role and identity of the healthcare executive.

The fundamental objectives of the healthcare management profession are to maintain or enhance the overall quality of life, dignity, and well-being of every individual needing healthcare service; and to create a more equitable, accessible, effective, and efficient healthcare system.

Healthcare executives have an obligation to act in ways that will merit the trust, confidence, and respect of healthcare professionals and the general public. Therefore, healthcare executives should lead lives that embody an exemplary system of values and ethics.

In fulfilling their commitments and obligations to patients or others served, healthcare executives function as moral advocates and models. Since every management decision affects the health and well-being of both individuals and communities, healthcare executives must carefully evaluate the possible outcomes of their decisions. In organizations that deliver healthcare services, they must work to safeguard and foster the rights, interests, and prerogatives of patients or others served.

The role of moral advocate requires that healthcare executives take actions necessary to promote such rights, interests, and prerogatives.

Being a model means that decisions and actions will reflect personal integrity and ethical leadership that others will seek to emulate.

I. The Healthcare Executive's Responsibilities
to the Profession of Healthcare Management

The healthcare executive shall:

A. Uphold the *Code of Ethics* and mission of the American College of Healthcare Executives;

B. Conduct all personal and professional activities with honesty, integrity, respect, fairness, and good faith in a manner that will reflect well upon the profession;

C. Comply with all laws and regulations pertaining to healthcare management in the jurisdictions in which the healthcare executive is located or conducts professional activities;

D. Maintain competence and proficiency in healthcare management by implementing a personal program of assessment and continuing professional education;

E. Avoid the exploitation of professional relationships for personal gain;

F. Avoid financial and other conflicts of interest;

G. Use this *Code* to further the interests of the profession and not for selfish reasons;

H. Respect professional confidences;

I. Enhance the dignity and image of the healthcare management profession through positive public information programs; and

J. Refrain from participating in any activity that demeans the credibility and dignity of the healthcare management profession.

II. The Healthcare Executive's Responsibilities to Patients or Others Served

The healthcare executive shall, within the scope of his or her authority:

A. Work to ensure the existence of a process to evaluate the quality of care or service rendered;

B. Avoid practicing or facilitating discrimination and institute safeguards to prevent discriminatory organizational practices;

C. Work to ensure the existence of a process that will advise patients or others served of the rights, opportunities, responsibilities, and risks regarding available healthcare services;

D. Work to ensure that there is a process in place to facilitate the resolution of conflicts that may arise when values of patients and their families differ from those of employees and physicians;

E. Demonstrate zero tolerance for any abuse of power that compromises patients or others served;

F. Work to provide a process that ensures the autonomy and self-determination of patients or others served; and

G. Work to ensure the existence of procedures that will safeguard the confidentiality and privacy of patients or others served.

III. The Healthcare Executive's Responsibilities to the Organization

The healthcare executive shall, within the scope of his or her authority:

A. Provide healthcare services consistent with available resources, and when there are limited resources, work to ensure the existence of a resource allocation process that considers ethical ramifications;

B. Conduct both competitive and cooperative activities in ways that improve community healthcare services;

C. Lead the organization in the use and improvement of standards of management and sound business practices;

D. Respect the customs and practices of patients or others served, consistent with the organization's philosophy;

E. Be truthful in all forms of professional and organizational communication, and avoid disseminating information that is false, misleading, or deceptive;

F. Report negative financial and other information promptly and accurately, and initiate appropriate action;

G. Prevent fraud and abuse and aggressive accounting practices that may result in disputable financial reports;

H. Create an organizational environment in which both clinical and management mistakes are minimized and, when they do occur, are disclosed and addressed effectively;

I. Implement an organizational code of ethics and monitor compliance; and

J. Provide ethics resources to staff to address organizational and clinical issues.

IV. The Healthcare Executive's Responsibilities to Employees

Healthcare executives have ethical and professional obligations to the employees they manage that encompass but are not limited to:

A. Creating a work environment that promotes ethical conduct by employees;

B. Ensuring that individuals may freely express ethical concerns and providing mechanisms for discussing and addressing such concerns;

C. Ensuring a work environment that is free from harassment, sexual and other; coercion of any kind, especially to perform illegal or unethical acts; and discrimination on the basis of race, ethnicity, creed, gender, sexual orientation, age, or disability;

D. Providing a work environment that promotes the proper use of employees' knowledge and skills;

E. Ensuring a safe work environment; and

F. Establishing appropriate grievance and appeals mechanisms.

V. The Healthcare Executive's Responsibilities to Community and Society

The healthcare executive shall:

A. Work to identify and meet the healthcare needs of the community;

B. Work to support access to healthcare services for all people;

C. Encourage and participate in public dialogue on healthcare policy issues, and advocate solutions that will improve health status and promote quality healthcare;

D. Apply short- and long-term assessments to management decisions affecting both community and society; and

E. Provide prospective patients and others with adequate and accurate information, enabling them to make enlightened decisions regarding services.

VI. The Healthcare Executive's Responsibility to Report Violations of the Code

An affiliate of ACHE who has reasonable grounds to believe that another affiliate has violated this *Code* has a duty to communicate such facts to the Ethics Committee.

From American College of Healthcare Executives (ACHE). (2003, November 10). *ACHE code of ethics*. Retrieved April 13, 2004, from http://www.ache.org/abt_ache/code.cfm. Used with permission from the American College of Healthcare Executives.

AMERICAN COLLEGE OF HEALTH CARE ADMINISTRATORS (ACHCA) CODE OF ETHICS

Preamble

The preservation of the highest standards of integrity and ethical principles is vital to the successful discharge of the professional responsibilities of all long-term health care administrators. This Code of Ethics has been promulgated by the American College of Health Care Administrators (ACHCA) in an effort to stress the fundamental rules considered essential to this basic purpose. It shall be the obligation of members to seek to avoid not only conduct specifically proscribed by the code, but also conduct that is inconsistent with its spirit and purpose. Failure to specify any particular responsibility or practice in this Code of Ethics should not be construed as denial of the existence of other responsibilities or practices. Recognizing that the ultimate responsibility for applying standards and ethics falls upon the individual, the ACHCA establishes the following Code of Ethics to make clear its expectation of the membership.

Expectation I

Individuals shall hold paramount the welfare of persons for whom care is provided.

Prescriptions: The Health Care Administrator shall:

- Strive to provide to all those entrusted to his or her care the highest quality of appropriate services possible in light of resources or other constraints.

- Operate the facility consistent with laws, regulations, and standards of practice recognized in the field of health care administration.

- Consistent with law and professional standards, protect the confidentiality of information regarding individual recipients of care.

- Perform administrative duties with the personal integrity that will earn the confidence, trust, and respect of the general public.

- Take appropriate steps to avoid discrimination on the basis of race, color, sex, religion, age, national origin, handicap, marital status, ancestry, or any other factor that is illegally discriminatory or not related to bona fide requirements of quality care.

Proscription: The Health Care Administrator shall not:

- Disclose professional or personal information regarding recipients of service to unauthorized personnel unless required by law or to protect the public welfare.

Expectation II

Individuals shall maintain high standards of professional competence.
Prescriptions: The Health Care Administrator shall:

- Possess and maintain the competencies necessary to effectively perform his or her responsibilities.

- Practice administration in accordance with capabilities and proficiencies and, when appropriate, seek counsel from qualified others.

- Actively strive to enhance knowledge of and expertise in long-term care administration through continuing education and professional development.

Proscriptions: The Health Care Administrator shall not:

- Misrepresent qualifications, education, experience, or affiliations.

- Provide services other than those for which he or she is prepared and qualified to perform.

Expectation III

Individuals shall strive, in all matters relating to their professional functions, to maintain a professional posture that places paramount the interests of the facility and its residents.
Prescriptions: The Health Care Administrator shall:

- Avoid partisanship and provide a forum for the fair resolution of any disputes which may arise in service delivery or facility management.

- Disclose to the governing body or other authority as may be appropriate, any actual or potential circumstance concerning him or her that might reasonably be thought to create a conflict of interest or have a substantial adverse impact on the facility or its residents.

Proscription: The Health Care Administrator shall not:

- Participate in activities that reasonably may be thought to create a conflict of interest or have the potential to have a substantial adverse impact on the facility or its residents.

Expectation IV

Individuals shall honor their responsibilities to the public, their profession, and their relationships with colleagues and members of related professions.
Prescriptions: The Health Care Administrator shall:

- Foster increased knowledge within the profession of health care administration and support research efforts toward this end.

- Participate with others in the community to plan for and provide a full range of health care services.

- Share areas of expertise with colleagues, students, and the general public to increase awareness and promote understanding of health care in general and the profession in particular.

- Inform the ACHCA Standards and Ethics Committee of actual or potential violations of this Code of Ethics, and fully cooperate with ACHCA's sanctioned inquiries into matters of professional conduct related to this Code of Ethics.

Proscription: The Health Care Administrator shall not:

- Defend, support, or ignore unethical conduct perpetrated by colleagues, peers or students.

From American College of Health Care Administrators (ACHCA). (2003). *Code of ethics.* Retrieved April 13, 2004, from http://www.achca.org/achca.asp?DP=content&FN=code_of_ethics.asp; reprinted by permission.

AMERICAN MEDICAL ASSOCIATION
PRINCIPLES OF MEDICAL ETHICS

Preamble

The medical profession has long subscribed to a body of ethical statements developed primarily for the benefit of the patient. As a member of this profession, a physician must recognize responsibility to patients first and foremost, as well as to society, to other health professionals, and to self. The following Principles adopted by the American Medical Association are not laws, but standards of conduct which define the essentials of honorable behavior for the physician.

Principles of Medical Ethics

I. A physician shall be dedicated to providing competent medical care, with compassion and respect for human dignity and rights.

II. A physician shall uphold the standards of professionalism, be honest in all professional interactions, and strive to report physicians deficient in character or competence, or engaging in fraud or deception, to appropriate entities.

III. A physician shall respect the law and also recognize a responsibility to seek changes in those requirements which are contrary to the best interests of the patient.

IV. A physician shall respect the rights of patients, colleagues, and other health professionals, and shall safeguard patient confidences and privacy within the constraints of the law.

V. A physician shall continue to study, apply, and advance scientific knowledge, maintain a commitment to medical education, make relevant information available to patients, colleagues, and the public, obtain consultation, and use the talents of other health professionals when indicated.

VI. A physician shall, in the provision of appropriate patient care, except in emergencies, be free to choose whom to serve, with whom to associate, and the environment in which to provide medical care.

VII. A physician shall recognize a responsibility to participate in activities contributing to the improvement of the community and the betterment of public health.

VIII. A physician shall, while caring for a patient, regard responsibility to the patient as paramount.

IX. A physician shall support access to medical care for all people.

From American Medical Association. (2001). *Principles of medical ethics.* Retrieved April 13, 2004, from http://www.ama-assn.org/ama/pub/category/print/2512.html; reprinted by permission.

AMERICAN MEDICAL ASSOCIATION
COUNCIL ON ETHICAL AND JUDICIAL AFFAIRS

Fundamental Elements of the Patient–Physician Relationship

From ancient times, physicians have recognized that the health and well-being of patients depend upon a collaborative effort between physician and patient. Patients share with physicians the responsibility for their own health care. The patient-physician relationship is of greatest benefit to patients when they bring medical problems to the attention of their physicians in a timely fashion, provide information about their medical condition to the best of their ability, and work with their physicians in a mutually respectful alliance. Physicians can best contribute to this alliance by serving as their patients' advocates and by fostering these rights:

1. The patient has the right to receive information from physicians and to discuss the benefits, risks, and costs of appropriate treatment alternatives. Patients should receive guidance from their physicians as to the optimal course of action. Patients are also entitled to obtain copies or summaries of their medical records, to have their questions answered, to be advised of potential conflicts of interest that their physicians might have, and to receive independent professional opinions.

2. The patient has the right to make decisions regarding the health care that is recommended by his or her physician. Accordingly, patients may accept or refuse any recommended medical treatment.

3. The patient has the right to courtesy, respect, dignity, responsiveness, and timely attention to his or her needs.

4. The patient has the right to confidentiality. The physician should not reveal confidential communications or information without the consent of the patient, unless provided for by law or by the need to protect the welfare of the individual or the public interest.

5. The patient has the right to continuity of health care. The physician has an obligation to cooperate in the coordination of medically indicated care with other health care providers treating the patient. The physician may not discontinue treatment of a patient as long as further treatment is medically indicated, without giving the patient reasonable assistance and sufficient opportunity to make alternative arrangements for care.

6. The patient has a basic right to have available adequate health care. Physicians, along with the rest of society, should continue to work

toward this goal. Fulfillment of this right is dependent on society providing resources so that no patient is deprived of necessary care because of an inability to pay for the care. Physicians should continue their traditional assumption of a part of the responsibility for the medical care of those who cannot afford essential health care. Physicians should advocate for patients in dealing with third parties when appropriate.

From Council on Ethical and Judicial Affairs of the American Medical Association. (1994). *Fundamental elements of the patient–physician relationship.* Retrieved April 13, 2004, from http://www.ama-assn.org/ama/pub/category/print/2510.html; reprinted by permission.

CODE OF ETHICS FOR NURSES
FROM THE AMERICAN NURSES ASSOCIATION (ANA)

1. The nurse, in all professional relationships, practices with compassion and respect for the inherent dignity, worth, and uniqueness of every individual, unrestricted by considerations of social or economic status, personal attributes, or the nature of health problems.

2. The nurse's primary commitment is to the patient, whether an individual, family, group, or community.

3. The nurse promotes, advocates for, and strives to protect the health, safety, and rights of the patient.

4. The nurse is responsible and accountable for individual nursing practice and determines the appropriate delegation of tasks consistent with the nurse's obligation to provide optimum patient care.

5. The nurse owes the same duties to self as to others, including the responsibility to preserve integrity and safety, to maintain competence, and to continue personal and professional growth.

6. The nurse participates in establishing, maintaining, and improving health care environments and conditions of employment conducive to the provision of quality health care and consistent with the values of the profession through individual and collective action.

7. The nurse participates in the advancement of the profession through contributions to practice, education, administration, and knowledge development.

8. The nurse collaborates with other health professionals and the public in promoting community, national, and international efforts to meet health needs.

9. The profession of nursing, as represented by associations and their members, is responsible for articulating nursing values, for maintaining the integrity of the profession and its practice, and for shaping social policy.

From American Nurses Association. (2001). *Code of ethics for nurses.* Washington, DC: Author; reprinted by permission.

SELECT BIBLIOGRAPHY

Ackermann, R.J. (2000, October 1). Withholding and withdrawing life-sustaining treatment. *American Family Physician, 62*, 1555–1560, 1562, 1564.

Ackoff, R.L. (1999). *Re-creating the corporation: A design of organizations for the 21st century*. New York: Oxford University Press.

Adler, M.J. (1978). *Aristotle for everybody: Difficult thought made easy*. New York: Macmillan.

Baily, M.A. (2003, January/February). Managed care organizations and the rationing problem. *The Hastings Center Report, 33*(1), 34–42.

Battin, M.P. (1995). *Ethical issues in suicide*. Upper Saddle River, NJ: Prentice Hall.

Beauchamp, T.L., & Childress, J.F. (2001). *Principles of biomedical ethics I* (5th ed.). New York: Oxford University Press.

Beauchamp, T.L., & Walters, L. (Eds.). (1999). *Contemporary issues in bioethics* (5th ed.). Belmont, CA: Wadsworth Group.

Boatright, J.R. (2003). *Ethics and the conduct of business* (4th ed). Upper Saddle River, NJ: Prentice Hall.

Buchanan, A. (1998, August). Managed care: Rationing without justice, but not unjustly. *Journal of Health Politics, Policy and Law, 23*(4), 616–634.

Callahan, D. (2003, March/April). Too much of a good thing: How splendid technologies can go wrong. *The Hastings Center Report, 33*(2), 19–22.

Chervenak, F.A., & McCullough, L.B. (2001, April). The moral foundation of medical leadership: The professional virtues of the physician as fiduciary of the patient. *American Journal of Obstetrics and Gynecology, 184*(5), 875–880.

Curtin, L.L. (1993, May). Damage control and the whistleblower. *Nursing Management, 24*, 33–34.

Deal, T.E., & Kennedy, A.A. (1982, reissued 2000). *Corporate cultures: The rites and rituals of corporate life*. New York: Perseus Books Group.

DeGeorge, R.T. (1990). *Business ethics* (3rd ed.). New York: Macmillan.

Dixon, N. (1998, September/October). On the difference between physician-assisted suicide and active euthanasia. *The Hastings Center Report, 28*(5), 25–29.

Doukas, D.J. (2003). Where is the virtue in professionalism? *Cambridge Quarterly of Healthcare Ethics, 12*, 147–154.

Emanuel, E.J. (2000, May/June). Justice and managed care: Four principles for the just allocation of health care resources. *The Hastings Center Report, 30*(3), 8–16.

Emanuel, L.L. (1996, January 15). A professional response to demands for accountability: Practical recommendations regarding ethical aspects of patient care. *Annals of Internal Medicine, 124,* 240–249.

Etzioni, A. (1999, March/April). Medical records: Enhancing privacy, preserving the common good. *The Hastings Center Report, 29*(2), 14–23.

Foley, K., & Hendin, H. (1999, May/June). The Oregon report: Don't ask, don't tell. *The Hastings Center Report, 29*(3), 37–42.

Frankena, W.K. (1973). *Ethics* (2nd ed.). Upper Saddle River, NJ: Prentice Hall.

Gallagher, E., Alcock, D., Diem, E., Angus, D., & Medves, J. (2002, March/April). Ethical dilemmas in home care case management. *The Journal of Healthcare Management,* 85–97.

Gallagher, J.A., & Goodstein, J. (2002). Fulfilling institutional responsibilities in health care: Organizational ethics and the role of mission discernment. *Business Ethics Quarterly, 12*(4), 433–450.

Gallagher, T.H., Waterman, A.D., Ebers, A.G., Fraser, V.J., & Levinson, W. (2003, February 26). Patients' and physicians' attitudes regarding the disclosure of medical errors. *Journal of the American Medical Association, 289*(8), 1001–1007.

Gert, H.J. (2002, September/October). Avoiding surprises: A model for informing patients. *The Hastings Center Report 32*(5), 23–32.

Goold, S.D. (2001, November/December). Trust and the ethics of health care institutions. *The Hastings Center Report 31*(6), 26–33.

Gunderman, R. (1998, January/February). Medicine & the pursuit of wealth. *The Hastings Center Report, 29*(1), 9–13.

Gunderson, M. & Mayo, D.J. (2001, November/December). Restricting physician-assisted death to the terminally ill. *The Hastings Center Report, 30*(6), 17–23.

Hall, R.T. (2000). *An introduction to healthcare organizational ethics.* New York: Oxford University Press.

Heitman, E. (1995). Institutional ethics committees: Local perspectives on ethical issues in medicine. In R.E. Bulger, E. Meyer Bobby, & H.V. Fineberg (Eds.), *Society's choices: Social and ethical decision making in medicine* (pp. 409–431). Washington, DC: National Academies Press.

Holleman, W.L., Edwards, D.C., & Mason, C.C. (1994, Summer). Obligations of physicians to patients and third-party payers. *Journal of Clinical Ethics, 5*(2), 113–120.

Hudson, T. (1994, February 20). Are futile care policies the answer? *Hospitals & Health Networks, 68,* 26–32.

Jansen, L.A., & Sulmasy, D.P. (2003, July/August). Bioethics, conflicts of interest, the limits of transparency. *The Hastings Center Report, 33*(4), 40–43.

Jennings, B., Gray, B.H., Sharpe, V.A., Weiss, L., & Fleischman, A.R. (2002, July/August). Ethics and trusteeship for health care: Hospital board service in turbulent times. *The Hastings Center Report, 32*(Suppl.), S1–S27.

Jonsen, A.R., & Toulmin, S. (1988). *The abuse of casuistry: A history of moral reasoning.* Berkeley: University of California Press.

Kelly, D.F., & Hoyt, J.W. (1996, January). Ethics consultation. *Medical Ethics, 12,*(1), 49–70.

Keown, J. (2002). *Euthanasia, ethics and public policy: An argument against legalization.* New York: Cambridge University Press.

Lauritzen, P., McClure, M., Smith, M.L., & Trew, A. (2001, January/February). The gift of life and the common good: The need for a communal approach to organ procurement. *The Hastings Center Report, 31*(1), 29–35.

Lee, D.E. (2003, January/February). Physician-assisted suicide: A conservative critique of intervention. *The Hastings Center Report, 33*(1), 17–19.

Loewy, E.H. (2001, February 12). Terminal sedation, self-starvation, and orchestrating the end of life. *Archives of Internal Medicine, 161*(3), 329–332.

Mastroianni, A., & Kahn, J. (2001, May/June). Swinging on the pendulum: Shifting views of justice in human subjects research. *The Hastings Center Report 31*(3), 21–28.

Miller, F.G., & Brody, H. (2003, May/June). A critique of clinical equipoise: Therapeutic misconception in the ethics of clinical trials. *The Hastings Center Report, 33*(3), 19–28.

Monagle, J.F., & Thomasma, D.C. (1994). *Health care ethics: Critical issues.* New York: Aspen Publishers.

Moreno, J.D. (2001, May/June). Goodbye to all that: The end of moderate protectionism to human subject research. *The Hastings Center Report 31*(3), 9–17.

Morreim, E.H. (1994, January/February). Profoundly diminished life: The casualties of coercion. *The Hastings Center Report, 24*, 33–42.

Morreim, E.H. (1995, November/December). Lifestyles of the risky and infamous. *The Hastings Center Report, 25*, 5–12.

Nelkin, D., & Andrews, L. (1998, September/October). *Homo economicus:* Commercialization of body tissues in the age of biotechnology. *The Hastings Center Report, 28*(5), 30–39.

Nuland, S.B. (1995). *How we die: Reflections on life's final chapter.* New York: Vintage Books.

Oakley, J., & Cocking, D. (2001). *Virtue ethics and professional roles.* New York: Oxford University Press.

Office of Inspector General of the U.S. Department of Health and Human Services and the American Health Lawyers Association. (2003, April 2). *Corporate responsibility and corporate compliance: A resource for health care boards of directors.* Retrieved March 9, 2004, from http://oig.hhs.gov/fraud/docs/complianceguidance/040203CorpRespRsceGuide.pdf

Panicola, M. (2001, November/December). Catholic teaching on prolonging life: Setting the record straight. *The Hastings Center Report 31*(6), 14–25.

Pellegrino, E.D. (1985). The virtuous physician and the ethics of medicine. In E.E. Shelp (Ed.), *Virtue and medicine: Exploration in the character of medicine.* Dordrecht, Holland: D. Reidel Publishing Company.

Pellegrino, E.D. (1994, Fall). Managed care and managed competition: Some ethical reflections. *Calyx, 4*(4), 1–5.

Pellegrino, E.D., & Thomasma, D.C. (1988). *For the patient's good: The restoration of beneficence in health care.* New York: Oxford University Press.

Pendola, C.J. (1992, Winter). Administrative ethics in health care resource allocation. *Review of Business, 14*, 20–22.

Phillips, L. (1997, January/February). A question of ethics. *Trustee,* 27–28.

President's Commission for the Study of Ethical Problems in Medicine and Biomedical and Behavioral Research. (1981). *Defining death: A report on the medical, legal and ethical issues in the determination of death.* Washington, DC: U.S. Government Printing Office.

President's Commission for the Study of Ethical Problems in Medicine and Biomedical and Behavioral Research. (1981). *Protecting human subjects: The adequacy and uniformity of federal rules and their implementation.* Washington, DC: U.S. Government Printing Office.

President's Commission for the Study of Ethical Problems in Medicine and Biomedical and Behavioral Research. (1981). *Whistleblowing in biomedical research: Policies and procedures for responding to reports of misconduct.* Washington, DC: U.S. Government Printing Office.

President's Commission for the Study of Ethical Problems in Medicine and Biomedical and Behavioral Research. (1982). *Compensating for research injuries: A report on the ethical and legal implications for programs to redress injured subjects. Volume 2.* Washington, DC: U.S. Government Printing Office.

President's Commission for the Study of Ethical Problems in Medicine and Biomedical and Behavioral Research. (1982). *Making health care decisions: A report on the ethical and legal implications of informed consent in the patient–practitioner relationship. Volume 1: Report.* Washington, DC: U.S. Government Printing Office.

President's Commission for the Study of Ethical Problems in Medicine and Biomedical and Behavioral Research. (1982). *Making health care decisions: A report on the ethical and legal implications of informed consent in the patient–practitioner relationship. Volume 2: Appendices, Empirical studies of informed consent.* Washington, DC: U.S. Government Printing Office.

President's Commission for the Study of Ethical Problems in Medicine and Biomedical and Behavioral Research. (1982). *Splicing life: A report on the social and ethical issues of genetic engineering with human beings.* Washington, DC: U.S. Government Printing Office.

President's Commission for the Study of Ethical Problems in Medicine and Biomedical and Behavioral Research. (1983). *Deciding to forego life-sustaining treatment: A report on the ethical, medical, and legal issues in treatment decisions.* Washington, DC: U.S. Government Printing Office.

President's Commission for the Study of Ethical Problems in Medicine and Biomedical and Behavioral Research. (1983). *Implementing human research regulations: Second biennial report on the adequacy and uniformity of federal rules and policies, and of their implementation, for the protection of human subjects.* Washington, DC: U.S. Government Printing Office.

President's Commission for the Study of Ethical Problems in Medicine and Biomedical and Behavioral Research. (1983). *Screening and counseling for genetic conditions: The ethical, social, and legal implications of genetic screening, counseling, and education programs.* Washington, DC: U.S. Government Printing Office.

President's Commission for the Study of Ethical Problems in Medicine and Biomedical and Behavioral Research. (1983). *Securing access to health care: A report on the ethical implications of differences in the availability of health services. Volume 1: Report.* Washington, DC: U.S. Government Printing Office.

President's Commission for the Study of Ethical Problems in Medicine and Biomedical and Behavioral Research. (1983). *Securing access to health care: A report on the ethical implications of differences in the availability of health services. Volume 2: Appendices, Sociocultural and philosophical studies.* Washington, DC: U.S. Government Printing Office.

President's Commission for the Study of Ethical Problems in Medicine and Biomedical and Behavioral Research. (1983). *Securing access to health care: A report on the ethical implications of differences in the availability of health services. Volume 3: Appendices, Empirical, legal, and conceptual studies.* Washington, DC: U.S. Government Printing Office.

President's Commission for the Study of Ethical Problems in Medicine and Biomedical and Behavioral Research. (1983). *Summing up: Final report on studies of the ethical and legal problems in medicine and biomedical and behavioral research.* Washington, DC: U.S. Government Printing Office.

Reiser, S.J. (1994, November/December). The ethical life of health care organizations. *The Hastings Center Report, 24,* 29–35.

Resnick, D. (2003, July/August). The Jesica Santillan tragedy: Lessons learned. *The Hastings Center Report, 33*(4), 15–20.

Salem, T. (1999, May/June). Physician-assisted suicide: Promoting autonomy—or medicalizing suicide? *The Hastings Center Report, 29*(3), 30–36.

Sandrick, K.M. (1993, March). Ethical misconduct in health care financial management. *Healthcare Financial Management,* 35–41.

Schneiderman, L.J., Fein, J.E., & Dubler, N. (2001, November/December). The limits of dispute resolution. *The Hastings Center Report, 31*(6), 10–12.

Spencer, E.M., Mills, A.E., Rorty, M.V., & Werhane, P.H. (2000). *Organization ethics in health care.* New York: Oxford University Press.

Stephens, B.J., Sinden, P.G., Ketcham, R.H., & Rzepkowski, N. (1995, Winter). The consequences of disclosure: One hospital's response to the presence of an HIV-positive physician. *Hospital & Health Services Administration,* 457–471.

Stern, A.L. (1999, June). When you hear that whistle blowing: How trustees can reduce the threat of "qui tam" lawsuits. *Trustee, 52*(6), 6–9.

Teisberg, E.O., Porter, M.E., & Brown, G.B. (1994, July/August). Making competition in health care work. *Harvard Business Review 72*(4), 131–141.

Sullivan, W.M. (1999, March/April). What is left of professionalism after managed care? *The Hastings Center Report, 29*(2), 7–13.

Swanton, C. (2003). *Virtue ethics: A pluralistic view.* New York: Oxford University Press.

Tomlinson, T., & Czlonka, D. (1995, May/June). Futility and hospital policy. *The Hastings Center Report, 25,* 28–35.

Vinten, G. (1994). *Whistleblowing: Subversion or corporate citizenship?* New York: St. Martin's Press.

Waisel, D.B., & Truong, R.D. (1995). The cardiopulmonary resuscitation-not-indicated order: Futility revisited. *Annals of Internal Medicine, 122*(4), 304–309.

Weber, L.J. (2001). *Business ethics in healthcare: Beyond compliance.* Bloomington: Indiana University Press.

Woolfrey, J. (1998, May/June). What happens now? Oregon and physician-assisted suicide. *The Hastings Center Report, 28*(3), 9–17.

Wu, A.W., Cavanaugh, T.A., McPhee, S.J., Lo, B., & Micco, G.P. (1997, December). To tell the truth: Ethical and practical issues in disclosing medical mistakes to patients. *Journal of General Internal Medicine, 12,* 770–775.

INDEX

Page numbers followed by *f, t,* or *n*
indicate figures, tables, or notes, respectively.

7-S Framework, 55, 56*f*

AAHSA, *see* American Association of
  Homes and Services for the
  Aging
AAN, *see* American Academy of
  Neurology
ABA, *see* American Bar Association
Academic accomplishments,
  misrepresentation of, 167,
  173*n*
Accepting gratuities and benefits,
  132–136
  cases, 132–133, 135
Access to treatment, 295–296
Acer case, implications for health care
  providers with human
  immunodeficiency virus
  (HIV), 198
ACHA, *see* American College of
  Hospital Administrators
ACHCA, *see* American College of
  Health Care Administrators
ACHE, *see* American College of
  Healthcare Executives
ACLU, *see* American Civil Liberties
  Union
Acquired immunodeficiency syndrome
  (AIDS), *see* Human
  immunodeficiency virus/
  acquired immunodeficiency
  syndrome (HIV/AIDS)
ACS, *see* American College of
  Surgeons
Active euthanasia, 244
Acute care hospitals
  futile treatment guidelines, 319
  institutional ethics committees, 95
Acute Physiology and Chronic Health
  Evaluation (APACHE) system,
  325

ADA, *see* American Dental
  Association; Americans with
  Disabilities Act of 1990 (PL
  101-336)
Administration model, 150, 151*f*
Administrative ethical issues, 37–39,
  121–122
Administrative institutional ethics
  committees (IECs), 96
  cases, 100–101
  membership, 98
Administrators, codes of ethics for,
  131–132, 365–367
Advance medical directives (AMDs),
  233–242, 312
  cases, 97–98, 247
  example, 235*f*–237*f*
  instructions from formerly
    competent patients, 247
  last wishes case, 97–98
Adverse selection, 291–292
Advertising, American Hospital
  Association (AHA) statement
  on, 286–287
Ageism, 335
AHA, *see* American Hospital
  Association
AHCA, *see* American Health Care
  Association
AHN, *see* Artificial hydration and
  nutrition
AIDS, *see* Human immunodeficiency
  virus/acquired
  immunodeficiency syndrome
  (HIV/AIDS)
Alcohol abuse, case involving staff,
  154–155
AMDs, *see* Advance medical directives
American Academy of Neurology
  (AAN), 233, 254*n*
American Academy of Pediatrics, 316

American Association of Homes and
Services for the Aging
(AAHSA), 83, 94
Membership Creed, 83
American Bar Association (ABA), 76,
233
Model Rules of Professional
Conduct, 76
American Civil Liberties Union
(ACLU), 69
American College of Health Care
Administrators (ACHCA),
79–80
Code of Ethics, 131–132, 133,
365–367
expectations for members, 79–80,
84
American College of Healthcare
Executives (ACHE), 77
Code of Ethics, 8, 77–79, 133, 146,
361–364
philosophical basis for, 84
use and enforcement, 85
Ethical Policy Statements, 79
American College of Hospital
Administrators (ACHA), 77
American College of Surgeons (ACS)
Principles of Patient Care, 224–225
Statements on Principles, 224
American Dental Association (ADA),
197
American Health Care Association
(AHCA), 83
American Hospital Association (AHA),
338, 340
Baby Doe regulations, 114
code of ethics, 77
conflict of interest statement,
127–129, 128f
guidelines for ethical conduct,
82–83
Management Advisory on Ethical
Conduct for Health Care
Institutions, 286–287
Patient's Bill of Rights, 69
policy statements about conflicts of
interest, 123
position on routine human
immunodeficiency virus (HIV)
testing of patients or staff, 162
recommendations for clinical
management of AIDS patients,
162
statement on advertising, 286–287

American Medical Association (AMA),
80–81, 233
Baby Doe regulations, 114
Council on Ethical and Judicial
Affairs, 81, 162, 212, 219, 224
Fundamental Elements of the
Patient–Physician
Relationship, 212, 219,
370–371
guidelines for research, 103
position on protecting patients and
community from staff with
human immunodeficiency
virus (HIV), 197
Principles of Medical Ethics, 80–81,
211–212, 219, 293, 368–369
philosophical basis for, 84
*Report of the Council on Ethical and
Judicial Affairs of the AMA*,
224
support for human
immunodeficiency virus (HIV)
testing, 160
Uniform Determination of Death
Act (UDDA), 232
American Nurses Association (ANA)
Code of Ethics for Nurses,
81–82, 157, 190, 372
philosophical basis for, 84
Americans with Disabilities Act (ADA)
of 1990 (PL 101-336), 159,
161, 315
Title II, 160
ANA, *see* American Nurses
Association
Anencephaly, case involving, 313–319
APACHE system, *see* Acute
Physiology and Chronic
Health Evaluation (APACHE)
system
Artificial hydration and nutrition
(AHN), 243
cases, 246, 249–250, 256n
Cruzan case, 249–250
goals of, 251
Schiavo case, 256n
Assessing quality of care, 191–195
cases, 192–193, 194
Assisted suicide, *see* Physician-assisted
suicide (PAS)
Association for Healthcare
Resources & Materials
Management, 134
Autonomy model, 95

Baby Boy Doe, 15, 30–32, 219, 233
  case description, 16
  regulations resulting from, 114,
    252–253
  related controversies, 94, 252
Baby K, 313–319
  aftermath of case, 316–317
  analysis of case, 317–319
  appeals court portion of case, 316
  clinical aspects of case, 314
  ethical and legal aspects of case,
    314–315
  summary of case, 319
  trial court portion of case, 315–316
*Belmont Report: Ethical Principles and
  Guidelines for the Protection of
  Human Subjects of Research*,
    102–103
Beneficence, 27–28
Benefits
  accepting, and conflicts of interest,
    132–136
  cases, 132–133, 135
  community benefit issues, 329–334
  measures of, as provided by
    hospitals to community, 340
Bills of rights, patient, 69–70
Biomedical ethical issues, 39–40, 209
  questions useful in identifying,
    39–40
Biomedical institutional ethics
    committees, 96
  membership, 98
  relationships, 99
Bouvia case, 269–270
Brain death, *see* Death 232, 254*n*
Brain injury, 322
Bribery, 130, 134

Cardiopulmonary resuscitation (CPR),
    335
Care, ethics of, 22–23
Caregivers
  codes of ethics for, 80–82
  see also specific types
Casuistry, 20–22
Categorical imperative, 18
CDC, *see* Centers for Disease Control
    and Prevention
Cedars of Lebanon Hospital case,
    130–131
Centers for Disease Control and
    Prevention (CDC)

definition of invasive procedures,
    196
  estimates of risk of transmission of
    human immunodeficiency
    virus (HIV), 198–199
  guidelines for human
    immunodeficiency virus (HIV)
    testing, 162
  guidelines for protecting patients
    and community from staff
    with human immunodeficiency
    virus (HIV), 198
  guidelines for universal precautions,
    162, 163
CEO, *see* Chief executive officer
Cerebral palsy, 269–271
Charity care, 338–339
Chief executive officer (CEO), 143,
    165
Child Abuse Prevention and
    Treatment Act Amendments
    of 1984 (PL 98-457), 32, 113,
    114, 253, 311, 319
Child Abuse Prevention and
    Treatment Act of 1974 (PL
    93-247), 32
Childress, James, theory of allocating
    lifesaving treatment, 307
CHP case, *see* Community Health
    Plan case
Christian Scientists, and consent,
    218–219, 221
Clear illegality, 183
Clinical activities, monitoring,
    178–182
Code of Hammurabi, 80
Codes of ethics, 75–91
  for administrators, 131–132,
    365–367
  American College of Health Care
    Administrators Code of Ethics
    (ACHCA), 131–132, 133,
    365–367
  American College of Healthcare
    Executives Code of Ethics
    (ACHE), 8, 77–79, 84, 85,
    361–364
  American Health Care Association
    (ACHA) code of ethics, 83
  American Hospital Association
    (AHA) code of ethics for
    hospitals, 77
  American Medical Association
    (AMA) Principles of Medical

Codes of ethics—*continued*
    Ethics, 80–81, 84, 211–212,
        219, 293, 368–369
    American Nurses Association
        (ANA) Code of Ethics for
        Nurses, 81–82, 84, 157, 190,
        372
    applying, 84–89
    Association for Healthcare
        Resources & Materials
        Management Code of Ethics
        and Professional Conduct, 134
    for caregivers, 80–82
    cases, 76
    and conflicts of interest, 131–132
    examples, 359–372
    for executives, 77–79, 361–364
    for hospitals, 77, 82–83
    for long-term care facilities, 83
    for managers, 77–80
    for nurses, 81–82, 84, 107, 157,
        190, 372
    for organizations, 82–83
    philosophical bases for, 84
    supplements to, example (Ethical
        Policy Statements), 79
    use and enforcement, 84–85
Coma, irreversible, 230
Comfort care
    Bouvia case, 269–271
    Miller case, 310–311
    morphia somnolence case, 242
    for premature infants, 310–311
Commonweal, 338–344
Communication issues
    cases, 152
    consent and, 144–145, 223–226
Community
    benefits, 329–334, 340
        cases, 329–330, 331
    ethical issues regarding, 175–207
    hospital associations, 65
    protecting from staff with human
        immunodeficiency virus
        (HIV), 195–203
        cases, 200–201
    relationships with, 63, 195–203
    responsibilities to, 364
    support, definition of, 340
Community Health Plan (CHP) case,
    100–101
Competent consent, 215, 218

Competent patients
    decision-making process, 245–247
    formerly competent patients,
        247–248
    noncompetent adult patients,
        248–252
    noncompetent patients, 248–252
Competition
    future of, 288–289
    hiring from, 289–290
    and human resources policy,
        289–290
Compliance, 190–191
Concern about ethics in health
    services, 3–4
Confidentiality, 27
    breach of, 147
    maintaining, 175–178, 200–203
        cases, 200–201
        ethical dimensions, 201–202
    misuse of insider information,
        148–150
    organizational information, 146–150
    professional, 146
    protecting the community, 200–201
    respect for professional confidences,
        146
    self-dealing, 147–148
    separating public actions from
        private actions, 85–86
Conflicts of duties, cause of, 154
Conflicts of interest
    American Hospital Association
        (AHA) statement, 127–129,
        128*f*
    cases, 125–127, 129–130, 130–131,
        137–138, 149, 166
    codes of ethics and, 131–132
    fiduciary duty and, 123–141
    minimizing, 296–298
    with no direct personal gain,
        137–138
Congruence of philosophies, 71–72
Consent, 211–227
    cases, 144–145, 218–219, 220, 222
    competent, 215, 218
    ethical aspects of, 217–219
    forms, 146
    general consent, 212, 213*f*
    informed, 215, 218
    legal aspects of, 212–217

in medical education, 144–145,
    223–226
role of organizations in, 219–223
special consent, 212, 214f
voluntary, 212–215, 217
Consultations
    "doorway consultations," and
        ethical issues 189–190
    for physician-assisted suicide (PAS),
        267
Corporate culture, 56–57
    barriers to establishing, 57–58
    cases, 86–87, 88
    essential elements of, 56
    and medical errors, 181–182
    and whistleblowing, 190–191
Corporate decisions, 8–9, 10f
Corporate directors, 125
Cost control, 329
    cases, 329–330
    and last-chance therapies, 338
    long-term savings, 298–299
CPR, see Cardiopulmonary
    resuscitation
Credentialing
    fraudulent, 167–170
    physicians and, 166–167
Cruzan case, 249–250, 313
Culture
    corporate, 56–57
    organizational, 86–89
    of patient, role in last wishes case,
        96–97
Custodial care, 342

Darsee case, 112–113
Data, falsification of, 112–113
Deal and Kennedy
    characteristics of successful
        companies, 55
    essential elements of a culture, 56
Death and dying, 229–257
    brain death, 232, 254n
    and competent patients, 245–247
    Cruzan case, 249–250
    cultural issues, 97–98
    definitions of, 230–233, 231t
    euthanasia, 242–245
    and formerly competent patients,
        247–248
    Henninger case, 245–247

in infants, 252–253
last wishes case, 97–98
and noncompetent adult patients,
    248–252
patient decision-making process
    regarding, 245–253
physician-assisted suicide (PAS),
    259–279
Quinlan case, 248–249
by starvation, 269–271
unequal treatment of, 336
Uniform Determination of Death
    Act (UDDA), 232
Death with Dignity Act (Oregon), 260
    results, 263
    steps to receive prescription, 263
    summary of findings, 264–265
Debt collection, and ethical issues,
    331–332
Decent minimum, definition
    regarding services, 337
Decision making
    about medical futility, 320–321
    guiding, 51–52
    patient process, 245–253
    surrogate, 238–239
Declaration of Helsinki,
    recommendations, 102, 212
Demand versus need, 283–288
Deming, W. Edwards, theories of, 59,
    164–165, 191
Deontology, 17–18
Department of Health and Human
    Services (DHHS), 240
    Baby Doe regulations, 252–253
    guidelines for infant care review
        committees (ICRCs), 113, 114
    infant care regulations, 32
    regulations for protection of human
        subjects in research, 103, 105,
        108, 113
    regulations for research warranting
        expedited review, 111–112
    requirements for institutional
        review boards (IRBs),
        103–104, 107
    research exempt from requirements
        of, 111–112
Department of Veterans Affairs (VA),
    104
    Patient Rights and Responsibilities,
        69–70

Descriptive ethics, 1
DHHS, *see* Department of Health and
    Human Services
Diagnosis-related groups (DRGs), 66,
    272
Difference principle, 20
Director,
    definition of, 125,
    ethical obligations of, 127–131
Disabilities, *see* Americans with
        Disabilities Act (ADA) of 1990
        (PL 101-336); Baby Boy Doe;
        Baby K; Formerly competent
        patients; Mental retardation,
        ethical issues for patients with;
        Noncompetent adult patients
Disclosure, 140
Disincentives for physicians, regarding
    managed care, 293–294
Disproportionate care, 243
Dispute resolution, 115–116
Do-not-resuscitate (DNR) orders,
    239–240, 312
    disparities in, 335, 336
    research findings about, 323
*Doe v. University of Maryland Medical
    System Corporation*, 172*n*
Double effect, rule of, 244–245
DRGs, *see* Diagnosis-related groups
Due care and attention, 267
Due process, 154–155
Duke University Hospital, *see*
    Santillan case
Durable powers of attorney, 239
Dying, *see* Death and dying

Economics
    approval of self-directed
        expenditures, and conflicts of
        interest, 136–137
    cost control, 329–330, 338
    fiduciary duty, 124–127
    investor-owned hospitals, 339, 340
    long-term cost savings of managed
        care, 298–299
    management of profits, 332–333
    of physician-assisted suicide (PAS),
        272–273
    stock ownership cases, 149

ECS, *see* Ethics Consultation Service
EDs, *see* Emergency departments
Egalitarianism, definition regarding
    health services, 20
Emergency departments (EDs),
    336–337
    cases, 337–338
Emergency medical services (EMS)
    and do-not-resuscitate (DNR)
        orders, 240
    reroute of ambulances, 337–338
Emergency Medical Treatment and
    Active Labor Act (EMTALA)
    of 1986 (PL 99-272), 315,
    316, 318, 343
Emerging ethical issues, 281
EMS, *see* Emergency medical services
EMTALA, *see* Emergency Medical
    Treatment and Active Labor
    Act of 1986 (PL 99-272)
Environmental Protection Agency
    (EPA), 104, 111
Epidemic, health, case, 200–201
Equity, in delivering health services,
    334–338
Ethical codes, *see* Codes of ethics
Ethical decision making
    committees for, 116–117
    guiding, 51–52
Ethical issues
    administrative, 37–39, 121–122
    biomedical, 39–40, 209
    in Bouvia case, 270–271
    emerging, 281
    in Miller case, 311
    obligations of trustees and directors,
        127–131
    regarding organization and staff,
        143–173
    regarding patients and community,
        175–207
    research principles, 102–103
Ethical problems
    identifying, 13, 35–40
    organizational responses to, 93–119
    resolving, 35–49
    solving, 13, 40–46
        schema for, 42–45, 43*f*
Ethicists, 115, 116
Ethics
    of care, 22–23
    versus compliance, 190–191

concern about, 3–4
of corporate decisions, 8–9, 10*f*
defined, 4–5
descriptive, 1
and law, 7–10, 9*f*
in marketing and managed care,
    283–302
normative, 1
personal
    developing, 46–48
    moral philosophy and, 29–33
    selecting principles to be included
        in, 47
in resource allocation, 303–328
virtue ethics, 23–25
Ethics committees, 94
Ethics Consultation Service (ECS),
    115, 116
Euthanasia, 242–245
    active, 244
    cases, 242
    hidden, 267
    involuntary, 244
    in the Netherlands, 265–269
    passive, 244
    required considerations, 266–267
    types of, 244–245
    voluntary, 244
Executives, *see* Health services
    executives
Expedited review, 111–112
Expenditures, self-directed, and
    conflicts of interest, 136–137
Extraordinary care, 31, 242–244, 312

Fairness, in providing services,
    334–338
False Claims Act, 183–184, 186
Falsification
    of medical records, 179–180
    of research data, 112–113
FDA, *see* Food and Drug
    Administration
Fidelity, as element of respect for
    persons, 27
Fiduciary duty, 124–127
Financial issues
    approval of self-directed
        expenditures, and conflicts of
        interest, 136–137
    cost control, 329–330, 338

economics of physician-assisted
    suicide (PAS), 272–273
fiduciary duty, 124–127
investor-owned hospitals, 339, 340
long-term cost savings of managed
    care, 298–299
management of profits, 332–333
stock ownership cases, 149
Focal virtues of health professionals,
    24
Food and Drug Administration (FDA)
    regulations for protection of human
        subjects in research, 105, 108
    requirements for institutional
        review boards (IRBs), 103–104
    requirements for reviewing research
        activities, 108
Formerly competent patients, 247–248
    instructions from, 247
Fraud
    falsification of medical records,
        179–180
    falsification of research data,
        112–113
    misrepresentation of academic
        accomplishments, 173*n*
Fraudulent credentials, 167–170
Fundamental Elements of the
    Patient–Physician
    Relationship, 212, 219,
    370–371
Futile treatment
    Baby K case, 313–319
    cases, 310–311, 313–319, 322
    guidelines for, 319–323
    Miller case, 310–311
    near-futile treatment, 310–311
    process for making decisions about,
        320–321
    research findings about, 323
    supplements to guidelines for,
        324–325
Futility theory, 312–325
    background, 312–313
    implications, 323–324
    qualitative aspect, 313
    quantitative aspect, 313

General powers of attorney, 239
George Washington University
    Medical Center

George Washington University
    Medical Center—*continued*
  Acute Physiology and Chronic
    Health Evaluation (APACHE)
    system, 325
  core principles, 355
  general consent form, 212, 213*f*
  mission statement, 354
  special consent form, 212, 214*f*
  statement of philosophy, 60,
    354–355
  vision statement, 354
Gifts, and ethical issues, 90, 132–136
Gilligan, Carol, comments on ethics
    of care, 22
Governance model, 150, 151*f*
Governing body relationships,
    150–153, 151*f*
  cases, 152
Gratuities, 90, 132–136
  accepting, 132–136
  cases, 132–133, 135
Guiding ethical decision making,
    51–52

Harvard Medical School, definition of
    irreversible coma, 230
Health, definition of, 285
Health care administrators, codes of
    ethics for, 131–132, 361–367
Health care agents, 239
  Virginia Advance Medical Directive
    form, 235*f*–237*f*
Health insurance, uninsured rates, 332
Health Insurance Portability and
    Accountability Act (HIPAA),
    176, 177
Health maintenance organizations
    (HMOs), 94–95, 290–291
Health service utilization, 292–293
Health services consultants, 76
Health services executives
  chief executive officers (CEOs), 143
  codes of ethics for, 77–79, 361–364
Health services managers
  cases, 147–148
  codes of ethics for, 77–80
  physician-assisted suicide issues
    (PAS), 271–273
  role of, 148

Henninger case, 245–247
Hermann Hospital case, 129–130
Heuristic model, 41
HHAs, *see* Home health agencies
Hierarchy of needs, Maslow's, 59
Hierarchy of relationships, 26*f*
HIPAA, *see* Health Insurance
    Portability and Accountability
    Act
Hippocratic oath, 80, 84, 293
Hiring the competition, ethical issues
    of, 289–290
HIV/AIDS, *see* Human
    immunodeficiency virus/
    acquired immunodeficiency
    syndrome (HIV/AIDS)
HMOs, *see* Health maintenance
    organizations
Home health agencies (HHAs), 63
Hospital ethics committees, 94
Hospital governance model, 150, 151*f*
Hospitals
  barriers to establishing strong
    corporate cultures for, 57–58
  California provision noncompliance
    for, 321
  codes of ethics for, 77, 82–83
  community benefits, 329–334, 340
  investor-owned, 339, 340
  not-for-profit, 339, 340
  quality measures for, 194–195, 195*t*
  teaching, 144–145, 146, 192–193
  uncompensated care, 338–339, 339,
    340
Human immunodeficiency virus/
    acquired immunodeficiency
    syndrome (HIV/AIDS),
    158–164
  Acer case, 198
  assessing and improving quality of
    care or, 192
  cases, 198, 199
  Centers for Disease Control and
    Prevention (CDC) estimates
    of risk of transmission of to
    patients, 198–199
  legal aspects of, 159–164
  maintaining confidentiality
    regarding, 200–202
  protecting patients and community
    from staff with, 195–203
  protecting staff from, 161–164

recommendations for preventing transmission of, 196, 206*n*
testing for, 160
Human resources policy, ethical issues regarding hiring, 289–290
Hydration, *see* Artificial hydration and nutrition (AHN)
Hyperegalitarianism, 304, 337
Hyperindividualism, 304
Hypermeritocracy, 337

ICRCs, *see* Infant care review committees
ICUs, *see* Intensive care units
IECs, *see* Institutional ethics committees
Illegal aliens, ethical issues in providing care
Santillan case, 340–342
uncompensated care for, 343–344
Illegality
clear, 183
potential, 183
Improving quality of care, 191–195
cases, 192–193, 194
In the Matter of Baby K, 313
Incentives for physicians, regarding managed care, 293–294
Incident reports, 154–155
Infant care
Baby Boy Doe, 15, 16, 30–32, 219, 233
Baby Doe controversies, 94, 252
Baby Doe regulations, 114, 252–253
Baby K case, 313–319
Department of Health and Human Services regulations for, 32
and near-futile treatment, 310–311
Infant care review committees (ICRCs), 113–114
Informed consent, 215, 218
cases, 106, 218–219
for physician-assisted suicide (PAS), 267
Insider information, misuse of, 148–150
Institutional ethics committees (IECs), 93–102, 300–301
administrative, 96, 98, 100–101
biomedical, 96, 98

cases, 97–98, 100–101
membership, 98
models for, 95–96
organization of, 95–96
possible roles for, 99, 99*t*
purpose and role of, 96–98
relationships, 98–101
Institutional review boards (IRBs), 102–113
cases, 104–105, 106
establishing, 103–107
membership and purpose, 107–108
pediatric research review, 106–107
requirements for reviewing research activities, 107, 108–111
Intensive care units (ICUs), 308–309
Invasive procedures
definition, 196
preventing transmission of human immunodeficiency virus (HIV) during, 206*n*
Investor-owned hospitals, 339, 340
Involuntary euthanasia, 244
IRBs, *see* Institutional review boards
Irreversible coma, Harvard Medical School definition, 230

Jehovah's Witnesses, and consent, 215
Johns Hopkins University, The, *see* Kennedy Krieger Institute case
Joint Commission on Accreditation of Healthcare Organizations
Patient Rights and Organization Ethics Standards, 69–70
patient safety and medical and health care error reduction standards, 181
requirements for advance medical directives (AMDs), 233–234
requirements for philosophy statements, 59, 61
requirements for resolving ethics issues, 95
Judgment, substituted, 239
Justice, 29, 31, 288

Kant, Immanuel, 15, 18
Kennedy Krieger Institute case, 111
Kevorkian, Jack, 259, 261, 274, 271

Last bed in the ICU dilemma, 308–309
Last wishes case, 97–98
Last-chance therapies, 338
Law
    ethics and, 7–10, 9f
    sources of, 5–7
    see also specific laws
Lee v. Harcleroad, 261
Legal considerations, 7–10, 9f
    in Baby K case, 314–315
    in Bouvia case, 270–271
    in consent, 212–217
    in corporate decisions, 8–9, 10f
    in human immunodeficiency virus/
        acquired immunodeficiency
        syndrome (HIV/AIDS) cases,
        159–164
    in physician-assisted suicide cases
        (PAS), 260–265
    powers of attorney, 239
    sources of law, 5–7
    theory of duty to warn, 161
Liberty principle, 20
Licensed independent practitioners
    (LIPs), definition, 3n
Licensure statutes, 89
Life-sustaining treatments, 230, 234
    see also Artificial hydration and
        nutrition (AHN)
LIPs, see Licensed independent
    practitioners, definition
Living wills, 234, 335
    cases, 246
    Virginia Advance Medical Directive
        form, 235f–237f
Long-term care facilities, codes of
    ethics, 83

Macroallocation, 304–306
    Santillan case, 340–342
Mailing lists case, 176–177
Malfeasance, 148
Managed care
    cases, 291–292
    ethics in, 283, 290–299
    long-term cost savings of, 298–299
    marketing, 291–292
Managed care organizations (MCOs),
    116, 289, 290–291

cases, 297
    constraints in, 295–296
    institutional ethics committees
        (IECs), 94–95
    minimizing conflicts of interest in,
        296–298
    service utilization in, 292–293
Management
    cases, 154–155
    model of, 150, 151f
    moral philosophy and, 32–33
    by objectives, 164–165
    personal ethics and, 32–33
Management Advisory on Ethical
    Conduct for Health Care
    Institutions, 286–287
Managers
    appraisal of, 164–166
    cases, 147–148, 166
    codes of ethics for, 77–80
    and physician-assisted suicide issues
        (PAS), 271–273
    role of, 148
Marketing
    demarketing to avoid bankruptcy,
        287–288
    ethics in, 283–302
    of managed care, 291–292
    responsible, 286–288
Maslow's hierarchy of needs, 59
Mauro v. Borgess Medical Center, 171n
Maximizing the minimum position
    (maximin), 20
Mayo Clinic
    core principles, 357
    mission statement, 357
    primary value, 357
    statement of philosophy, 60, 357
McGregor's Theories X and Y, 59
McKinsey 7-S Framework, 55, 56f
MCOs, see Managed care
    organizations
Medical education, consent issues
    regarding, 144–145, 223–226
Medical errors, 181
    cases, 179–180, 340–342
    organizational culture and, 181–182
    Santillan case, 340–342
Medical morals committees, 94
Medical records, 175–178
    falsification of, 179–180
Medical staff

managers' relationships with,
  153–156
new, 164
nonphysician staff, 156–158
nurses, 156–157
Medical staff–hospital (MeSH)
  concept, *see* MeSH concept
Medically indicated treatment, 253
Medicare
  fraud, 186, 187, 205*n*
  Medicare Payment Advisory
    Commission, 339
Mental retardation, ethical issues for
    patients with
  Baby Boy Doe, 15, 16, 30–32, 219,
    233
  children at Willowbrook State
    Hospital, 109
MeSH (medical staff–hospital)
    concept, 164
Microallocation, 306–311, 338
  cases, 307, 308–309, 340–342
Mill, John Stuart, 16–17
Miller case, 310–311
Minimizing conflicts of interest,
    296–298
Minimum position, maximizing, 20
Miriam Hospital case, 137–138
Misrepresentation
  of academic accomplishments, 173*n*
  of credentials, 167–170
  see also Fraud
Mission, organizational, 53–74
Mission statements, 54, 55
  for community hospital associations,
    65
  developing, 64–66
  examples, 65, 349–358
Misuse of insider information,
    148–150
Model Rules of Professional Conduct,
    76
Monitoring clinical activities, 178–182
Moral philosophies, 16–25
  application of, 30–32
  bases for codes of ethics, 84
  congruence of, 71–72
  considerations for, 15–34
  and personal ethic, 29–33
Moral reasoning methodology, 40–41
Morphia somnolence case, 242, 243,
    244, 246

National Commission for the
    Protection of Human Subjects
    of Biomedical and Behavioral
    Research, 102–103
National Conference on Uniform
    State Laws, 232
National Institutes of Health (NIH),
    113, 335
National Society of Patient
    Representatives, 94
Natural law, 18–19
Near-futile treatment, 310–311
  Miller case, 310–311
Needs
  versus demand, 283–288
  Maslow's hierarchy of, 59
New York University Committee on
    Human Experimentation, 109
Nightingale Pledge, 81
NIH, *see* National Institutes of Health
Nonacute care organizations, 96
Noncompetent adult patients,
    248–252
Noncompliance, 321, 343
Nonfeasance, 148
Nonmaleficence, 28
  cases, 222
  principle of, 243
Nonphysician staff, relations with
    administration, 156–158
Normative ethics, 1
Not-for-profit hospitals, 339, 340
Nuremberg Code, 102
Nurses
  codes of ethics for, 81–82, 84, 107,
    157, 190, 372
  relationships with, 156–157
Nursing facilities, 94–95
Nursing facility administrators, 79–80
Nursing supervisors, 179–180
Nutrition, *see* Artificial hydration and
    nutrition (AHN)

Objectives, as part of mission
    statements
  examples, 65
  statements of, 64
Occupational Safety and Health Act
    of 1970 (OSHA), 160

Occupational Safety and Health Administration (OSHA), 162
Office of Government Ethics (OGE), 75
Operational efficiency, 329–330
Ordinary care, 31, 242–244, 312
Organizational context, 143–146
Organizational culture, 86–89
  cases, 86–87, 88
  and medical errors, 181–182
  and whistleblowing, 190–191
Organizational information, 146–150
Organizational philosophy
  cases, 66–67
  as concept, 2n
  developing, 54–64
  examples, 349–358
  reconsidering, 66–68
Organizational responses, 93–119
Organizational social policy, 183
Organizational values, vision, and mission, 53–74
Organizations
  codes of ethics for, 82–83
  ethical issues regarding, 143–173
  healthcare executive's responsibilities to, 363
  role in consent, 219–223
  successful characteristics, 55
  suicide and, 269–271
Original position, as part of Rawls's theory, 19–20
OSHA, see Occupational Safety and Health Act of 1970; Occupational Safety and Health Administration

Parens patriae, 30–32
Parochialism, 334
PAS, see Physician-assisted suicide
Passive euthanasia, 244
Paternalism, 26, 211, 216
Patient(s)
  autonomy, 259–279
  benefit model, 96
  bills of rights, understanding, 69–70
  decision-making process, 245–253
    with competent patients, 245–247
    with formerly competent patients, 247–248
  Henninger case, 245–247
  with infants, 252–253
  with noncompetent adult patients, 248–252
  definition, 1n
  education, 144–145, 223–226
  records, 175–178
Patient Rights and Organization Ethics Standards, 69–70
Patient Rights and Responsibilities, 69–70
Patient Self-Determination Act (PSDA), 233
Patients
  communication with, 144–145, 223–226
  ethical issues regarding, 175–207
  Fundamental Elements of the Patient–Physician Relationship, 212, 219, 370–371
  protecting from human immunodeficiency virus (HIV) transmission, 195–203
  relationships with, 60–61
Patient's Bill of Rights, 69
Pediatric research, 108–109
  cases, 106–107, 109
Performance appraisal, managerial, 164–166
Persistent vegetative state (PVS), 42, 239
  Cruzan case, 249–250
  terminology of permanent versus persistent, 239n
  Schiavo case, 256n
  Wanglie case, 313
Personal ethics
  developing, 46–48
  moral philosophy and, 29–33
  selecting principles to be included in, 47
Philosophy statements, 54–55
  content of, 59–64
  organizational content, 59–60
PHOs, see Physician–hospital organizations
Physical restraints, and consent, 222
Physician-assisted suicide (PAS), 259–279
  alternatives, 267
  in Belgium, 265, 273

Bouvia case, 269–271
consultation for, 267
criteria for, 266–267
economics of, 272–273
in Germany, 276
issues for health services managers,
    271–273
issues for physicians, 274–275
Kevorkian, Jack, 259, 261, 274, 271
laws in New Jersey, 270
laws in New York, 270
Lee v. Harcleroad, 261
legal aspects of, 260–265
in Michigan, 261, 273, 274
in the Netherlands, 264–265,
    265–269, 273, 275
in Oregon, 262–265, 274
    Death with Dignity Act, 260
    economics of physician-assisted
        suicide (PAS) in, 272–273
    insurance issues, 263
and organizations, 269–271
patient characteristics, 263–264
physician characteristics, 264
physician concerns for, 274, 275
process for receiving, 262–263
public support of, 271
Vacco v. Quill, 260, 261
voluntary, 266
Washington v. Glucksberg, 260, 261
see also Euthanasia
Physician–hospital organizations
    (PHOs), 164
Physician(s)
    California noncompliance provision
        for, 321
    codes of ethics for, 80–81
    credentialing, 166–167
    definition of, 3*n*
    Fundamental Elements of the
        Patient–Physician
        Relationship, 212, 219,
        370–371
    human immunodeficiency virus
        (HIV) testing for, 160
    incentives and disincentives,
        regarding managed care,
        293–294
    physician-assisted suicide (PAS)
        issues, 274–275
    protecting patients and community
        from staff with human

immunodeficiency virus
    (HIV), 195–203
traditional role as guardians of life,
    274
in training, 144–145, 223–224
Plato, 5–6, 23
PL 93-112, *see* Rehabilitation Act of
    1973
PL 93-247, *see* Child Abuse
    Prevention and Treatment Act
    of 1974
PL 98-272, *see* Emergency Medical
    Treatment and Active Labor
    Act (EMTALA) of 1986
PL 98-457, *see* Child Abuse
    Prevention and Treatment Act
    Amendments of 1984
PL 101-336, *see* Americans with
    Disabilities Act (ADA) of 1990
Potential illegality or danger, 183
Powers of attorney, 239
    durable, 239
    general, 239
    principal, definition, 239
Practice acts, 89
Premature infants
    Baby K, 313–319
    near-futile treatment for, 310–311
President's Commission for the Study
    of Ethical Problems in
    Medicine and Biomedical and
    Behavioral Research, 94, 97,
    211, 216
Principal, definition of, regarding
    powers of attorney, 239
Principles of Medical Ethics, 80–81,
    211–212, 219, 293, 368–369
    philosophical basis for, 84
Principles of Patient Care, 224–225
Private versus public actions,
    regarding health services
    managers, 85–86
Problem solving, 13, 35–49
    heuristic model of, 41
    rational model of, 41
    schema for, 42–45, 43*f*
    types of, 41
Profits, management of, 332–333
Prognosis committees, 94
Proportionate care, 243
PSDA, *see* Patient Self-Determination
    Act

Public relations, 342–343
Publications, physician
　　misrepresentation of, 173*n*
PVS, *see* Persistent vegetative state

Quality
　of care, 288
　　assessing and improving, 191–195
　　cases, 192–193, 194
　　equity in, 334–338
　　ordinary versus extraordinary
　　　care, 242–244
　　commitment to, 357
　　measures, 194–195, 195*t*
Quality-of-life criteria, 233
qui tam actions, 184
　example cases, 186, 187, 189–190,
　　205*n*
Quinlan case, 94, 248–249, 313

Ramsey, Paul, lottery approach to
　　services, 308
Rational model, 41
Rawls, John, 15, 19–20
RDE, *see* Rule of double effect
Records, 175–178
Rehabilitation Act of 1973 (PL
　　93-112), 161, 315
　Section 504, 160, 252, 315
Relationships
　cases, 63, 152, 166
　with community, 63
　Fundamental Elements of the
　　Patient–Physician
　　Relationship, 212, 219,
　　370–371
　with governing body, 150–153, 151*f*
　hierarchy of, 26*f*
　with medical staff, 153–156, 164
　with nonphysician staff, 156–158
　with nurses, 156–157
　organizational context of, 143–146
　with other institutions, 63–64
　with patients, 60–61
　with staff, 61–62
*Report of the Council on Ethical and
　　Judicial Affairs of the AMA,*
　　224
Reporting violations, 364

Rescher, Nicholas, theory of
　　allocating lifesaving treatment,
　　307
Research
　cases, 104–105, 106, 109
　as core principle, 357
　equity in, 335
　ethical principles in, 102–103
　exempt, 111–112
　falsification of data, 112–113
　nontherapeutic, 106, 109
　warranting expedited review,
　　111–112
Residents, and medical education
　　issues in consent, 144–145,
　　223–224
Resource allocation
　Baby K case, 313–319
　cases, 305–306, 307, 308–309,
　　313–319, 340–342
　core principle of, 357
　ethics in, 303–328
　last bed in the ICU dilemma,
　　308–309
　macroallocation, 304–306, 340–342
　microallocation, 306–311, 338,
　　340–342
　Santillan case, 340–342
Respect, 18
　cases, 88
　for persons, 26–27, 88
　for professional confidences, 146
Responsibility, social, 329–347
Responsible marketing, 286–288
Restraints, and consent, 222
Right to due process, 154–155
Right to refuse treatment, 215–216,
　　249
Risk management
　cases, 179–180
　higher-risk procedures, 192–193
Roe v. Wade, 7, 93–94, 261
Rule of double effect (RDE), 244–245
Rules of conduct, model, 76

Santillan case, 340, 341–342
Schiavo case, 256*n*
*School Board of Nassau County, Florida
　　v. Arline,* 161
*Scoles v. Mercy Health Corporation of
　　Southeastern Pennsylvania,* 171*n*

Section 504, *see* Rehabilitation Act of 1973 (PL 93-112)
Self-dealing, 130, 147–148
  cases, 147–148, 149
Self-directed expenditures, and conflicts of interest, 136–137
Self-regulation, 75
Service utilization, 292–293
Sexual abuse/exploitation, case involving, 185–186
Sexual harassment, case involving, 88
Sibley Memorial Hospital, 125–127
  mission statement, 356
  statement of philosophy, 60, 356
  Stern et al. v. Lucy Webb Hayes National Training School of Deaconesses and Missionaries et al., 125–127
  values, 356
  vision statement, 356
Social justice, 352
  model, 95
Social policy, organizational, 183
Social responsibility, 329–347
  as core principle, 357
  implications for hospitals, case, 332–333
  Santillan case, 340–342
Societal responsibilities, 364
Solving problems, 40–46
Specialized assistance, 114–116
Spiritual needs, 97–98, 358
St. Joseph Hospital case, 68
Staff
  ethical issues regarding, 143–173
  protecting patients and community from staff with human immunodeficiency virus (HIV), 199
  protecting staff from patients with human immunodeficiency virus (HIV), 161–164
  relationships, 61–62, 153–156, 156–158
  see also Physician(s)
State statutes, 234–238, 235f–237f
Statement of philosophy, 54–55
  content of, 59–64
  examples, 349–358
Statements of objectives, 64
Sterling County Hospital, objectives, 65, 66

Stern et al. v. Lucy Webb Hayes National Training School of Deaconesses and Missionaries et al., 125–127
Stock ownership, and ethical issues, 149
Strategic management, 70–71
Study to Understand Prognoses and Preferences for Outcomes and Risks of Treatment (SUPPORT), 323–324
Substituted judgment, 239
Suicide, *see* Physician-assisted suicide (PAS)
Sunrise Senior Living
  core values, 358
  foundational belief, 358
  mission statement, 358
  principles of service, 358
  statement of philosophy, 60, 358
SUPPORT, *see* Study to Understand Prognoses and Preferences for Outcomes and Risks of Treatment
Surrogate decision making, 238–239
Survey of Income and Program Participation, 332
Sutter Health
  mission statement, 351
  statement of philosophy, 59, 351
  vision, 351
Systems conflicts, 138–140

Tarasoff v. Regents of the State of California, 161
Teaching hospitals, 146
  cases, 144–145, 192–193
Technology, allocation of resources for, 305–306
Terminal care, 97–98
Theories X and Y, 59
Theory, linking to action, 25–29
Therapeutic privilege, 216–217
Third-party payers, 300, 302n
Training
  equity in, 335
  of residents, 144–145, 223–224
Transplantation
  recipients, 307
  Santillan case, 340–342

Transplantation—*continued*
United Network for Organ Sharing
(UNOS), 341, 342
Traumatic brain injury, 322
Trinity Health
core values, 352–353
futile treatment guidelines, 320–321
futility guidelines for, 319–320
mission statement, 352
statement of philosophy, 59–60,
352–353
vision statement, 353
Trustees, 125, 127–131
Tube feeding, 336

UDDA, *see* Uniform Determination
of Death Act
Uncompensated care, 338–339, 339,
340
cases, 342–343
for illegal aliens, 343–344
Uniform Determination of Death Act
(UDDA), 232
Uninsured rates, in various U.S.
states, 332
United Network for Organ Sharing
(UNOS), 341, 342
*United States ex rel. Brandimarte v.
Wurtzel*, 205n
Universal precautions, 162, 163
University of California–Irvine
Medical Center,
whistleblowing example, 186
UNOS, *see* United Network for
Organ Sharing
Utilitarianism, 2, 16–17
Utilization review committees, 106

VA, *see* Department of Veterans
Affairs

Vacco v. Quill, 260, 261
Values, organizational, 53–74
Vegetative state, *see* Persistent
vegetative state
Veterans Affairs, Department of, *see*
Department of Veterans
Affairs (VA)
Violations, reporting, 364
Virginia Advance Medical Directive
form, 235f–237f
Virtue ethics, 23–25
Virtues
application of, 30–32
focal, 24
Vision, organizational, 53–74
Vision statements, 64
Visioning, 53
Voluntary consent, 212–215, 217
Voluntary euthanasia, 244

Wanglie case, 313
Washington v. Glucksberg, 260, 261
Waste, as an ethical issue, 330
Whistleblowing, 182–191
cases, 184–185, 189–190
courses of action, 188
examples, 184–187
negative aspects of, 187–188
organizational culture and, 190–191
place of, 189
Whole brain death, 232, 254n10
Willowbrook State Hospital case,
109–111
Withholding or withdrawing
treatment
Miller case, 311
in the Netherlands, 265
see also Euthanasia
Work atmosphere, 357
World Health Organization, 159, 285
Writs of capias, 331n